# COGNITION, RISK, AND RESPONSIBILITY IN OBSTETRICS

# The Anthropology of Obstetrics and Obstetricians: The Practice, Maintenance, and Reproduction of a Biomedical Profession

Editors:
Robbie Davis-Floyd, Rice University
Ashish Premkumar, Northwestern University

Obstetricians are the primary drivers of the research on and the implementation of interventions in the birth process that have long been the subjects of anthropological critiques. In many countries, they are also primary drivers of violence, disrespect, and abuse during the perinatal period. Yet there is little social science literature on obstetricians themselves, their educational processes, and their personal rationales for their practices. Thus, this dearth of social science literature on obstetricians constitutes a huge gap waiting to be filled. These groundbreaking edited collections seek to fill that gap by officially creating an "anthropology of obstetrics and obstetricians" across countries and cultures—including biopolitical and professional cultures—so that a broad and deep understanding of these maternity care providers and their practices, ideologies, motivations, and diversities can be achieved.

**Volume I**
*Obstetricians Speak:*
*On Training, Practice, Fear, and Transformation*
Edited by Robbie Davis-Floyd and Ashish Premkumar

**Volume II**
*Cognition, Risk, and Responsibility in Obstetrics:*
*Anthropological Analyses and Critiques of Obstetricians' Practices*
Edited by Robbie Davis-Floyd and Ashish Premkumar

**Volume III**
*Obstetric Violence and Systemic Disparities:*
*Can Obstetrics Be Humanized and Decolonized?*
Edited by Robbie Davis-Floyd and Ashish Premkumar

# Cognition, Risk, and Responsibility in Obstetrics

## Anthropological Analyses and Critiques of Obstetricians' Practices

Edited by
*Robbie Davis-Floyd and Ashish Premkumar*

berghahn
NEW YORK · OXFORD
www.berghahnbooks.com

First published in 2023 by
Berghahn Books
www.berghahnbooks.com

**Library of Congress Cataloging-in-Publication Data**

A C.I.P. cataloging record is available from the Library of Congress
Library of Congress Cataloging in Publication Control Number: 2023001062


**British Library Cataloguing in Publication Data**

A catalogue record for this book is available from the British Library


ISBN 978-1-80073-831-7 hardback
ISBN 978-1-80073-833-1 paperback
ISBN 978-1-80073-832-4 ebook


https://doi.org/10.3167/9781800738317

From Robbie Davis-Floyd:
*I dedicate this book to my dear friend and colleague Nia Georges,*
*who has helped me in more ways than she will ever know, including*
*the support that she has given to me at various times in my life*
*when I have deeply needed that support.*

From Ashish Premkumar:
*I dedicate this book to my former attendings and to my residents,*
*who have helped me to develop a critical eye toward obstetric knowledge*
*and ways to rethink the current paradigm of practice.*

# Contents

# Illustrations

## Figures

## Tables

# Acknowledgments

We thank our chapter authors for their dedication and perseverance in conducting and writing up the research projects on which their chapters are based and for sticking with us throughout our sometimes-extensive chapter editing processes. We also thank our Berghahn Books editor Tom Bonnington and Keara Hagerty for responding to our endless questions and for shepherding this book through to production. And profound thanks go to Charles D. Laughlin for taking the time and trouble to create the index for this volume.

# Introduction
## An Overview of This Volume and of Significant Concepts Used

*Robbie Davis-Floyd and Ashish Premkumar*

This book is Volume II of the three-volume series *The Anthropology of Obstetrics and Obstetricians: The Practice, Maintenance, and Reproduction of a Biomedical Profession*, co-edited by medical/reproductive anthropologist Robbie Davis-Floyd and perinatologist and medical anthropologist Ashish Premkumar. Volume I is entitled *Obstetricians Speak: On Training, Practice, Fear, and Transformation* (Davis-Floyd and Premkumar 2023a); Volume III is *Obstetric Violence and Systemic Disparities: Can Obstetrics Be Humanized and Decolonized?* (Davis-Floyd and Premkumar 2023b). In all of these volumes, we have left the decision about what words to apply to people who are pregnant or are in the process of giving birth to the individual chapter authors. These terms include "women," "childbearers," "pregnant people," and others; sometimes they are culture-specific.

In this Introduction to Volume II—the book you are now holding in your hands—we provide a brief overview of its chapters. We also note here the relevance to the entire series of Chapter 1 of this volume, as some of our chapter authors make use of its schema of the "4 Stages of Cognition" and "Substage." And since some of these chapters utilize Robbie Davis-Floyd's (2001, 2018, 2022) delineations of the technocratic, humanistic, and holistic paradigms of birth and health care (described more fully in our Series Overview at the beginning of Volume I), we first present a brief overview of these paradigms, just as we also have done in the Introduction to Volume III.

## The Technocratic, Humanistic, and Holistic Paradigms of Birth and Health Care: A Brief Overview

The hegemonic technocratic paradigm, or model, is based on the *principle of separation*—of mind and body, practitioner and patient, body parts from the bodily whole. Its practitioners metaphorize the human body as a machine, view the female body as a defective machine, teach other practitioners to objectify their patients and their disorders ("the gall bladder in room 212"; "the cesarean in 314"), and rely on multiple technologies to manage, surveil, control, and intervene in the normal physiology of birth. This over-management and over-intervention exemplify the *obstetric paradox*: intervene in birth to keep it safe, thereby causing harm (Cheyney and Davis-Floyd 2019:8). These authors (Cheyney and Davis-Floyd 2020a, 2020b, 2021) have argued for the humanistic replacement of TMTS (too much too soon) and TLTL (too little too late) forms of care (see Miller et al. 2016) with RARTRW care—the right amount at the right time *in the right way*—for *how* care is provided matters as much or more than what care is provided and when.

The humanistic model, toward which many maternity care providers strive, is based on the *principle of connection*—the connections of mind to body, person to person, body part to body whole. This paradigm heavily emphasizes this "right way," because its practitioners define the body as what it is: an organism that responds well to kind and compassionate treatment and poorly and defensively to what the organism perceives as unkind and hurtful treatment. Davis-Floyd (2018, 2022) has been careful to distinguish between *superficial humanism*—in which compassionate treatment, including allowing the presence of a partner and/or doula, is often just an overlay on multiple and usually unnecessary technological interventions in labor and birth—and *deep humanism*, in which the "deep physiology" (2018, 2022) of birth is understood, honored, and facilitated. Deeply humanistic maternity care practitioners recognize, for example, that the uterus is responsive to the environment and can function well, or poorly, depending on how the body/organism it inhabits is treated. Thus Davis-Floyd (2022) has re-defined her "technocratic–humanistic–holistic" spectrum as "technocratic–superficially humanistic–deeply humanistic–holistic."

The holistic paradigm that lies on the far end of this spectrum defines the body as more than an organism; its practitioners view the body as an energy system in constant interaction with all other energy systems around it. And this holistic model is based on the *principles of connection and integration*—of mind, body, and spirit, of practitioner and "client" (a much more egalitarian word than "patient," often used by holistic practitioners of all types). Within this model, unlike in the other two, spirit and energy are brought into play, for example, by having the parent(s) "call the spirit" of an unresponsive baby (before and/or while a practitioner performs neonatal resuscitation) to ask that spirit to choose come into its body, as many midwives and some neonatologists do, and/or by following the holistic maxim *Change the energy, change the outcome.* This can mean keeping what Brazilian obstetrician Ricardo Jones (2009) calls the "psychosphere" of birth clear and clean, perhaps by asking people with fear- or tension-filled "negative energy" to leave the birthing room.

We stress that these paradigms lie across a *spectrum*, as they can elide into one another in practice: for example, highly technocratic obstetricians (obs) trained to keep emotional distance from their patients can choose to take the emotional risk of developing personal relationships with those patients when they become aware of the value such relationships have for the perinatal process. Or humanistic obs might bring some elements of holism into their practices, perhaps by having the parents "call the baby" as described above, while they call a neonatologist. In fact, a neonatologist once approached Robbie at a medical conference and earnestly asked her what homebirth midwives do when a baby is not breathing when it is born. To his great relief, Robbie responded that all US homebirth midwives are trained in neonatal resuscitation—but, wanting to give him more, Robbie also explained that homebirth midwives have the parents call the baby. She told him that first, it can do no harm; second, it gives the parents a sense of agency; and third, it just might work! Thrilled with this information, around four months later, this neonatologist sent Robbie a letter saying that ever since he had started asking parents to call their non-breathing babies, those babies began breathing right away, making resuscitation unnecessary. In holism, the interpretation is that babies' spirits or souls are often hovering, trying to make the decision to be or not to be (!) born, and that the assurance of truly being wanted that they feel when their parents call them will help the spirit to decide to come into its newborn body, or if that soul feels unwanted, perhaps it will decide to pass back through the gateway to "the other side." (Most holists are deeply spiritual, and many believe in reincarnation.)

Having briefly described these paradigms, we now turn to a presentation of the chapters in this volume.

## An Overview of the Chapters in This Volume

In Chapter 1, which series lead editor Robbie Davis-Floyd has constructed as a "think-piece," she offers a conceptual framework within which various ways of cognizing and believing can be fruitfully understood, including those utilized by obstetricians of all types. She describes the differences between "open" and "closed" ways of thinking, and delineates "4 Stages of Cognition," correlating each with an anthropological concept. She correlates Stage 1—rigid or concrete thinking—with *naïve realism* ("Our way is the only way, or the only way that matters"), *fundamentalism* ("Our way is the only right way"), and *fanaticism* ("Our way is so right that everyone who disagrees with it should be assimilated or eliminated"). She correlates Stage 2 thinking with *ethnocentrism* ("There are other ways out there, but our way is best") and demonstrates that technocratic obstetrics is a relatively rigid Stage 1 or Stage 2 system, depending on how it is practiced.

The next two Stages represent more fluid types of thinking—Robbie correlates Stage 3 thinking with *cultural relativism* ("All ways have value, and individual behaviors must be understood within their sociocultural contexts") and suggests that obstetricians should seek to understand the cultures within which they practice and should demonstrate cultural competence and provide Cultural Safety[1] in their care via what Robbie terms "informed relativism" (see Davis-Floyd et al. 2018). She relates Stage 4 thinking to *global humanism* ("We must search for better ways that honor the human rights of all individuals") and insists that obstetricians should always honor women's rights in their care, even in cultures that devalue women and do not honor their human rights in daily life.

Robbie then categorizes various types of birth practitioners, especially obstetricians, within these 4 Stages and shows how each Stage affects and influences practice. She goes on to show how ongoing stress can cause even the most fluid of thinkers to shut down cognitively and operate at a Stage 1 level or to degenerate into "Substage"—a condition of cognitive breakdown, or "losing it," which can include treating birthing people and other practitioners with disrespect, violence, and abuse. She describes how the performance of rituals can help such practitioners to ground themselves at least at a Stage 1 level and offers ways in which they may move beyond rigidity and rejuvenate and inspire themselves to think and practice more openly and fluidly. She also describes the ongoing battles between fundamentalists and global humanists, and the persecutions that Stage 4 globally humanistic birth practitioners, including obstetricians, often experience from fundamentalist or fanatical Stage 1 obstetricians and officials—often referred to as the "global witch hunt" from which humanistic and holistic practitioners frequently suffer, as some of them describe in their chapters in Volume I (Davis-Floyd and Premkumar 2023a).

In Chapter 2, authors Margaret Dunlea, Martina Hynan, Jo Murphy-Lawless, Magdalena Ohaja, Malgorzata Stach, and Jeannine Webster describe the culture of Irish obstetrics and obstetricians. They begin with the characterization of Irish society not only as a "man's world" but also as one where the "patriarchal dividend" continues to underpin widespread cultural acceptance of male authority as entirely appropriate. The Irish government unquestioningly accepts the mainstreaming of this obstetric authority, funding maternity services on this basis. These authors describe the international hegemony of the Irish text *Active Management of Labour: The Dublin Experience*, now in its 4th edition (O'Driscoll, Meagher, and Robson 2004) and the *National Maternity Strategy* of 2016, wherein a woman's "care pathway" is determined by obstetric risk criteria. They conclude with arguments about the need to take women's activism in more fruitful directions to reach obstetricians directly and to effect positive changes in their practices.

In Chapter 3, "Becoming an Obstetrician in Greece: Medical Training, Informal Scripts, and the Routinization of Cesarean Births," medical anthropologist Eugenia (Nia) Georges begins by showing that in Greece, the vast majority of women give birth in private or public hospitals under the exclusive care of obstetricians, with highly trained professional midwives mostly relegated to obstetrician-subservient roles. Greece currently has the highest cesarean birth (CB) rate in the European Union and in the world. Despite a growing public awareness that many, if not most, cesareans are unnecessary, Greece's CB rate remains at its long-standing 65%.

Over the course of her long-term ethnographic research on pregnancy and birth in Greece, Nia has often heard obstetricians themselves bemoan the high cesarean rate. To date, however, there have been no qualitative studies that explore their points of view—a gap that Georges' study fills. In her chapter, she complements her prior research on the experiences of pregnant women with interviews with obstetricians to explore their understandings of their profession and their perspectives on cesarean births. To examine the "hidden curriculum" (Dixon, Smith-Oka, and El Kotni 2019) that implicitly informs their understandings, Georges also draws on the perspectives and experiences of adjacent medical doctor (MD) care providers, such as neonatologists, who are increasingly called upon to attend to the unintended consequences of the large number of Greek babies born by cesarean. These consequences include many preterm births, as Greek obs often schedule CBs at or before 37 weeks of pregnancy, as Georges describes.

Chapter 4, by Michelle Sadler, a medical anthropologist, and Gonzalo Leiva, a practicing midwife in Chile with a Master's in Health Administration, explores obstetricians' explanations for the high rates of cesareans in Chile, especially considering the extreme differences among health insurance systems. In the Chilean public health insurance system in 2017, cesarean births were at 28%; in the private system, 62%; and in the PAD (Pago Asociado a Diagnóstico) Birth system—public insurance until the 37th week of gestation followed by transfer to the private system—72%. In this latter subsystem, only women with full-term healthy pregnancies can be attended, and therefore this sector should have the lowest rates of cesarean births. Instead, it has the highest.

When trying to explain these extreme differences, Sadler and Leiva's ob/gyn interlocutors acknowledged that economic incentives are primary. In private care, fees are paid per birth, and therefore, a greater number of births—a number that can be optimized by performing cesareans—translates into higher income. In the PAD Birth system, the institutional and practitioners' fees are much lower than in the private system; thus, the volume of procedures is privileged, leading to the 72% CB rate. Obstetricians take different positions on this problem, ranging from a defense of these options in a free market framework to a profound criticism that highlights the violations of women's human rights and of biomedicine's ethical core values. In addition to financial incentives, the interlocutors mentioned other factors that weighed differently, depending on their approaches to childbirth. Those more closely aligned with a technocratic view of birth identified causes that they considered "external" to their own practices, such as maternal request and fear of lawsuit, and were less critical of their own influences on the high cesarean rates. Those ascribing to a humanistic approach placed greater weight on economic incentives and on obs' general ignorance of how to attend vaginal births. Since cesareans are decided on mainly by obstetricians, Sadler and Leiva argue that understanding the factors and incentives that drive these surgical interventions is vitally important for the effective design of humanistic birth models.

In Chapter 5, social anthropologists Caroline Chautems and Irene Maffi begin by noting that Switzerland ranks among the European countries with the highest cesarean rates (32.3% in 2017)—around the same as that in the United States. Those obstetricians who recognize the adverse consequences of unnecessary CBs face difficulties in inversing the current trend. Although some public hospitals are trying to modify standard practices that contribute to increasing CB rates, such as frequent induction and systematic active management of labor, in situ decisions frequently lead to cesarean instead of vaginal deliveries. However, most obstetricians conceive of "normal birth" as vaginal, and the majority of parents want to limit medical interventions during childbirth. In this context, the recent introduction into some Swiss hospitals of "gentle cesareans"—a technique mimicking vaginal delivery—appears to be an attempt to reconcile the natural childbirth model with surgical birth. "Gentle cesareans" are intended to favor parents' participation in childbirth within the constraints of the hospital environment—for example, by allowing them to see the baby's extraction and for the mother to have her baby on her chest immediately after birth. (Our readers can see a photo of a gentle cesarean on the cover of this volume. Just after this photo was taken, the baby was passed directly to the mother.)

This chapter is primarily based on an in-depth, lengthy interview with one of the two obstetricians, Alexandre Farin, who introduced the "gentle cesarean" technique in French-speaking Switzerland, which has become the default protocol in the maternity ward where he practices. The interview focused on his professional trajectory, his conceptions of normal childbirth and surgical birth, and the reasons for his commitment to "gentle" cesareans. More broadly, this interview investigated Farin's opinions on obstetrics in Switzerland, including medical training, protocols, obstetric cultures in public hospitals and private clinics, and couples' attitudes toward childbirth.

In Chapter 6, obstetrician/gynecologist Nicholas Rubashkin provides a historically and ethnographically grounded overview of the emergence and rise to dominance of the Maternal Fetal Medicine Network (MFMU) VBAC (vaginal birth after cesarean) Success Calculator in the United States. The "VBAC calculator" was designed to assist providers and women to make more informed mode-of-birth decisions. Drawing from interviews with clinician users and non-users of the VBAC calculator as well as with pregnant and postpartum women, all of whom had a prior cesarean, Rubashkin demonstrates how certain uses of the VBAC calculator circumscribed VBAC-interested women's decision-making capacities, because the calculator put forth cesarean surgery as the best and only treatment for a predicted low probability of success. Importantly, the MFMU VBAC calculator used race/ethnicity to predict a score and, as a result, assessed Black and Hispanic women to be, on average, 5 to 15 points less likely to achieve a VBAC compared to white women with similar risk factors. Because the VBAC calculator explicitly factored in race/ethnicity, as opposed to racism, as an intrinsic risk factor for poor individual health, the calculator put VBAC-interested Black and Hispanic women at risk for cesareans they didn't desire or need. Rubashkin also examines how some maternity care providers—more often midwives but also some obstetricians—challenged the calculator's approach and supported women wishing to have VBACs in a range of birth options. In his concluding remarks, Rubashkin discusses how, through the selective sharing of information, the calculator drew from and perpetuated the authoritative status of obstetrics as the modern science supposedly best equipped to deal with risks in childbirth through invasive procedures, and describes the development of a new VBAC calculator that does not include race/ethnicity as a variable but has its own set of problems, in that this new calculator is not "preference-sensitive"—it does not include women's preferences and commitments to achieving a VBAC, *yet it should.*

In Chapter 7, medical anthropologists Vania Smith-Oka and Lydia Z. Dixon also address risk and responsibility in obstetrics, this time among Mexican obstetricians. They begin by noting that there has been a growing body of literature on women's experiences with obstetric care, yet less attention has been paid to the ways in which obstetricians themselves have come to behave, believe, and practice as they do. This chapter draws on the authors' combined years of research on childbirth in Mexico to specifically examine the perspectives of Mexican obstetricians. Using rich ethnographic data from obstetricians, obstetric residents, and midwives, Smith-Oka and Dixon focus on how changing narratives about risk, maternal mortality, and obstetric violence in Mexico are interpreted by obstetricians and ultimately impact patients. These narratives at times motivate changes in patient care, while at other times such changes are framed as unrealistic, unnecessary, or even undesirable.

Smith-Oka and Dixon's analysis highlights the roles that medical hierarchies, defensive medicine, social inequalities, and structural inadequacies play in the decisions obstetricians make. The extent to which obs embrace changes in their field (such as humanizing their practices and working with midwives) depends on more than individual willingness; it also depends on the socio-structural contexts within which Mexican obstetricians work. Building on the well-known trope of the need to "listen to women" during maternity care, these authors insist that ultimately, "If we hope to see change in obstetric practice, we have to *listen to obstetricians.*" They show that ethnography is a powerful and effective tool for achieving this goal.

Chapter 8 by Vania Smith-Oka, the medical anthropologist who co-authored the preceding chapter, and Megan K. Marshalla, an obstetrics and gynecology resident, keeps us in Mexico to investigate how class, ethnic, and gender differences are reproduced in biomedical training in that country. These authors begin with the premise that bodies are useful instruments for understanding the reproduction of inequalities. They go on to investigate why and how bodily, social, intimate, and physical boundaries are crossed in biomedical practice in general, and specifically in obstetric practice, and what this can tell us about individual and social bodies. Smith-Oka and Marshalla unpack how seeing and being seen, touching and being touched, and feeling and being felt are conditioned in very particular ways by obstetric training and by the broader political economy. Ob participants in the authors' ethnographic research in Mexico used the term *manitas* to describe how they trained their sensory organs (hands, ears, eyes) during medical practice; how they learned through practice on the bodies of less-agentive populations (female, raced, impoverished); and how they crossed intimate, structural, and physical boundaries through what these authors term "somatic translation": seeing others' bodies through their own. *Manitas* were developed unconsciously by obstetricians, were never explicitly taught or learned in practice (but rather were part of obstetrics' "hidden curriculum"), and (re)produce social differences. As Smith-Oka and Marshalla demonstrate, these forms of learning highlight the friction between the "violence of knowing" and the importance of touch as a legitimate mode of care. This tactile and sensorial learning not only entails a form of boundary crossing that is medically useful but also highlights social inequalities by taking advantage of them.

In Chapter 9, "The Limitations of Understanding Structural Inequality: Obstetricians' Accounts of Caring for Substance-Using Patients in the United States," Katharine McCabe, who works in law, gender, and health care, shares findings from a study examining obstetricians' attitudes and responses to substance-using patients to demonstrate that these providers already engage in a process of "social diagnosis," by which signs of social precarity and disadvantage are identified and incorporated into clinical decision-making. However, as McCabe shows, the ability of obstetricians to identify disadvantages does not necessarily improve patient care or outcomes; rather it creates a new set of iatrogenic effects. Patients identified as "problematic" due to their substance use and positionality (i.e., poverty, lack of access to opportunities) are less likely to be treated in a clinically normative manner and are often referred to coercive and punitive social systems to address structural and social risks deemed outside of the scope of obstetricians' expertise. McCabe concludes with a discussion of the limitations of approaches that seek to resolve health inequalities through consciousness or awareness raising. Instead, she encourages a more complete understanding of "biomedicine as a structure of inequality in and of itself" and argues that actors working within this structure—especially obstetricians—must be morally and politically committed to transforming biomedicine from the inside out to generate effective humanistic changes.

In Chapter 10, Melissa Goldin Evans, a community health researcher, addresses "Contraceptive Provision by Obstetricians/Gynecologists in the United States: Biases, Misperceptions, and Barriers to an Essential Reproductive Health Service." Evans begins by noting that unintended pregnancies occur in nearly one out of every two (45%) pregnancies in the United States and that unintended pregnancies and short interpregnancy intervals are associated with adverse health and social outcomes for the infant and the mother. She continues by affirming that the risks of unintended pregnancies and short interpregnancy intervals are significantly reduced when women use long-acting reversible contraceptives (LARCs)—intrauterine devices and implants. Evans emphasizes that ob/gyns play important roles in patient uptake of LARCs—whether or not they provide routine unbiased contraceptive counseling that preserves patient autonomy in choice, have the training to insert LARCs, and can provide LARCs by removing on-site barriers such as multiple-day protocols for insertions. Additionally, although the American College of Obstetricians and Gynecologists (ACOG) and the CDC (Centers for Disease Control and Prevention) state that LARCs are safe and effective for the majority of women, many reproductive healthcare providers consider certain populations to be inappropriate LARC candidates. Since LARC insertion is a procedure that requires a trained healthcare provider, any bias against LARCs for women with certain demographics and gynecologic histories can prevent equitable access and uptake of LARCs.

The objective of Evans's chapter is to describe contraceptive provision practices, particularly LARCs, among ob/gyns to both the general population at risk of unintended pregnancies and to postpartum women. She delineates ob/gyns' fundamental duty to help women achieve their reproductive goals through unbiased, woman-centric contraceptive counseling and, for contextualization, includes descriptions of historical and present-day efforts to control the reproductive autonomy of low-income women and Women of Color. She follows up with a discussion on system-level barriers that restrict LARC provision with suggestions for overcoming these barriers.

In Chapter 11, "Cognition, Risk, and Responsibility: Home Birth and Why Obstetricians Fear It," obstetrician Amali U. Lokugamage—who herself gave birth at home—and midwife and researcher Claire Feeley describe home births as "physiologic births that take place under the social, deeply humanistic, and holistic models of birth" and note that these tend to be rare in hospitals—meaning that obstetricians have little experience in attending them. Therefore, obstetricians traditionally have been very fearful of home births, cognizing them as "extremely risky." Lokugamage and Feeley demonstrate that normal physiologic births contribute to improving public health and that obstetricians are often not aware of the extent of these benefits, which include adaptive physiologic functions in the baby, better mother and baby bonding, and higher breastfeeding rates, which in turn lead to better lifelong emotional and physical health for infants. Normal birth affirms health, promotes empowerment in mothers, and is linked to promoting positive emotional qualities in society via the hormone oxytocin—often referred to as "the hormone of love." Training within the technocratic model constrains obstetricians' ability to value normal birth, especially when it occurs outside of hospitals. Experiences of complications and a lack of awareness of the evidence surrounding home birth—compounded by their lack of training in normal physiologic birth—perpetuate fear of home birth among obstetricians, as this chapter illustrates.

In the Conclusions to this volume, we describe the theoretical concepts and frameworks used by the chapter authors and the key points made in their chapters.

**Robbie Davis-Floyd,** Adjunct Professor, Department of Anthropology, Rice University, Houston, and Fellow of the Society for Applied Anthropology is a cultural/medical/reproductive anthropologist interested in transformational models of maternity care, and an international speaker who has given more than 1,000 talks at universities and obstetric and midwifery conferences over the course of her long career. She is also a Board member of the International MotherBaby Childbirth Organization (IMBCO), in which capacity she helped to wordsmith the *International Childbirth Initiative: 12 Steps to Safe and Respectful MotherBaby-Family Maternity Care* (www.ICIchildbirth.org). E-mail: davis-floyd@outlook .com.

**Ashish Premkumar** is an Assistant Professor of Obstetrics and Gynecology at the Pritzker School of Medicine at The University of Chicago and a doctoral candidate in the Department of Anthropology at The Graduate School at Northwestern University. He is a practicing maternal-fetal medicine subspecialist. His research focus is on the intersections of the social sciences and obstetric practices, particularly surrounding the issues of risk, stigma, and quality of health care during the perinatal opioid use disorder epidemic of the 21st century. E-mail: premkumara@ bsd.uchicago.edu.

## Note

1. According to the authors of Chapter 6 in Volume III of this series (Lokugamage, Ahillan, and Pathberiya 2023), Māori nurse and educator Irihapiti Ramsden of New Zealand recognized that midwifery and nursing education needed to incorporate the concept of *Cultural Safety*—which, as she and the Māori insist, should always be capitalized; not to do so is considered a subtle insult. In their chapter, these authors state that "It is vital to distinguish *Cultural Safety* from *cultural competence*. 'Cultural Safety' acknowledges the inherent power imbalances between clinician and patient, requiring practitioners to use critical self-reflection on their own beliefs, values, biases and assumptions, but 'cultural competence' does not include this important reflexivity on power." Amali Lokugamage (personal correspondence with Robbie, February 2022) adds to this that: "Cultural competence is deficient due to the perpetuation of racial stereotypes as it depends on Western interpretations of other cultures; it doesn't include co-creation of health policies through patient/public engagement; and, again, doesn't include reflexivity or power imbalances" (see Lokugamage et al. 2021).

## References

Cheyney M, Davis-Floyd R. 2019. "Birth as Culturally Marked and Shaped." In *Birth in Eight Cultures*, eds. Davis-Floyd R, Cheyney M, 1–16. Long Grove IL: Waveland Press.

———. 2020a. "Birth and the Big Bad Wolf: A Biocultural, Co-Evolutionary Perspective, Part 1." *International Journal of Childbirth* 9(4): 177–192.

———. 2020b "Birth and the Big Bad Wolf: A Biocultural, Co-Evolutionary Perspective, Part 2." *International Journal of Childbirth* 10(2): 66–78.

———. 2021. "Birth and the Big Bad Wolf: Biocultural Evolution and Human Childbirth." In *Birthing Techno-Sapiens: Human-Technology Co-Evolution and the Future of Reproduction*, ed. Davis-Floyd R, 15–46. Abingdon, Oxon: Routledge.

Davis-Floyd R. 2001. "The Technocratic, Humanistic, and Holistic Paradigms of Childbirth." *International Journal of Gynecology & Obstetrics* 75, Supplement 1: S5–S23.

———. 2018. "The Technocratic, Humanistic, and Holistic Paradigms of Birth and Health Care." In *Ways of Knowing about Birth: Mothers, Midwives, Medicine, and Birth Activism*, Davis-Floyd R and Colleagues, 3-44. Long Grove IL: Waveland Press.

———. 2022. *Birth as an American Rite of Passage*, 3rd edn. Abingdon, Oxon: Routledge.

Davis-Floyd R, with Matsuoka E, Horan H, Ruder B, Everson CL. 2018. "Daughter of Time: The Postmodern Midwife." In *Ways of Knowing about Birth: Mothers, Midwives, Medicine, and Birth Activism*, Davis-Floyd R and Colleagues, 221–264. Long Grove IL: Waveland Press.

Davis-Floyd R, Premkumar A. 2023a. *Obstetricians Speak: On Training, Practice, Fear, and Transformation*. New York: Berghahn Books.

————. 2023b. *Obstetric Violence and Systemic Disparities: Can Obstetrics Be Humanized and Decolonized?* New York: Berghahn Books.

Dixon LZ, Smith-Oka V, El Kotni M. 2019. "Teaching about Childbirth in Mexico: Working across Birth Models." In *Birth in Eight Cultures*, eds. Davis-Floyd R, Cheyney M, 17–48. Long Grove IL: Waveland Press.

Jones R. 2009. "Teamwork: An Obstetrician, a Midwife, and a Doula in Brazil." In *Birth Models That Work*, eds. Davis-Floyd R, Barclay L, Daviss BA, Tritten J, 271–304. Berkeley: University of California Press.

Lokugamage AU, Rix EL, Fleming T, et al. 2021. "Translating Cultural Safety to the UK." *Journal of Medical Ethics* Jul 19: medethics-2020-107017. Epub ahead of print. PMID: 34282043.

Lokugamage A, Ahillan T, Pathberiya SDC. 2023. "Decolonizing Ideas of Healing in Medical Education." In *Obstetric Violence and Systemic Disparities: Can Obstetrics Be Humanized and Decolonized?* eds. Davis-Floyd R, Premkumar A. Chapter 6. New York: Berghahn Books.

Miller S, Abalos E, Chamillard M, et al. 2016. "Beyond Too Little, Too Late and Too Much, Too Soon: A Pathway Towards Evidence-Based, Respectful Maternity Care Worldwide." *Lancet* 388(10056): 2,176–2,192.

O'Driscoll K, Meagher D, Robson M. 2003. *Active Management of Labour: The Dublin Experience.* London: Mosby.

# CHAPTER 1

# Open and Closed Knowledge Systems, the 4 Stages of Cognition, and the Obstetric Management of Birth

*Robbie Davis-Floyd*

## Introduction

This chapter is a "think-piece" focused on seeking to make sense of how people in general—and birth practitioners, especially obstetricians—cognize the world around them by analyzing the differences between open and closed knowledge systems. It stems from my anthropological work on belief systems, myths, paradigms, and the rituals that enact them (Davis-Floyd and Laughlin 2016, 2022), from my more than 30 years of exploring issues in childbirth, midwifery, obstetrics, and reproduction, and also from information shared by physicians of all types. Much of that work has focused on knowledge systems—ways of knowing about birth and health care (see for examples Davis-Floyd and Sargent 1997; Davis-Floyd and St John 1998; Davis-Floyd and Colleagues 2018; Davis-Floyd and Cheyney 2019). During my years of research, I have had many chances to observe what happens when these knowledge systems are "closed"—excluding all other ways of knowing—or "open" to new learning.

## Ways of Thinking and Knowing: Open and Closed Systems

> *We cannot solve our problems with the same thinking we used when we created them.*
> —Albert Einstein[1]

This think-piece is loosely based on the cognitive model of the "4 Stages of Cognition" developed by Harold Schroder, Michael Driver, and Siegfried Streufert (1967), which I have expanded upon greatly herein.[2] I take a broad look at ways of thinking and knowing—of *cognizing*—the world around us. I focus specifically on the differences between two types of knowledge systems: those that are relatively open and those that are relatively closed. Why? Because to avoid battles large and small—among nations, religions, or professional groups such as midwives and obstetricians—and to achieve global peace and sustainable societies in this rapidly changing world, people must be open to absorbing new information and adapting their knowledge systems to it. Battles of all types occur when closed knowledge systems confront and compete with others. But for positive change to occur, people must first recognize the belief system they adhere to *as* a belief system. You can't change your belief and knowledge system, or paradigm, unless you see it as such and recognize its limitations—something people locked into a rigid knowledge/belief system are generally unwilling to do. If you are already sure you have all the answers, why look beyond in search of better ones? To achieve an open knowledge system, the kind that is most fitting for this fluid world and that is also essential to achieve better births—births that are safe, physiologic, and childbearer-centered—one must first understand what it means for a knowledge system to be "closed."

## Relatively Closed Knowledge Systems: Stages 1 and 2

### Stage 1 Thinking

If children grow up in one culture and are exposed for the first 20 or so years of life only to the rhythms, patterns, language, and belief system of that culture, their neural networks will become more or less set in those terms. After that, learning something that does not fit well with what they have already internalized becomes increasingly difficult over time because integrating new information always requires the formation of entirely new neural pathways in the brain. For a child whose brain is still developing, forming millions of new neural networks every day, that process is effortless; for adults whose neural structures are already largely set, that process requires *enormous amounts of time, energy, and concentrated effort* to create new neural networks to absorb and process new information. If you have tried to learn a new language later in life, you will know exactly what I mean.

Individuals, including obstetricians (obs) who are never required to "think beyond" the belief systems of the cultures or subcultures in which they are raised or trained can over time become resistant to processing new information and can become neurocognitively "rigid" or "concrete" in their thinking—placing them in the cognitive arena of what Schroder, Driver, and Streufert (1967) have called Stage 1 thinking. For Stage 1 thinkers, there is only one possible set of interpretations of reality, and that set of interpretations *is* reality to them; their knowledge system is closed. According to ritual specialist John McManus (1979:217, 220), "Stage 1 thinkers tend to be oriented toward external standards, authority, and categorical thinking (right/wrong, good/bad) and tend to avoid ambiguity and conflict within the cognitive system. In Piagetian terms, the adaptive balance is toward assimilating reality to the [person's] own standards, needs, and structure"—in other words, toward cognitively constructing "reality" as you want it to be rather than as it is. Many obstetricians are experts at accomplishing that goal, using technology to alter biology in ways that suit their personal ideologies (Davis-Floyd 2022; Diamond-Brown 2023).

*Three Types of Stage 1 Thinking: Naïve Realism, Fundamentalism, Fanaticism*

Expanding on Schroder, Driver, and Streuferts's concept of Stage 1 "closed thinking," I here identify three types of Stage 1 thinking in anthropological terms (please see Table 1.1 below for an overview of all 4 Stages of Cognition and of "Substage"):

1. **Naïve realism:** The certainty that "Our way is the only way there is—or the only way that matters." Anthropologists have long applied this term to isolated, small-scale societies whose members, before their massive exposure to Western culture, had no or little notion that other ways even existed. And yet, in a way, naïve realism is an anthropological construct—humans have always moved around, and cross-cultural contacts have been occurring for millennia. Thus, to speak of naïve realism in the sense of small-scale societies who have had no, or very little, contact with outsiders is misleading; there are few, if any, such societies left—if, in fact, such societies ever existed. In contrast, there are many small-scale societies who do have the certainty that "Our way is the only way that matters to us." And, as we will see below, many religious groups raise their children to be naïve realists, and obstetricians who never think beyond what they are taught can be coded as naïve realists as well.

   I must stress that I am not taking any sort of evolutionary perspective here—I reject any notion that naïve realists are less intelligent than others and that the rest of us have "evolved" beyond naïve realism. Both rigid and fluid thinkers exist in every type of society. It is not intelligence but rather the degrees of *socialization and habituation* and a *lack of exposure to other ways* that have the greatest effects on how deeply individuals, including obstetricians, will internalize the core beliefs of their society—or their profession.

2. **Fundamentalism:** The certainty that "Our way is the only right way and should be the only way for everyone." First called "true believers" by Eric Hoffer (1951), most fundamentalists try hard to shut out all conflicting information, especially from their children, whom they seek to raise as naïve realists, often by not allowing them to engage with social media or the internet or watch television shows, read books, or attend schools that do not confirm their parents' belief system, worldview, and/or religion's tenets (see Rose 1988). Fundamentalists usually do not harm others or try to coerce them—rather, they generally just feel sorry for them and often try to proselytize in the hope that they will convert on their own to the one true way to "save their souls." But the punishment for those who leave that "one true way" can be severe, often involving an extremely traumatizing "shunning" process practiced, for brief examples, by Jehovah's Witnesses, by the members of full-fledged cults, and by fundamentalist professionals, such as obstetricians who shun, bully, and often actively persecute other obstetricians who practice outside the Stage 1 technocratic box. (See for profound examples the chapters in Volume I of this series (Davis-Floyd and Premkumar 2023a) by former obstetrician Ricardo Jones [2023] and by former obstetrician and midwife Ágnes Geréb and her colleague Katalin Fábián [2023]).

3. **Fanaticism:** The deep certainty that "Our way is so right that those who do not adhere to it should be either assimilated or eliminated." Religious and other types of fanatics play increasingly frightening roles in today's world, terrorizing the rest of us with the constant threat of acts designed to bring about an end to the world as we know it and re-create it in the image they seek. In this contemporary world, where people of many beliefs and cultures live in close proximity, fanatics can be extraordinarily dangerous in their efforts to either coerce or destroy those who do not share their completely closed belief systems. It might be a jump for some readers to consider that obstetricians can be fanatics too. Yet around the world, technocratic obstetric fanatics seek to shut out the possibility of incorporating evidence-based

information about how to facilitate normal physiologic birth that refutes their dominant paradigm. And many seek to discredit and/or eliminate humanistic and holistic practitioners who do act on that information—by taking away their licenses—as happened to Ricardo Jones and Ágnes (Agi) Geréb, and sometimes imprisoning them, as Agi was, for 77 days followed by more than three years of house arrest (Geréb and Fábián 2023).

### The Roles of Ritual in Stage 1 Thinking

I have long defined *rituals* as patterned, repetitive, and symbolic enactments of cultural (or individual) beliefs and values (Davis-Floyd [1992] 2003, 2018a; Davis-Floyd and Laughlin 2022). Rituals play critical roles in the creation and preservation of Stage 1 thinking. Through rhythmic repetition and the use of powerful core symbols, rituals work to imprint or "penetrate" these core beliefs and the behaviors that accompany them into the minds and bodies of ritual participants—a process that Charles D. Laughlin and I have described in depth in *Ritual: What It Is, How It Works, and Why* (2022). For indoctrination in or conversion to a particular belief system, rituals are the most powerful tools, as rituals are experiential and embodied. As Brigitte Jordan (1993, 1997) has shown, experiential learning through the body and the emotions is the deepest and most effective way to learn. *We tend to believe most deeply what we feel and experience most deeply.* Understanding the power of experiential learning, fundamentalist and fanatical preachers, totalitarian dictators, cult leaders, and obstetricians who train residents use the intense experiential practice of rituals (routine procedures) to draw their followers in and keep the boundaries tight. The more hours their followers spend performing rituals that enact the belief systems of their ritual leaders, the less time they have to think beyond those systems to examine whether they even want to believe what they are continually being taught.

All cultures and societies, all religions and belief systems, employ rituals to enact and display their beliefs and celebrate and continue their traditions. Rituals can be used to socialize people into a certain worldview (from early childhood on or later during adulthood) and stabilize them in it, and can also be used to trap people in that worldview and create an "us" versus "them" mentality in their true believers. In technocratic obstetrics, the "good patients" are compliant and accepting of technocratic rituals/standard procedures, while the "bad patients" are those who reject those rituals and the technocratic paradigm that underlies them, asking "too many questions" and refusing rituals/standard procedures that are TMTS (too much too soon [Miller et. al. 2016]). In her chapter in Volume III of this series (Davis-Floyd and Premkumar 2023c), medical anthropologist Lauren Diamond-Brown (2023) demonstrates that US obstetricians often call such "bad" patients via gendered tropes that include "misinformed" childbearers, "control freaks," and "selfish" mothers who put their own interests before those of their babies.

### Stage 2 Thinking: Ethnocentrism

Schoder, Driver, and Streufert described Stage 2 thinking as "the emergence of alternate perceptions of the same dimensions" (quoted in McManus 1979:217). Anthropologically, I code Stage 2 thinkers as what anthropologists call *ethnocentric*. Ethnocentrists know that other ways exist and are generally willing to acknowledge that it's ok for others to think differently. But they are entirely certain that "Our way is best." Stage 2 thinkers may feel scorn or pity for "others" who do not comprehend how much better "our way" is. Stage 2 ethnocentrism, while broader than Stage 1 cognitive systems, is also a relatively closed system, constantly reinforced by the rituals that enact and sustain it. Ethnocentrists are often very willing to explore and learn about other cultures, other ways of thinking and being, out of curiosity and a desire to expand their horizons—yet generally remain convinced that their way is best.

For example, ethnocentric obs may watch midwives attend normal births out of curiosity or view a video about how to attend breech births, but are unlikely to actually adopt such practices. A more powerful example is the fact that many Americans are so ethnocentric that they believe the United States must be Number 1 in all things and must remain the most powerful country in the world. Their ethnocentrism, along with that of many Russians, Chinese, Europeans, and others, is the reason we will likely never have a world government with any actual power—few if any countries would be willing to surrender their sovereignty, even if actually having a world government might stop wars and limit climate change, or might pass enforceable laws against environmental pollution, ethnic "cleansing," and human trafficking. Instead of seeing a world government as a potentially good thing, people in general are too afraid of subordinating whatever power their own countries have, too afraid of the very real possibility that a world government might turn into a dictatorship ruled perhaps by corporations or power-hungry technocrats. Instead, we have the United Nations—an organization with lofty goals but with little power to achieve them—yet which does offer the possibility of world "governance" (government by consensus among sovereign nations). But to make that work, we must move beyond ethnocentrism to more open systems that work for the good of all.

## Open Knowledge Systems: Stages 3 and 4

### Stage 3 Thinking: Cultural Relativism

Schroder, Driver, and Streufert described Stage 3 thinking as "complex rules for simultaneously comparing and relating perspectives." In other words, and in dramatic contrast to Stage 1 and 2 thinkers, Stage 3 thinkers are very open. They realize at some point in their lives that every culture and religion has created its own story about the nature and structure of reality, and that no one has the authority to say which story is right. In anthropological terms, I code Stage 3 thinkers as *cultural relativists* who come to see every story about reality as relative to every other story ("All ways have value; individual behavior should be understood within its sociocultural context.") No one has a lock on "truth," and every belief system must be understood in terms of its own cultural, ecological, historical, ideological, and political context, and must be respected as legitimate in its own right. And, again, all individual behaviors must be understood and interpreted within their sociocultural context. Where cultural relativism can be useful in birth is in what I have called *informed relativism* (Davis-Floyd et al. 2018:226), by which I mean the ability to be familiar with various birth knowledge systems, including Indigenous and traditional knowledge systems, to pick and choose among them what works best in a particular perinatal situation, and to provide culturally competent and culturally safe care—as I will discuss later on in this chapter.

Many anthropologists are cultural relativists who understand that comparing a given culture with others is the best way to comprehend that culture and its ways, for cross-cultural comparisons highlight otherwise invisible aspects of every culture. Certainly, every culture's customs, rituals, and the value and belief systems they enact are worth description, interpretation, and understanding. Thus, cultural relativism can sound ideal—it entails respect for, appreciation for, and understanding of every story that every culture or religion tells, and of the laws and traditions of each and every society. Such tolerance! No bigotry, no racism, no ethnocentrism, no judgment.

And yet cultural relativism, especially when confused with or equated to *moral relativism*—the notion that the same thing that is considered immoral in one culture may be considered moral in another— has severe limitations, as it can and has been used to justify behaviors that are fully acceptable within their cultural contexts yet also violate human rights. For examples, in some cultures and subcultures, such as those of US law enforcement personnel, racialized police brutality has long been normalized (though that is now changing); in rural Pakistan, men are entitled to beat their wives every night just to remind them who is boss (Jalil, Zakar, and Qureshi 2013; Zakar, Zakar, and Abbas 2016). In some cultures, as we all know from the news media, gay men or adulterous women are stoned to death, torture of prisoners is normal, what outsiders call "female genital mutilation" is mandatory, and female fetuses are often aborted due to a higher cultural value on sons (see Ghosh 2012; Bongaarts and Guilmoto 2015). In most large-scale technocratic societies, gender, class, racial, ethnic, and socioeconomic discrimination are systemic—systematic and endemic—and environmental pollution is normative, especially when it is profitable in the short term. And in hospitals around the world, most predominantly in low-resource countries, treating birthing women with disrespect and abuse is so culturally normative that it has been officially named by those who critique it—*obstetric violence* (see Sadler et al. 2016 and Volume III of this series, Davis-Floyd and Premkumar 2023a). Given that all such practices are part of their cultures, a true cultural relativist would simply seek to understand them within their cultural context, respecting the cultural beliefs that lead to such practices. Is that ok? By what standards can cultural relativists say that it is not?

### Stage 4 Thinking: Global Humanism

> It would seem that the world has come far enough so that it is
> only by starting from relativism and its tolerations that we may
> hope to work out a new set of absolute values and standards,
> if such are attainable at all or prove to be desirable.
> —Alfred Kroeber (1949:320)

The dilemmas posed by cultural relativism have led to an increased international focus on the development of *global humanism*, which I link to Stage 4 thinking. (Schroder, Driver, and Streufert described Stage 4 thinking as the "generation of complex relationships among rules of comparison" [quoted in McManus 1979: 217]). I suggest that Stage 4/ global humanist thinkers ("All individuals have rights that should be honored, not violated") recognize the intrinsic integrity and value of every cultural and religious story; every set of customs, beliefs, and the rituals that enact them; yet these thinkers seek higher standards that can be applied in every context to ensure the honoring of the *human rights of individuals*, most particularly the poorer and weaker members of society. No one should be discriminated against, beaten, tortured, raped, abused, or murdered in the name of any cause, sociocultural hierarchy, or belief system. Everyone should have access to clean water, good nutrition, effective health care, and fair pay for their work. Daughters should be viewed as intrinsically valuable as sons. And obstetricians should practice in ways that honor the human rights, and thus the protagonism, of the birthing people they attend.

Such seemingly desirable goals can often go deeply against the grain of a given culture—as in South Africa before the end of apartheid; as in those cultures whose members believe that uncircumcised women are unclean and must be socially excluded; and as in the culture of technocratic obstetrics with its maxim "the doctor knows best" and its general disregard of childbearers' rights and of local cultural birth customs. Thus, many global humanists (sometimes also called "universalists") seek to think beyond the limitations of cultural relativism, *searching for universal standards that work for everyone*. They want to validate and legitimate every culture *and* every individual, while devaluing and discouraging specific cultural practices that hurt people who do not deserve to be hurt in this higher, human rights sense (see Table 1.1.). Stage 4 humanistic obs do not harm their patients with TMTS or TLTL (too little too late [Miller et al. 2016]) practices; rather, they provide RAR-TRW (the right amount at the right time in the right way [Cheyney and Davis-Floyd 2020]) evidence-based care that is culturally safe and respectful and offers fully informed choice and shared decision-making.

Global humanists tend to be acutely aware of the structural inequities that pervade technocratic societies and often do their best to address and work to find solutions for them. Global humanists are also aware that they are on an almost impossible set of missions—how can you work to preserve a culture while also working to change key aspects of it?—such as ending the poverty caused by colonialism and the global culture of the capitalistic technocracy, fostering the births and education of girls and women in nations where they are devalued, or honoring women's rights in childbirth within an obstetric culture that routinely disregards and denies those rights and is full of racial and ethnic bias. Those working in maternity-related fields know well that such systemic inequities are largely responsible for the high maternal and perinatal mortality and prematurity rates of Black women in the US (Davis 2019a, 2019b) and in low-resource nations, where effective care is often provided for the wealthy but not for the poor. Yet such missions must be attempted anyway for the good of all. Global humanists understand that they must keep their knowledge systems open to new information and engage in bioethical discussions and debates, trying to figure out what works best

Table 1.1. The Stages of Cognition and Their Anthropological Equivalents. (I created this Table with the help of Charles D. Laughlin; it originally appeared in *The Power of Ritual* [2016], on which we hold the copyright, so I reprint it here with Charlie's permission. This Table also appears in the recently abridged version of that book, called *Ritual: What It Is, How It Works, and Why* [2022].) © Davis-Floyd and Laughlin.

| Stages of Cognition | Anthropological Equivalents |
|---|---|
| Stage 4: Fluid, open thinking | **Global humanism:** "All individuals have rights that should be honored, not violated." |
| Stage 3: Relative, open thinking | **Cultural relativism:** "All ways have value; individual behavior should be understood within its sociocultural context." |
| Stage 2: Self- and culture-centered semi-closed thinking | **Ethnocentrism:** "Other ways may be ok for others, but our way is best." |
| Stage 1: Rigid/concrete closed thinking, intolerance of other ways of thinking | **Naïve realism:** "Our way is the only way, or the only way that matters." **Fundamentalism:** "Our is way is the only *right* way"; **Fanaticism:** "Our way is so right that all others should be assimilated or eliminated." |
| +Substage: Non-thinking; inability to process information; lack or loss of compassion for others. | **Cognitive regression:** Intense egocentrism, irritability, inability to cope, burnout, breakdown, hysteria, panic, "losing it," abusing or mistreating others. |

+I will discuss "Substage" later on in this chapter.

to preserve everyone's rights without necessarily assuming superiority for any one system, such as that of technocratic obstetrics.

For example, many global humanists work to lower maternal and perinatal mortality rates in low- to middle-income countries without buying into the biomedical notion that traditional midwives (aka traditional birth attendants [TBAs]) should be eliminated because "biomedical facility births are always better," no matter how low-quality and TLTL that facility care may be (Miller, Cordero et al. 2003; Miller and Lalonde 2015; Miller, Abalos et al. 2016). Some Indigenous and traditional birthways, such as laboring and birthing in upright or all-fours positions, are far better than those of hospital birth, and vice versa. So in birth, in the practice of "informed relativism"—which they share with cultural relativists, along with open and fluid ways of thinking—global humanists look for what *actually* works best, rather than what is simply *assumed* to work best in pregnancy, birth, and the postpartum period.

Stage 4 thinkers do develop and perform rituals; such rituals are usually very fluid attempts to express and enact humanistic values. For example, in *Imagery in the Rituals of Birth: Ontology between the Sacred and the Secular* (2019:88), Anna Hennessey writes that she collected a wide variety of birth images prior to her labor:

> looking at them and visualizing what was happening to my body and to the baby so as to encourage birth. . . . All the images, some of which stem from religious traditions, are now sacred to me. Two midwives, a doula, and my husband were part of a supportive social circle that encouraged my ritual visualization practices. Yet this sacredness is of a non-religious and humanistic nature.

Since the beliefs of Stage 4 globally humanistic thinkers are open to flux and change, the rituals they create tend to constantly change as well, or they are spontaneous enactments of something going on in the moment, such as the rituals that homebirthing families often spontaneously create—for example, lighting candles and symbolically throwing their fears into the candle flames (Cheyney 2011; Davis-Floyd 2022)—or birth activists and midwives singing songs about love and peace at the end of conferences, with everyone forming a circle and holding hands. One such song is:

> *Circle round for freedom, circle round for peace*
> *For all of us in prison, circle for release*
> *Circle for the planet, circle for each soul*
> *For the children of our children, keep the circle whole!*

Freedom and peace are two core values of global humanism, as is the salvation of our planetary environment to ensure a viable life for ourselves and our descendants—whose future welfare is also a core value of global humanism. The "prison" to which the song refers can mean literal prison, or the conceptual prison of psychological issues that keep us isolated, or the rigid and often racist ideologies that keep us apart.

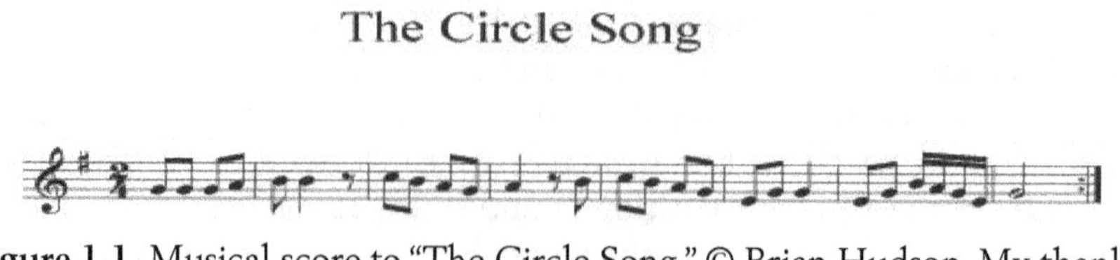

## The Circle Song

**Figure 1.1.** Musical score to "The Circle Song." © Brian Hudson. My thanks to my beloved godson Brian Hudson for creating this musical score for me.

Another one, often sung at the end of Midwifery Today conferences in particular, again, forming a circle and holding hands:

*Humble yourself in the sight of your sister*
*You need to bow down low (everyone bows) and*
*Humble yourself in the sight of your brother*
*You need to know what he knows (all stand up straight) and*
*We shall lift each other u-u-u-up (all arms are raised)*
*We shall lift each other up!*

## Humble Yourself

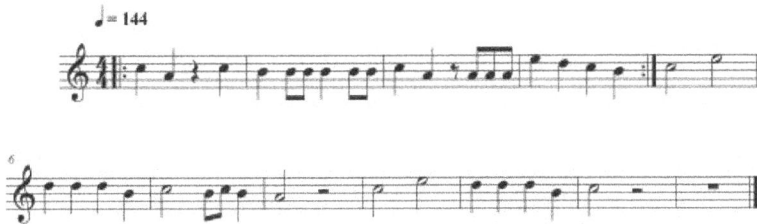

**Figure 1.2.** Musical score to "Humble Yourself." © Brian Hudson. My thanks to my beloved godson Brian Hudson for creating this musical score for me.

This song, "Humble Yourself," is also an apt example of globally humanistic thinking, as it expresses another core value of global humanism—that every individual knows something of value and everyone's knowledge should be honored, sought, and shared. And in keeping with two of the primary characteristics of ritual—repetition and redundancy—such songs are usually sung or chanted at least four times in a row, which aids their repetitive messages to more deeply penetrate the psyches of the singers.

## Stage 1 versus Stage 4 Thinkers: The Ongoing Battles

*There is no greater challenge to Stage 1 fundamentalists and fanatics than global humanism*—and vice versa. Global humanism says that there can be *many* right ways as long as everyone's individual rights are preserved; fundamentalists and fanatics say that there is only *one* right way, and that only their leaders and/or their authoritative texts get to decide who has which rights. Fundamentalists and fanatics seek to build temples of isolation, rigid silos within which their rules can prevail—where cults and sects can practice their belief systems without interference—and including silos designed to protect the turf of a given profession (e.g., obstetrics) against others with overlapping claims to parts of that turf (e.g., midwives). Fundamentalists and fanatics hold tight to their concrete silos, standing firm against the swirling, constantly changing cultural forms of our late modern technocracies. True cultural relativists would have no grounds for criticizing these cultural and professional silos—which have their own subcultures—whereas true global humanists would want to ensure that everyone within them chooses freely to be there and has their rights as human beings honored, even when they step outside the silo box—which is so often not the case. Thus, Stage 1 fundamentalists and fanatics abhor global humanists, in life and in birth, and global humanists abhor the efforts of Stage 1 fundamentalist and fanatical thinkers to take away individual rights and freedom of choice. Below, we will see obstetric fanaticism at work in the examples I provide of the ongoing persecutions of humanistic and holistic midwives and obstetricians by the obstetric establishments in their regions or countries, in what many are calling the contemporary "global witch hunt" of birth practitioners who choose to let childbearers be the protagonists of their own births.

## Human Rights

The concept that *individuals have rights* is relatively new in human history. Its early roots in the Western world can be traced to the *Magna Carta*, signed in 1215 by King John of England, guaranteeing for the first time that the king did not have absolute power, but had to acknowledge the sovereign rights of the nobility—the dukes, barons, earls—to own their own lands and generally rule them as they saw fit. Yet the concept that serfs, peasants, and the poor in general had rights too did not gain much traction until the American Revolution of 1776 with its *Declaration of Independence*, which acknowledged the rights of white males—that was a start—and the French Revolution of 1789, and later the Russian Revolution of 1917 that overthrew the Czar and brought in the communist system, in which every individual was supposed to have rights—until Stage 1 totalitarian dictators took over and that notion went back to the back burner. Hitler's defeat in World War II allowed a huge step forward in the defining and promotion of human rights; one of its many consequences was the development of Ethical Guidelines for Research (Chalmers 2019). And then came the United Nations, which took on the issue of global human rights in a very powerful way, formalizing in key documents for the first time in the world the concept that *every human being has certain rights*.

The fact that some Islamic nations have long criticized the 1948 UN *Universal Declaration of Human Rights* as biased in favor of Western values demonstrates just how hard it is to enumerate rights that every individual and government in the world can agree on. And the granting of those rights seemed to apply mostly to men, until the UN's 4th World Congress on Women (Beijing, 1995), where Hillary Clinton so powerfully stated that "Women's and children's rights are human rights." (Actually, this concept was first promoted at the World Conference on Human Rights in Vienna in 1993, yet it was Clinton's statement at the 1995 Beijing conference that drew the most global attention.) And that concept opened the way for childbearers, social scientists, and birth activists to use human rights language to claim that their human rights must be honored, in birth as in daily life.

There are many documents that charter the honoring of human rights in childbirth; a primary one is the White Ribbon Alliance *Charter on the Universal Rights of Childbearing Women* (2011). Yet the one I wish to call attention to here is the *International Childbirth Initiative* (ICI): *12 Steps to Safe and Respectful MotherBaby-Family Maternity Care.* The ICI's 12 Steps provide a rights-based, globally humanistic template for high quality, evidence-based, mother- and family-friendly maternity care (see Lalonde et al. 2019; Lalonde 2023; and *International Childbirth Initiative*[3]). The ICI has been translated into multiple languages and has been or is being implemented in many birthing facilities, both large and small, around the world. Researchers are needed to study the implementation process and its outcomes and to identify barriers to implementation and suggest ways to overcome them. (For a list of the ICI implementation sites and the countries in which they are located, see Lalonde's [2023] chapter in Volume I of this series.) If you are interested in conducting such research, please contact me at davis-floyd@outlook.com. I strongly encourage all birth practitioners to implement these 12 Steps and their underlying philosophy—the MotherBaby-Family Model of Care—in their facilities and practices.

Since women's rights in perinatal care are not obvious to many obstetricians and not recognized by them, feminist activists have managed to get legislation passed in Venezuela, Argentina, Panama, and Mexico guaranteeing women the right to have companions during their labors and births and protecting them from obstetric violence, disrespect, and abuse. These are positive steps forward, yet to date there have been no mechanisms in place to enforce these laws. So technocratic, fundamentalist, silo-oriented obs in these countries simply ignore the laws and continue their traditional ritual practices, often forcing women to labor without companionship; using harmful maneuvers such as Kristeller (heavy fundal pressure applied by a practitioner); cutting episiotomies on all who do not have cesareans because they are taught that "the perineum will explode" if an episiotomy is not performed (see Davis-Floyd and Georges 2023); treating laboring women disrespectfully and often abusively; and denying their protagonism in birth and their supposedly informed freedom of choice (see Miller and Lalonde 2015; Sadler et al. 2016; Liese et al. 2021; Davis-Floyd and Premkumar 2023c, and the other chapters in this volume). Liese and colleagues (2021) have identified a UHDVA *spectrum of obstetric iatrogenesis*, with unintentional harm (UH) caused by the performance of standard obstetric procedures/rituals at one end of the spectrum and overt obstetric disrespect, violence, and abuse (DVA) at the other.

In previous works, I have answered the question of *why* obstetricians so often deny women's protagonism in birth in my analyses of the intense socialization of obstetricians into the technocratic model of birth via their many years of training, during which they are both bodily and psychologically habituated to the fear-based rituals of hospital birth (Davis-Floyd 1987, 2018b). According to the epidemiologists I have spoken with, and many of my physician interlocutors as well, the intensity and longevity of this socialization generates "narrow-mindedness" and "tunnel vision" (Stage 1). Here is a direct verbal quote—also provided in the Series Overview in Volume I (Davis-Floyd and Premkumar 2023d)—from one of those (highly frustrated) epidemiologists who works for PAHO (Pan American Health Organization, a branch of the World Health Organization [WHO]):

> Why don't obstetricians get it? We epidemiologists understand that the vast majority of what they do during labor and birth is just plain wrong ... Lots of pediatricians do too ... So why don't obs act according to the evidence, as we have long been insisting that they do? Instead they just blindly follow obstetric traditions—why can't they learn to think for themselves?

**Again please note:** The 4 Stages of Cognition as I describe them here have *nothing to do with intelligence levels nor are necessarily replicated in all areas of cognition*—it is possible to be a rigid thinker in one or several areas while being a fluid thinker in many others. For example, a quantum physicist studying ambiguities in the universe with a completely open mind to the existence of other universes, string theory, the "multiverse," and other dimensions may also be a devout religious practitioner, choosing in this uncertain world to find certainty via faith. An obstetrician with a cesarean rate of 75%, who knows nothing about normal birth and has no desire to learn how to support it, can also run a charitable foundation serving the poor with a full understanding of how social stratification and systemic disparities work to hold them in poverty. How fundamentalist or fanatical you are tends to depend on your level of socialization and embodied habituation into the areas in which your thinking becomes rigidified—the deeper the socialization and habituation, and the more rituals associated with them, the "truer believer" (Hoffer 1951) you are likely to be. The "true believer" phenomenon is fairly well understood, but *why some people become open and fluid thinkers is not*; thus, this is a subject ripe for further research.

I should also note here that seemingly Stage 4 global humanists can themselves become fundamentalist or fanatical in the new beliefs they come to hold—for example, I have witnessed many (highly fanatical) homebirth activists discounting evidence that does not uphold their particular views, just as many obstetricians do. In my view, Stage 4 thinking is about keeping your belief system open to new learning, not about learning a new way and then becoming entrenched in it.

## Birth Practitioners and the 4 Stages of Cognition

### Stages 1 and 2 Birth Knowledge Systems

Most traditional midwives, and many professional midwives, nurses, and obstetricians are Stage 1 or 2 thinkers in terms of maternity care. Stage 1 naïve realist practitioners can work within their settings, whether community- or facility-based, for their lifetimes, without ever questioning their practices and the beliefs that underlie them, because they simply know no other way. But there are few obs, at least in the higher-resource nations, who do not know that their practices are constantly scrutinized and criticized by thousands of birth activists in many countries, by many of their patients, by the more humanistically inclined midwives and nurses who may work with them, and by the doulas who increasingly attend to the support needs of the laboring people under their care. Doulas, like humanistic midwives and labor and delivery nurses, often suggest (quietly) that their clients should reject the ritual interventions they are receiving—sometimes causing obstetricians to resent these doulas mightily. These obs may become fundamentalists, carefully guarding their epistemic boundaries, or fanatics who seek to destroy humanistic and holistic obstetricians and midwives. For example, in Puerto Rico, when demand for community births rose during the coronavirus pandemic, obstetricians launched a vicious media campaign against the 24 community midwives on that island, who in general attend less than 1% of the more than 200,000 annual births (Reyes 2021).

Ethnocentric obstetricians (who simply think that their way is best) who feel themselves under siege in their practices have choices:

1. They can move beyond curiosity to actually examine the evidence, listen to women, and ultimately choose to grow beyond the limitations of their training and make a paradigm shift to the more fluid thinking that humanistic or holistic practice requires (Davis-Floyd 2001, 2018c). A few do take this path, like the Stage 4 (self-named and woman-centered) "good guys and girls" of Brazil, who work with midwives and doulas and have very low cesarean birth (CB) rates (see the chapter by Davis-Floyd and Georges 2023 in Volume II of this three-volume series (Davis-Floyd and Premkumar 2023a, 2023b, 2023c)—and also suffer various forms of persecution from the obstetric establishments in their cities.

2. They can take refuge in their Stage 1 silos, developing a fundamentalist attitude and performing their rituals/standard procedures as they always have—choosing to ignore both the scientific evidence and the growing criticisms and efforts of others to encourage them to change.

3. They can go deeper into Stage 1, "circling the wagons" by becoming highly defensive, even fanatical, critiquing and imposing harsh punishments on their colleagues who "go rogue"/step out of the silo by humanizing their practices. I could provide hundreds of examples here, but will confine myself to two (see also the chapters in Volume I of this series: Davis-Floyd and Premkumar 2023a):

   • In Brazil in 2012, a well-respected obstetric professor, Dr. Jorge Kuhn, during a nationally broadcast television interview, declared that he supported home birth—as long as the birth was attended by a skilled professional and transport arrangements were in place. In an extremely fanatical overreaction, the medical council of Rio de Janeiro (CREMERJ) immediately called for Kuhn's medical license to be revoked, completely refusing to even look at the irrefutable evidence on which he had based his statement. (See Anderson, Daviss, and Johnson [2021], and Daviss, Anderson, and Johnson [2021] for compilations of that evidence.) These actions led to a major series of marches in the streets by women and others demanding the rights to home birth, companionship during labor, and other issues, to which CREMERJ, again fanatically, responded by forbidding *any* doctor to attend home births, forcing all of Brazil's "good guys and girls" to stop doing so, and leaving homebirth attendance to the professional midwives, who are few in number in Brazil while obs are many.

- The closure of the Albany Midwifery Practice (which had served an all-risk population) by King's Hospital in London. For decades, the Albany was touted as one of the best midwifery practices in Europe. Yet, after reaching a 43% homebirth rate (the UK homebirth rate was only 2% at the time), they were suddenly shut down by their hospital for trumped up reasons. Despite their excellent outcomes, marches in the streets, and other forms of protest from their former clientele, they were never allowed to re-open. (For the story of the Albany practice, how well it worked, and how its midwives achieved such a high homebirth rate with excellent outcomes, see Reed and Walton 2009. For an analysis of its excellent statistical outcomes, see Homer et al. 2017. For the story of its closure, see Reed and Edwards, in press).

Such "witch hunts" of Stage 4 birth practitioners take place all over the world.[4] The closed technocratic obstetric system, when fanatically applied as Stage 1, has ruined many of the lives of those who oppose it and will likely seek to continue to do so for years to come as its hegemony is increasingly challenged, both by scientific research and by humanistic and holistic practitioners who put the childbearer, not the system, first.

Technocratic obstetrics is a relatively closed Stage 1 fundamentalist system, often degenerating into fanaticism when challenged, as we have just seen. Its practitioners tend to incorporate only the kinds of new information that fit within their pre-existing knowledge system. Obstetricians who read a study comparing epidurals with other types of pain medication can easily process that kind of information, for example, but the same obstetricians presented with multiple studies that demonstrate the benefits of midwives, doulas, being in water, massage, eating and drinking at will, and frequent changes in position for labor facilitation will be likely to discount this kind of non-silo information. Entrenched, they see no reason to exert the much greater amounts of energy it would take to assimilate information from outside their technocratic paradigm. Hence what my former student Kyra Kramer (2002) named "the evidence-discourse-practice gap": obstetricians often know that the evidence exists, and sometimes talk about it, but do not implement it because that would take them out of their Stage 1 comfort zone. This is also true of thousands of professional midwives around the world, who work hard to learn accepted biomedical ways and then are thrust into busy practices.

Often overworked, overstressed, and underpaid, they too are unwilling to open their cognitive systems to process information that contradicts the technocratic approaches they are taught. Birth is not a good catalyst for change in such cases, as the birth process is resilient, and most babies come out alive and relatively healthy most of the time anyway—though the negative psychological and physical effects on the mother and the baby of mistreatment during birth can be extreme (see Liese et al. 2021; Davis-Floyd 2022). So the more practitioners attend births in their habitual ritual ways, the more these ways become the only ways they can imagine for attending births—an all-too-common tautology.

It is ironic that science, which was supposed to be the foundation of obstetrics, does not support most standard obstetric practices. Yet "science" has been used by obstetricians for 150 years to justify the interventions they invented and then increasingly performed. *Science used ethnocentrically for Stage 1 or 2 technomedical thinkers is a blinder for what is really biomedical ritual and tradition*, passed down from teacher to student through apprenticeship/experiential learning—again, the most powerful learning mode.

### Stage 3/Cultural Relativist and Stage 4/Global Humanist Birth Knowledge Systems

Of all the birth practitioners I have spoken with during my more than 30 years of research, I can't think of any cultural relativists who base their decisions on no standards at all just because they can't choose between the many viable care standards out there. Pregnant women will die of eclampsia if they do not receive effective prenatal care. Postpartum hemorrhages must be stopped if at all possible. Babies who don't breathe at birth must be resuscitated—and, in the Stage 4 holistic approach, which involves energy and spirit, the parents can "call the baby," inviting the spirit to come into the body—a practice that, according to many of the midwives I have interviewed over time, and also to some perinatologists who have learned about this practice from midwives, often actually works, precluding the need for actual resuscitation. (See Davis-Floyd 2022 and the Introduction to this volume for descriptions of the technocratic, superficially humanistic, deeply humanistic, and holistic paradigms of birth and health care.) In addition to informed relativism, where cultural relativism can be helpful in birth is when respect for every culture encourages practitioners to become *culturally competent* enough to generate *Cultural Safety*[5] for childbearers by understanding what in fact makes marginalized childbearers, and/or those who come from traditional or Indigenous societies, feel safe: communicating with them in their own language or having a translator present; honoring their cultural value on modesty, for example, by refraining from exposing their genitals and allowing them to eat and drink at will; and supporting them to labor and birth in the upright, deeply physiologic (and evidence-based) positions they tend to value; allowing the presence of supportive members of their own family and/or community; providing care in their communities—something all childbearers want—and treating them with dignity and respect instead of with racial or ethnic discrimination. All these can stem from a culturally relativistic approach that includes informed relativism, just as they can from a globally humanistic approach. It seems clear that Stage 3 and 4 ways of thinking can elide into each other, as cultural relativists are also often humanistic practitioners. Yet it is also possible for Stage 3 cultural relativists to perform TMTS interventions while respecting some cultural customs and values, whereas globally humanistic Stage 4 practitioners keep their focus on honoring women's rights and providing culturally appropriate RARTRW (the right amount at the right time in the right way) care.

When not overstressed (see below), Stage 3 and 4 birth practitioners will frequently expose themselves to new information, whether it comes from science, traditional midwifery, a book they happened to read, or a workshop they attended the day before. For example, Turkish obstetrician Hakan Çoker changed his entire practice style after sneaking into a childbirth education workshop out of sheer ethnocentric curiosity, eventually developing a Stage 4 model called "Birth with No Regret" that includes a birth psychologist along with a midwife/doula and obstetrician (see Çoker, Karabekir and Varlık 2021; Çoker 2023 in Volume I of this series). The birth psychologist's responsibility is to process the emotions of the laboring woman and her family, as well as those of the obstetrician and midwife, before, during, and after the birth, to ensure that the *psychosphere* (Jones 2009) of the birth stays clean and clear, and that no one regresses into "Substage" (see below). For many other examples of Stage 4 models, see Davis-Floyd et al. (2009); Daviss and Davis-Floyd (2021); and Gutschow, Davis-Floyd, and Daviss (2021).

In today's rapidly changing and highly fluid world, to be truly effective, Stage 3 and 4 practitioners must remain open to the new information that is constantly emerging from actual science and from the increasing availability of birth knowledge from multiple systems—allopathic, Indigenous, holistic, integrative. Sometimes the best option for a birth complication might be emotional support, a homeopathic remedy, or an acupressure treatment; sometimes it might be a position used by traditional midwives, such as hands-and-knees (which widens the pelvic outlet to its maximum capacity [see Bruner et al. 1998]); sometimes it might be a cesarean birth. Humanistic practitioners will keep their knowledge systems open to new learning from many sources in highly postmodern ways (as I and my colleagues describe in "Daughter of Time: The Postmodern Midwife" [Davis-Floyd et al. 2018])—sometimes by going back to the past to recover helpful traditional knowledge and bring it into the future. They will practice informed relativism and will base their Stage 4 practices on viable scientific evidence and on the highest moral and ethical standards, which involve giving compassionate, woman-centered care responsive to the needs of individuals and honoring their human rights. Yet humanistic practitioners, or those who would like to become so, must be careful to distinguish between *superficial* and *deep* humanism in birth. In superficial humanism, the labor rooms may be pretty, partners and doulas may be present, and the practitioners are kind as they continue to perform TMTS interventions. In contrast, deeply humanistic practitioners honor what I call the *deep physiology of birth* (Davis-Floyd 2018c, 2022), working to facilitate that physiology rather than to interfere with it.

### Why Many Birth Attendants Do Not Give Stage 4 Care: Tunnel Vision and "Substage"

Cognitive openness and humane standards are not easy to maintain, especially in a busy and stressful practice. Even those Stage 4 practitioners who want to remain open to new learning and new ways of thinking find that the more stress they are under, the less able and willing they are to process new information. *Persistent stress can reduce even highly fluid, Stage 4 thinkers to Stage 1 levels* by causing cognitive overload and the development of "tunnel vision"—the need to shut out most stimuli and focus on one thing only. In other words, stress can make fluid thinkers become rigid, if only for a while. How often have you thought on an especially stressful day, "I can't deal with any more information—just don't tell me one more thing!"? Usually rest or a vacation will restore Stage 4 thinkers to their normal fluid state. But if the stress continues for too long or becomes too intense, anyone can disintegrate into what Charles Laughlin and I (2022) call *Substage* (which Schroder, Driver, and Streufert [1967] termed "Sub-1")—intense irritability, anxiety, anger, burnout, breakdown, hysteria, panic. This might also be termed "losing it"—a highly self-centered condition in which it is very hard to feel compassion and very easy to abuse others below you in the status hierarchy—especially if they are socially marginalized via race, ethnicity, or socioeconomic status. Again, ongoing stress can lower one's cognitive level from Stage 4 to Stage 1—a conceptual space in which you don't have to think—you just go on "automatic pilot." And the more stress you are under, the harder it becomes to "think beyond" and the more likely you are to "lose it" and cognitively regress into Substage.

## Rituals as "Life-Hacks"

Performing rituals can stabilize individuals under stress at Stage 1, thereby preventing them from degenerating into Substage—or bring them back out of it. Ritual researcher Dimitris Xygalatas calls rituals both "mechanisms of resilience" and "life-hacks," meaning that people use them to relieve stress and anxiety and to create a sense of calm. He notes that rituals actively work in the human brain to achieve those goals, explaining: "The mechanism that we think is operating here is that ritual helps reduce anxiety by providing the brain with a sense of structure, regularity, and predictability." He recommends the performance of rituals as an effective way to cope with anxiety, noting that ritual is a powerful "mental technology" that we can use "to trick ourselves into [calming down]. That is what these rituals do—they act like life hacks . . . that have been with and have served us well since the dawn of our kind" (quoted in the *University of Connecticut Science News* 2020:1). Thus, when practitioners—or anyone—find themselves overwhelmed and about to regress into Substage, I suggest that they use the "mental technology" of ritual to "life-hack" themselves back to cognitive stability.

For example, stressed out practitioners can intentionally perform rituals that calm and comfort—perhaps practicing yoga or Tai Chi; taking time every day to exercise, meditate, pray; returning to church, synagogue, temple, mosque. *Ritual stands as a buffer between cognition and chaos*, between Stage 1 and Substage, and again, its power can be used to keep people out of Substage, or to bring them back from it. The ob who is about to yell at a nurse or a laboring person can use the ritualistic anger management technique of leaving the room to take ten deep breaths to avoid abusing others. Yet instead, most technomedical obstetric practitioners rely on the rituals of hospital birth to comfort and calm them, as those rituals/standard procedures, despite their often-negative effects on the normal physiology of birth, work well to keep fear at bay for practitioners and also often for birthing people (see Davis-Floyd 2022).

### Stage 1 Rituals: Restoring a Sense of Control

When labor slows or fetal heart tones drop, rather than operationalizing the virtue of patience or suggesting a position change, obstetricians may administer Pitocin or rush to perform a cesarean. Such Stage 1 rituals can generate a sense that everything is under control (even if it isn't). Again, ritual stands as a buffer between cognition and chaos. Obstetricians facing what they see as constant potential crises in childbirth often use such Stage 1 rituals preventatively, so that things at least feel or seem to be under control. They practice defensively to avoid accusations of malpractice and to conform to institutional systems and protocols rather than taking the time and energy (and the risks to their careers) to try to change them, because it's just easier that way and because of our general Stage 1 belief that technologically intervening in birth makes it safer—when in fact, such interventions often cause more harm than good. This is the *obstetric paradox*: intervene in birth to keep it safe, thereby causing harm (Cheyney and Davis-Floyd 2019:8).

## How Obstetricians Can Foster Stage 4 Thinking: Resocialization

In her chapter in Volume III of this series, "'Selfish Mothers,' 'Misinformed' Childbearers, and 'Control Freaks': Gendered Tropes in US Obstetricians' Justifications for Delegitimizing Patient Autonomy in Childbirth," Lauren Diamond-Brown (2023) notes the ever-present possibility that obstetricians can *resocialize* themselves into Stage 4, globally humanistic practices. I suggest that possibilities for such resocializations include:

### 1. Attendance at Midwifery Conferences
Again, moving from technocratic to humanistic or holistic practice (from Stage 1 to Stage 4) requires a tremendous amount of new learning, which in turn requires a great deal of time, attention, and energy. At conferences, obs are free to put in that time and energy to develop new neural networks as they are exposed to differing ways of thinking, knowing, and practicing. Yet at obstetric conferences, obstetricians tend to learn more of what they already know—their belief systems are not challenged as they would be at a midwifery conference where "the midwifery model of care" (described in Rooks 1999 and Davis-Floyd 2018d), with its woman-centered focus and its many accompanying hands-on skills, is taught and demonstrated in lectures and workshops. When obs show up at midwifery conferences, they generally receive a great deal of support from the midwives they meet for their efforts to learn and change. And if they have already learned and changed, they can present the practice models they have developed and receive feedback on them that can help them improve. For example, in her chapter

in Volume I of this series (Davis-Floyd and Premkumar 2023a), Rosana Fontes (2023:103) described:

> In 2014, I attended the first SIAPARTO São Paulo, Brazil, annual international normal childbirth conference, organized by well-known holistic homebirth midwife Ana Cristina Duarte. This is one of the few conferences here in Brazil where an obstetrician can come into direct contact with evidence-based information about birth assistance and the people who are practicing it. This first conference changed my views of childbirth, women's power, corporate power, and the work of doulas and midwives. I intensely embraced this new universe I hadn't encountered in medical school, and it satisfied all my needs for the ability to make a professional change.

Over the years, I have attended hundreds of midwifery conferences and have watched how both midwives and the few obs who attend "get their juice" by being there. Every such conference has offered its participants many ways to "think beyond" established paradigms and practices; thus I encourage every practicing and student midwife, obstetric nurse, doula, and obstetrician to attend as many such conferences as they possibly can—especially those put on by a small organization called Midwifery Today, which are always holistic in nature. And those larger conferences put on by, for examples, the American College of Nurse-Midwives, the International Confederation of Midwives, and Women Deliver, also offer many talks and workshops that are humanistically and holistically oriented.

## 2. Learning from Women

Obs who practice the same way for many years have usually stopped—or never started—*listening to women*. Every woman whom practitioners attend during labor and birth can bring something new to their knowledge and practices. I have often been struck by the changes in practice that can result from listening carefully to and learning from even one woman, who perhaps is unusual but can teach the obstetrician and other practitioners something new about how best to provide woman-centered care.

## 3. Learning from Midwives

From listening to obs hanging out in groups, I know that the birth stories they tell usually focus on pathologies that they find intrinsically interesting because of the intellectual puzzles they present or crises in which they saved, or failed to save, a life. In dramatic contrast, midwives tend to tell stories of normal births or of how they figured out how to help a birth that could have become pathological stay normal—a process I call *normalizing uniqueness* (Davis-Floyd and Davis 2018:212). For example, one such story, told by homebirth midwife Kate Bowland of Santa Cruz, California, was about a laboring woman who was having trouble moving the baby down, until the doula present suggested that they all do the "Hula-Hula Stomp-Stomp"—which involved putting hula hoops around their waists, circling them a few times, and then lifting each leg and then stomping it down. After several repetitions of this exercise, accompanied by peals of laughter, the woman sank down on her knees and gave birth.

Much midwifery lore and knowledge are encoded in such stories. If you want to understand the normal physiology of birth in its wide variations, listen to midwives' stories and read their many books, which tell such stories. From a US perspective, these books include:

- Ina May Gaskin's *Spiritual Midwifery* ([1975, 1980, 1990] 2002) and *Ina May's Guide to Childbirth* (2003)—both books are full of fascinating birth stories that illustrate how Ina May, arguably the most famous midwife in the world, and her midwifery colleagues acquired their birth wisdom and skills;
- Penfield Chester's *Sisters on a Journey: Portraits of American Midwives* (1997).
- *A Midwife's Tale: The Life of Martha Ballard Based on Her Diary 1785–1812* by Laurel Thatcher Ulrich (1990). This book tells the story of white pioneer midwife Martha Ballard, who kept a diary and careful records of each birth she attended, showing the outstanding outcomes she achieved before the advent of modern medicine. A movie has been made based on this book.
- *Diary of a Midwife: The Power of Positive Childbearing* by Juliana van Olphen-Fehr (1998);
- *Breech Birth, Woman Wise* by New Zealand midwife Maggie Banks (2004 [1998]);
- Patricia Harman's *The Blue Cotton Gown: A Midwife's Memoir* (2008);
- Carol Leonard's *Lady's Hands, Lion's Heart: A Midwife's Saga* (2008);
- Jennifer Worth's famous *Call the Midwife: A True Story of the East End in the 1950s* (2008) on which the popular TV series is based;
- Sister Morningstar's *The Power of Women: Instinctual Birth Stories* (2009);
- Geradine Simkins's *Into These Hands: Wisdom from Midwives* (2011);

—and many others, most of which can be found listed in an Annotated Bibliography that I and others have created.[6] These include a
whole raft of wonderful books (too many to list here) telling the
stories of revered "Black granny midwives" like Gladys Milton (see
Milton and Bovard 1993; Milton and Fulwylie 1997) and Margaret
Charles Smith (see Smith and Holmes 1996), who attended births
in the US South at a time when Black women were not admitted
to hospitals, so their midwives had to deal with any complications
that arose as best they could, developing many skills as they went
along (see also Lee 1996; Susie 1998). Such midwives, almost all of
whom were phased out of practice once biomedical hospitals began
accepting Black women, are now called by the Stage 4 honorific term
"Grand Midwives."

Continuing the trope of what obstetricians can learn from midwives,
I provide some examples from Australian ob Andrew Bisits's (2023)
chapter in Volume I of this series (Davis-Floyd and Premkumar 2023a),
in which he described how the midwives he worked with "taught me an
enormous amount about childbirth." As he started to think more about
vaginal breech birth, after reading New Zealand midwife Maggie Bank's
book *Breech Birth, Woman Wise* (1998), he discussed via emails with her
about women adopting upright positions for the births of breech babies.
Bisits also described learning far more about attending vaginal breech
births from midwives than from obstetricians or obstetric textbooks,
noting that the best descriptions of how to attend vaginal breech births
come from midwife Anne Frye's (2005) textbook on holistic midwifery
(in which, as Bisits states in his chapter, she "provides a comprehensive description of normal and abnormal breech birth mechanics that
is far superior to that in any obstetric textbook") and from Betty-Anne
Daviss's (2014) manual *Re-Thinking the Physiology of Vaginal Breech
Birth: Evidence-Based Guide to Upright Delivery*, which includes detailed
descriptions and photos of appropriate techniques. Bisits additionally
recommends the book chapter that he co-authored with Betty-Anne
(Daviss and Bisits 2021), which also provides extensive details about
how to safely attend breech births.

I can truthfully say that I have witnessed even deeply humanistic obs
go into shock when they hear about midwives' techniques for vaginal
breech births; for external versions (turning the baby in utero; see Davis-
Floyd et al. 2018); and for stopping hemorrhages without Pitocin or
Cytotec/misoprostol. Professional community midwives in the United
States and other countries do carry Pitocin and know how to administer it via an injection or an IV, which they are trained to insert, but in
the United States, such midwives, most of whom are CPMs—certified

professional midwives—are still illegal in 13 states and cannot carry IV equipment in those states, lest they be caught and accused of "practicing medicine without a license," which could land them in jail. So they have other methods of stopping hemorrhages. According to renowned homebirth midwife Sister Morningstar CPM (personal communication, October 2021), these include "using many time-tested herbs—such as Shepherd's Purse, strong red raspberry, synergistic blends of the cohoshes, and others" (see Falcon and Contreras 2009). Of course, homebirth midwives also perform bimanual compression of the uterus. Additionally, they often use what homebirth midwife Janneli Miller CPM (personal communication, 2015) has called "midwives' magical speech"—which consists of grabbing the new mother by the shoulders, looking deep into her eyes, and commanding her to "STOP BLEEDING NOW!"—which often actually works, according to the reports of midwives whom I have interviewed over the years, and in accordance with the holistic tenet of "mindbody integration." Sister Morningstar put it this way:

> I have simply said to a mother pouring out her life force like a faucet, "Tell your body to stop bleeding" while I look deep into her eyes and hold that gaze till she turns her attention to her body. Mothers can have many distractions right after birth, including husbands, other children, or a newborn with halting first breaths. And it doesn't hurt to bleed to death, so she may not realize the severity of the situation. So sometimes she needs to bring her own awareness back to self and get calm and focused. (Unless its effect is immediate, such word medicine is always accompanied with the supportive actions described above.) Also extremely effective for stopping a hemorrhage is taking a bite of the hormone-filled placenta. (Personal communication, October 2021)

### 4. Attention to the Scientific Evidence

The body of scientific evidence supporting the many traditional and professional midwifery practices that facilitate normal, physiologic birth is ever-growing and includes meta-analyses from the renowned *Cochrane Database of Systematic Reviews* (n.d.) and *The Lancet Series on Midwifery* (2014), for two examples. Every birth attendant should keep up with this evidence, as so much of it reinforces the midwifery model of care. *Real science differs fundamentally from biomedical tradition.* All Stage 4 RARTRW practitioners should have science at their command—all references ready to counteract every technomedical objection to the kind of care they wish to give.

**5. Attention to Other Healing Philosophies and Modalities**
Naturopathy, chiropractic, homeopathy, Reiki, breath therapy, massage therapy, pre- and perinatal psychology, Ayurveda, Chinese medicine, acupuncture, acupressure, and many other types of "alternative," "complementary," "holistic," "integrative," or "functional" health care, as well as many Indigenous knowledge systems, have much to offer the contemporary birth practitioner. It is not possible for everyone to know all of these systems, but it is possible to be open to what they can offer by learning about them and incorporating one or some of them, and finding practitioners to whom clients can be referred. For examples, some chiropractors and osteopaths are experts in positioning the baby properly for birth and/or in healing or correcting post-birth injuries or traumas to the baby's neck or spine; some acupuncturists have holistic ways to jump-start labor; some psychologists and other birth practitioners are experts in helping women to release their pre-birth fears, to "psychically connect" with their unborn babies, whom they regard as conscious beings, and to heal post-birth traumas.[7]

## Conclusion:
## Social Scientists and Birth Practitioners in the 21st Century

To recap, in this chapter I have made a clear distinction between rigid and fluid ways of thinking, described 4 Stages of Cognition originally explicated by others, and correlated them with what I suggest are their anthropological equivalents. Stage 1 (rigid, concrete) thinking incorporates *naïve realism* ("Our way is the only way that matters to us"), *fundamentalism* ("Our way is the only right way"), and *fanaticism* ("Our way is so right that those who do not adhere to it should be either assimilated or eliminated"). I correlated Stage 2 thinking to *ethnocentrism* ("We know there are other ways, and that's ok for others, but our way is best!"). I correlated Stage 3 thinking with *cultural relativism*—a very fluid way of thinking ("All ways are equal in relative value and individual behavior must be understood within its cultural and societal context"), yet one that offers no way of thinking above and beyond the limitations of "culture" in general. Thus, I went on to correlate Stage 4 fluid thinking with *global humanism*—while respecting each culture, we must seek and establish standards that put the human rights of each individual above cultural mores and traditions that dishonor such rights.

I explained each of these 4 Stages of Cognition in relation to each other in terms of open and closed knowledge systems, and noted that, importantly, *ritual can stand as a barrier between cognition and chaos*. Ritual can be employed to reinforce each of these ways of thinking; it can also be used to reduce many kinds of stress by giving birth practitioners and others a sense of safety and stability in an uncertain world. And ritual can keep practitioners from "losing it" by regressing into Substage or can help to bring them back into functionality by getting them out of Substage. Ritual can also be employed to effect change: *to change your paradigm, change the rituals* to those that enact the core value and belief system you wish to adopt. (For more information on how to accomplish this kind of paradigm shift, see *From Doctor to Healer: The Transformative Journey* [Davis-Floyd and St John 1998]; "The Paradigm Shifts of Humanistic and Holistic Obstetricians: The 'Good Guys and Girls' of Brazil" [Davis-Floyd and Georges 2018, 2023]; *Ritual: What It Is, How It Works, and Why* [Davis-Floyd and Laughlin 2022]; and many of the chapters in Volume I of this series [Davis-Floyd and Premkumar 2023a], in which ten obstetricians describe their own paradigm shifts and how they accomplished them).

Around the world, midwives who practice the midwifery model of care—a judicious combination of the humanistic and holistic models that includes multiple technical skills (see Davis-Floyd 2018d, 2022)—and humanistic and holistic obs are under siege as the power of techno-medicine grows. Traditional midwives in many countries are in danger of extinction, having already been pushed out of practice or simply died off; professional midwives are too often either naïve or ethnocentric servants to technocratic ways of knowing and practicing; and many practitioners, including some professional midwives and obstetricians, who reject those ways are often persecuted and punished by "the system." Yet in almost every country, there are dozens and sometimes hundreds of birth practitioners, both traditional and professional, who are Stage 4 global humanists striving to think beyond established paradigms and practices to eliminate TMTS (too much too soon) and TLTL (too little too late) in favor of RARTRW (the right amount at the right time in the right way) care. Again, see Volume I of this series (Davis-Floyd and Premkumar 2023a) for some of their stories.

Such practitioners, when not under too much stress, are practicing informed relativism, constantly working to combine the best of pre-modern Indigenous techniques, modern allopathic, and complementary/holistic/integrative knowledge systems to create fluid and open Stage 4 birth knowledge systems (see Davis-Floyd et al. 2018). These approaches are responsive to childbearers' needs and desires, to ideas and information from others, to scientific evidence, and to "whatever works" from wherever it can be learned in globally humanistic ways that honor individual human rights.

If you are a social scientist, it might be well to consider what roles the social sciences might play in facilitating the expansion of Stage 4, globally humanistic thinking and related practices within healthcare systems, as well as in policy. Social scientists are accustomed to working in a "grey area" where life is acknowledged as complex, changing, and fluid. Nevertheless, as the chapters in this volume and in Volumes II and III of this series (Davis-Floyd and Premkumar 2023b, 2023c) illustrate, social scientists tend to be very good at describing, analyzing, and critiquing closed systems like that of technocratic obstetrics—not stopping at critiques, but moving forward to provide "thick" interpretations (Geertz 1973) of why such systems and their practitioners are as they are, think and act as they do. This approach might be further facilitated by increased interdisciplinary work, participation in public health education and events, and greater involvement in multidisciplinary policy and protocol development. Perhaps we anthropologists could also educate the public about the power of ritual both to stabilize us cognitively and to effect change. I ask, in what other ways could anthropology in particular, and social science in general, facilitate the kinds of Stage 4 systems that would make our world a safer place? And I encourage social scientists to respond.

If you are a practitioner in the 21st century, you have two brand new advantages that your historical counterparts did not: (1) access to information from a rich variety of sources, including Indigenous knowledge that has been documented by Indigenous people themselves, or in collaboration with social scientists (see, for example, Falcon and Contreras 2009) and solid science, such as the Cochrane meta-analyses (which support many Indigenous birth practices, such as movement, upright and all-fours positions, and nourishment during labor); and (2) strength in local, national, and international organizations. I ask birth practitioners to utilize these strengths, acknowledge their limitations (remember that stress can take you down while ritual, spiritual, and bodily nourishment can bring you up), and strive to keep their knowledge systems open to the rich learning that this new, digitally interconnected, and increasingly complex world can provide.

## Acknowledgments

This chapter, which appears here in greatly improved and expanded form, was first published by the same title in *Frontiers in Sociology* 3(23): 12–22. I thank Frontiers for permission to reprint the parts of that article that I use herein. Additionally, some portions of this chapter are adapted from my earliest iteration of some of these ideas in my article "Ways of Knowing: Open and Closed Systems," *Midwifery Today* 69 (2004): 9–13, copyright Robbie Davis-Floyd and *Midwifery Today*. I thank *Midwifery Today* for constantly supporting and publishing my work, and its founder Jan Tritten for consistently inviting me to speak (from 1995 to 2019) at the Midwifery Today conferences she and her team organize around the world, and for the knowledge, energy, and inspiration those conferences always provide. Thanks also to Charles D. Laughlin, my co-author for *The Power of Ritual* (2016) and for its abridged version, *Ritual: What It Is, How It Works, and Why* (2022), for helping me flesh out my anthropological interpretations of the 4 Stages of Cognition, which also appear in different forms in those books.

**Robbie Davis-Floyd,** Adjunct Professor, Department of Anthropology, Rice University, Houston, Fellow of the Society for Applied Anthropology, and Senior Advisor to the Council on Anthropology and Reproduction, is a cultural/medical/reproductive anthropologist interested in transformational models of maternity care. She is also a Board member of the International MotherBaby Childbirth Organization (IMBCO), in which capacity she helped to wordsmith the *International Childbirth Initiative: 12 Steps to Safe and Respectful MotherBaby-Family Maternity Care* (www.ICIchildbirth.org). The ICI has been translated into over 30 languages and has been implemented in birth facilities, small and large, around the world, showing that transformative change is indeed possible. Researchers are needed to study the processes and effects of ICI implementation in multiple sites; if you are interested, please contact Robbie at davis-floyd@outlook.com.

## Notes

1. This is a verbal quote from Albert Einstein. "Albert Einstein Quotes." *BrainyQuote*. Retrieved 28 October 2022 from https://www.brainyquote.com/quotes/albert_einstein_121993.
2. The combination of this schema with the anthropological concepts of naïve realism/fundamentalism/fanaticism, ethnocentrism, cultural relativism, and global humanism is entirely my own.
3. *International Childbirth Initiative* (ICI)*: 12 Steps to Safe and Respectful Mother-Baby-Family Maternity Care.*" Retrieved 28 October 2022 from www.ICIchildbirth.org.
4. Canadian midwife and social scientist Betty-Anne Daviss, US midwifery attorney Hermine Hayes-Klein, and I are presently designing a book on that subject,

to be called *The Global Witch Hunt Plaguing Birth: Practitioner Persecution and Restorative Resistance*.

5. The authors of Chapter 6 in Volume III of this series (Lokugamage, Ahillan, and Pathberiya 2023) explain that Māori nurse and educator Irihapiti Ramsden of New Zealand recognized that midwifery and nursing education needed to incorporate the concept of *Cultural Safety*—which, as she and the Maori insist, should always be capitalized; not to do so is considered a subtle insult. These authors stress the importance of distinguishing Cultural Safety from "cultural competence." "Cultural Safety" acknowledges the inherent power imbalances between patient and practitioner, requiring care providers to use critical self-reflection on their own values, beliefs, assumptions, and biases; "cultural competence" does not include this important reflexivity on power.

6. "An Annotated Bibliography of Selected Books in the Anthropology of Reproduction." *Google Docs*. Retrieved 28 October 2022 from https://docs.google.com/document/d/17GJD6lQh7CoJVRdRPaZAoET7WD74aKElcNrK8hZ7Eao/edit?usp=sharing.

7. The Association of Prenatal and Perinatal Psychology and Health. "Birth Psychology." Retrieved 28 October 2022 from https://birthpsychology.com/.

## References

Anderson D, Daviss BA, Johnson KC. 2021. "What If Another 10% of Deliveries in the United States Occurred at Home or in a Birth Center? Safety, Economics, and Politics." In *Birthing Models on the Human Rights Frontier: Speaking Truth to Power*, eds. Daviss BA, Davis-Floyd R, 205–228. Abingdon, Oxon, UK: Routledge.

Banks M. 1998. *Breech Birth, Woman Wise*. Hamilton NZ: Birthspirit Books.

Bisits A. 2023. "Attempting to Maintain a Positive Awareness about Vaginal Breech Birth in Australia." In *Obstetricians Speak: On Training, Practice, Fear, and Transformation*, eds. Davis-Floyd R, Premkumar A, Chapter 11. New York: Berghahn Books.

Bongaarts, J, Guilmoto, CZ. 2015. "How Many More Missing Women? Excess Female Mortality and Prenatal Sex Selection, 1970–2050." *Population and Development Review* 41(2): 241–269.

Bruner JP, Drummond SB, Meenan AL, Gaskin IM. 1998. "All-Fours Maneuver for Reducing Shoulder Dystocia during Labor." *Journal of Reproductive Medicine* 43(5): 439–43.

Chalmers B. 2019. "The Medical Manipulation of Reproduction to Implement the Nazi Genocide of Jews." *Conatus* 4(2): 127–147.

Chester P. 1997. *Sisters on a Journey: Portraits of American Midwives*. New Brunswick NJ: Rutgers University Press.

Cheyney M. 2011. "Homebirth as Ritual Performance." *Medical Anthropology Quarterly* 25(4): 519–542.

Cheyney M, Davis-Floyd R. 2019. "Birth as Culturally Marked and Shaped." In *Birth in Eight Cultures*, eds. Davis-Floyd R, Cheyney M, 1–16. Long Grove IL: Waveland Press.

———. 2020. "Birth and the Big Bad Wolf: A Biocultural, Co-Evolutionary Perspective, Part 2." *International Journal of Childbirth* 10(2): 66–78.

*Cochrane Database of Systematic Reviews*. Retrieved 28 October 2022 from https://www.cochranelibrary.com/cdsr/about-cdsr.

Çoker H. 2023. "'Birth with No Regret' in Turkey: The Natural Birth of the 21st Century." In *Obstetricians Speak: On Training, Practice, Fear, and Transformation*, eds. Davis-Floyd R, Premkumar A, Chapter 10. New York: Berghahn Books.

Çoker H, Karabekir N, Varlık S. 2021. "Birth with No Regret in Turkey." In *Birthing Models on the Human Rights Frontier: Speaking Truth to Power*, eds. Daviss BA, Davis-Floyd R, 347–358. Abingdon, Oxon, UK: Routledge.

Davis DA. 2019a. "Obstetric Racism: The Racial Politics of Pregnancy, Labor, and Birthing." *Medical Anthropology* 38(7): 560–573.

Davis DA. 2019b. *Reproductive Injustice: Racism, Pregnancy, and Premature Birth*. New York: New York University Press.

Davis-Floyd R. 1987. "Obstetric Training as a Rite of Passage." *Medical Anthropology Quarterly* 1(3): 288–318.

———. 2001. "The Technocratic, Humanistic, and Holistic Models of Birth." *International Journal of Gynecology & Obstetrics* 75, Supplement 1: S5–S23.

———. (1992) 2003. *Birth as an American Rite of Passage*, 2nd edn. Berkeley: University of California Press.

———. 2004. "Ways of Knowing: Open and Closed Systems." *Midwifery Today* 69: 9–13.

———. 2018a. "The Rituals of Hospital Birth: Enacting and Transmitting the Technocratic Model." In *Ways of Knowing about Birth: Mothers, Midwives, Medicine, and Birth Activism*, Davis-Floyd R and Colleagues, 45–70. Long Grove IL: Waveland Press.

———. 2018b. "Medical Training as Technocratic Initiation." In *Ways of Knowing about Birth: Mothers, Midwives, Medicine, and Birth Activism*, Davis-Floyd R and Colleagues, 107–140. Long Grove IL: Waveland Press.

———. 2018c. "The Technocratic, Humanistic, and Holistic Paradigms of Birth and Health Care." In *Ways of Knowing about Birth: Mothers, Midwives, Medicine, and Birth Activism*, Davis-Floyd R and Colleagues, 3–44. Long Grove IL: Waveland Press.

———. 2018d. "The Midwifery Model of Care: Anthropological Perspectives." In *Ways of Knowing about Birth: Mothers, Midwives, Medicine, and Birth Activism*, Davis-Floyd R and Colleagues, 323–338. Long Grove IL: Waveland Press,

———. 2022. *Birth as an American Rite of Passage*, 3rd edn. Abingdon, Oxon, UK: Routledge.

Davis-Floyd R, Barclay L, Daviss BA, Tritten J. 2009. *Birth Models That Work*. Berkeley: University of California Press.

Davis-Floyd R, Cheyney M, eds. 2019. *Birth in Eight Cultures*. Long Grove IL: Waveland Press.

Davis-Floyd and Colleagues. 2018. *Ways of Knowing about Birth: Mothers, Midwives, Medicine, and Birth Activism*. Long Grove IL: Waveland Press.

Davis-Floyd R, Davis E. 2018. "Intuition as Authoritative Knowledge in Midwifery and Homebirth." In *Ways of Knowing about Birth: Mothers, Midwives, Medicine, and Birth Activism*, Davis-Floyd R and Colleagues, 189–220. Long Grove IL: Waveland Press.

Davis-Floyd R, Georges E. 2018. "The Paradigm Shifts of Humanistic and Holistic Obstetricians: The 'Good Guys and Girls' of Brazil." In *Ways of Knowing about Birth: Mothers, Midwives, Medicine, and Birth Activism*. Davis-Floyd R and Colleagues, 141–161. Long Grove IL: Waveland Press.

———. 2023. "The Paradigm Shifts of Humanistic and Holistic Obstetricians: The 'Good Guys and Girls' of Brazil." In *Obstetric Violence and Systemic Disparities: Can Obstetrics Be Humanized and Decolonized?* eds. Davis-Floyd R, Premkumar A, Chapter 9. New York: Berghahn Books.

Davis-Floyd R, Laughlin CD. 2016. *The Power of Ritual*. Brisbane, Australia: Daily Grail Press.

———. 2022. *Ritual: What It Is, How It Works, and Why*. New York: Berghahn Books.

Davis-Floyd R, with Matsuoka E, Horan H, Ruder B, Everson CL. 2018. "Daughter of Time: The Postmodern Midwife." In *Ways of Knowing about Birth: Mothers, Midwives, Medicine, and Birth Activism*, Davis-Floyd R and Colleagues, 221–264. Long Grove IL: Waveland Press.

Davis-Floyd R, Premkumar A, eds. 2023a. *Obstetricians Speak: On Training, Practice, Fear, and Transformation*. New York: Berghahn Books,

———. 2023b. *Cognition, Risk, and Responsibility in Obstetrics: Anthropological Analyses and Critiques of Obstetricians' Practices*. New York: Berghahn Books.

———. 2023c. *Obstetric Violence and Systemic Disparities: Can Obstetrics Be Humanized and Decolonized?* New York: Berghahn Books.

———. 2023d. "The Anthropology of Obstetrics and Obstetricians: The Practice, Maintenance, and Reproduction of a Biomedical Profession." In *Obstetricians Speak: On Training, Practice, Fear, and Transformation*, eds. Davis-Floyd R, Premkumar A., Series Overview. New York: Berghahn Books.

Davis-Floyd R, Sargent C, eds. 1997. *Childbirth and Authoritative Knowledge: Cross-Cultural Perspectives*. Berkeley: University of California Press.

Davis-Floyd R, St John G. 1998. *From Doctor to Healer: The Transformative Journey*. New Brunswick NJ: Rutgers University Press.

Daviss BA. 2014. *Re-Thinking the Physiology of Vaginal Breech Birth: Evidence-Based Guide to Upright Delivery*. Ottawa ON: Informed Descent Publishing. Retrieved 28 October from www.understandingbirthbetter.com.

Daviss BA, Anderson DA, Johnson KC. 2021. "Pivoting to Childbirth at Home or in Freestanding Birth Centers in the US during COVID-19: Safety, Economics and Logistics." *Frontiers in Sociology* 6: 618210.

Daviss BA, Bisits A. 2021. "Bringing Back Breech: Dismantling Hierarchies and Re-Skilling Practitioners." In *Birthing Models on the Human Rights Frontier: Speaking Truth to Power*, eds. Daviss BA, Davis-Floyd R, 145–183. Abingdon, Oxon, UK: Routledge.

Daviss BA, Davis-Floyd R, eds. 2021. *Birthing Models on the Human Rights Frontier: Speaking Truth to Power*. Abingdon, Oxon: Routledge.

Diamond-Brown L. 2023. "'Selfish Mothers,' 'Misinformed' Childbearers, and 'Control Freaks': Gendered Tropes in US Obstetricians' Justifications for Delegitimizing Patient Autonomy in Childbirth." In *Obstetric Violence and Systemic*

*Disparities: Can Obstetrics Be Humanized and Decolonized?* eds. Davis-Floyd R, Premkumar A, Chapter 3. New York: Berghahn Books.

Falcon, AG, Contreras E. 2009. *Medicina Tradicional: Doña Queta y El Legado de Los Habitantes de las Nubes.* Las Palmas de Gran Canarias: Hamalgama Editorial.

Fontes R. 2023. "Repercussions of a Paradigm Shift in the Professional and Personal Life of a Brazilian Obstetrician." In *Obstetricians Speak: On Training, Practice, Fear, and Transformation,* eds. Davis-Floyd R, Premkumar A, Chapter 6. New York: Berghahn Books.

Frye A. 2005. *Holistic Midwifery: A Comprehensive Textbook for Midwives in Home-birth Practice. Volume 2, Care During Labor and Birth.* Portland OR: Labrys Press.

Gaskin, Ina May. (1975, 1980, 1990) 2002. *Spiritual Midwifery,* 4th ed. Summertown TN: The Book Publishing Company.

———. 2003. *Ina May's Guide to Childbirth.* New York: Bantam Dell.

Geertz C. 1973. *The Interpretation of Cultures.* New York: W.W. Norton.

Geréb Á, Fábián K. 2023. "Hungarian Birth Models Seen through the Prism of Prison: The Journey of Ágnes Geréb." In *Obstetricians Speak: On Training, Practice, Fear, and Transformation,* eds. Davis-Floyd R, Premkumar A, Chapter 8. New York: Berghahn Books.

Ghosh P. 2012. "Abortions of Female Fetuses Creating Widening Gender Imbalance in India." *International Business Times,* 18 September. Retrieved 28 October 2022 from https://www.ibtimes.com/abortions-female-fetuses-creating-widening-gender-imbalance-india-790122.

Gutschow K, Davis-Floyd R, Daviss BA. 2021. *Sustainable Birth in Disruptive Times.* Cham, Switzerland: Springer Nature.

Harman P. 2008. *The Blue Cotton Gown: A Midwife's Memoir.* Boston: Beacon Press.

Hennessey A. 2019. *Imagery, Rituals, and Birth: Ontology between the Sacred and the Secular.* New York: Lexington Books.

Hoffer, Eric. 1951. *The True Believer: Thoughts on the Nature of Mass Movements.* New York: Harper and Row, Perennial Classics.

Homer, C, Leap M, Edwards N, Sandall J. 2017. "Midwifery Continuity of Carer in an Area of High Socio-Economic Disadvantage in London: A Retrospective Analysis of Albany Midwifery Practice Outcomes Using Routine Data (1997–2009)." *Midwifery* 48: 1–10.

Jalil A, Zakar R, Qureshi S. 2013. "Physical Wife Abuse in Rural Sindh, Pakistan: Prevalence, Protective and Risk Factors." *Journal of the Research Society of Pakistan* 50: 171–193. http://pu.edu.pk/images/journal/history/PDF-FILES/Article%2009%20Aisha.pdf.

Jones R. 2009. "Teamwork: An Obstetrician, a Midwife, and a Doula." In *Birth Models That Work,* eds. Davis-Floyd R, Barclay L, Daviss BA, Tritten J, 271–304. Berkeley: University of California Press.

———. 2023. "The Bullying and Persecution of a Humanistic/Holistic Obstetrician in Brazil: The Benefits and Costs of My Paradigm Shift." In *Obstetricians Speak: On Training, Practice, Fear, and Transformation,* eds. Davis-Floyd R, Premkumar A, Chapter 7. New York: Berghahn Books.

Jordan B. 1993. *Birth in Four Cultures: A Cross-Cultural Investigation of Childbirth in Yucatan, Holland, Sweden, and the United States.* Long Grove IL: Waveland Press.

———. 1997. "Authoritative Knowledge and Its Construction." In *Childbirth and Authoritative Knowledge: Cross-Cultural Perspectives*, eds. Davis-Floyd R, Sargent C, 55–79. Berkeley: University of California Press.

Kramer K. 2002. Class paper, Southern Methodist University, unpublished.

Kroeber A. 1949. "An Authoritarian Panacea." *American Anthropologist* 51(2): 318–320.

Lalonde A. 2023. "How an Obstetrician Promoted Respectful Care in Canada and in the World." In *Obstetricians Speak: On Training, Practice, Fear, and Transformation*, eds. Davis-Floyd R, Premkumar A, Chapter 13. New York: Berghahn Books.

Lalonde A, Herschderfer K, Pascali Bonaro D, Hanson C, Fuchtner C, Visser GHA. 2019. "The International Childbirth Initiative: 12 Steps to Safe and Respectful MotherBaby-Family Maternity Care." *International Journal of Gynecology and Obstetrics* 146: 65–73.

Lee V. 1996. *Granny Midwives and Black Women Writers: Double-Dutched Readings*. New York: Routledge.

Leonard C. 2008. *Lady's Hands, Lion's Heart: A Midwife's Saga*. Hopkinton NH: Bad Beaver Publishing.

Liese K, Davis-Floyd R, Stewart L, Cheyney M. 2021. "Obstetric Iatrogenesis in the United States: The Spectrum of Unintentional Harm, Disrespect, Violence, and Abuse." *Anthropology & Medicine* 28(2): 1–16.

Lokugamage A, Ahillan T, Pathberiya SDC. 2023. "Decolonizing Medical Education in the UK." In *Obstetric Violence and Systemic Disparities: Can Obstetrics Be Humanized and Decolonized?* eds. Davis-Floyd R, Premkumar A, Chapter 6. New York: Berghahn Books.

McManus J. 1979. "Ritual and Human Social Cognition." In *The Spectrum of Ritual*, eds. d'Aquili E, Laughlin CD, McManus J, 216–248. New York: Columbia University Press.

Meeks M. (1998) 2004. *Breech Birth, Woman Wise*, 3rd ed. Auckland NZ: Birthspirit Ltd.

Miller S, Abalos E, Chamillard M et al. 2016. "Beyond Too Little, Too Late and Too Much, Too Soon: A Pathway Towards Evidence-Based, Respectful Maternity Care Worldwide." *Lancet* 388(10056): 2176–2192.

Miller S, Lalonde A. 2015. "The Global Epidemic of Abuse and Disrespect during Childbirth: History, Evidence, Interventions, and FIGO's *Mother-Baby Friendly Birthing Facilities Initiative*." *International Journal of Gynecology and Obstetrics* 131(Sl): S49–52.

Miller S, Cordero M, Coleman AL, Figueroa J, Brito-Anderson S, Dabash R et al. 2003. "Quality of Care in Institutionalized Deliveries: The Paradox of the Dominican Republic." *International Journal of Gynecology and Obstetrics* 82(1): 89–103.

Milton G, Bovard W. 1993. *Why Not Me? The Story of Gladys Milton, Midwife*. Summertown TN: The Book Publishing Company.

Milton G, Fulwylie C. 1997. *Beyond the Storm: An Extraordinary Journey*. Pensacola FL: Boaz Fulwylie Press.

Morningstar S. 2009. *The Power of Women: Instinctual Birth Stories*. Eugene OR: MotherBaby Press.

Reed B, Edwards N. In press. *Closure*. London: Pinter and Martin.

Reed B, Walton C. 2009. "The Albany Midwifery Practice." In *Birth Models That Work*, eds. Davis-Floyd R, Barclay L, Daviss BA, Tritten J, 141–158. Berkeley: University of California Press.

Reyes E. 2021. "Born in Captivity: The Experiences of Puerto Rican Birth Workers and Their Clients in Quarantine." *Frontiers in Sociology* 6: 613831.

Rooks J. 1999. "The Midwifery Model of Care." *Journal of Nurse-Midwifery* 44(4): 370–374.

Rose SD. 1988. *Keeping Them Out of the Hands of Satan: Evangelical Schooling in America*. New York: Routledge.

Sadler M, Santos MJ, Ruiz-Berdún D et al. 2016. "Moving beyond Disrespect and Abuse: Addressing the Structural Dimensions of Obstetric Violence." *Reproductive Health Matters* 24(47): 47–55.

Schroder HM, Driver MJ, Streufert S. 1967. *Human Information Processing*. New York: Holt, Rinehart, and Winston.

Simkins G. 2011. *Into These Hands: Wisdom from Midwives*. Traverse City MI: Spirituality and Health Books.

Smith MC, Holmes LJ. 1996. *"Listen to Me Good": The Life Story of an Alabama Midwife*. Columbus: Ohio State University Press.

Susie DA. 1998. *In the Way of Our Grandmothers: A Cultural View of Twentieth-Century Midwifery in Florida*. Athens: University of Georgia Press.

*The Lancet Series on Midwifery*. 2014. Retrieved 28 October 2022 from https://www.thelancet.com/series/midwifery.

Ulrich LT. 1990. *The Life of Martha Ballard, Based on Her Diary, 1785–1812*. New York: Vintage Books.

United Nations (UN). 1948. *Universal Declaration of Human Rights*. Retrieved 7 January 2023 from https://www.un.org/en/about-us/universal-declaration-of-human-rights.

*University of Connecticut Science News*. 2020. "Life-Hack: Rituals Spell Anxiety Relief." *Science Daily*, 30 June. Retrieved 28 October 2022 from https://www.sciencedaily.com/releases/2020/06/200630111504.htm.

van Olphen-Fehr J. 1998. *Diary of a Midwife: The Power of Positive Childbearing*. Westport CT: Bergin and Garvey.

White Ribbon Alliance. 2011. *Charter on Respectful Maternity Care: The Universal Rights of Childbearing Women*. Retrieved 7 January 2023 from http://www.healthpolicyproject.com/index.cfm?ID=publications&get=pubID&pubID=46.

Worth J. 2008. *Call the Midwife: A True Story of the East End in the 1950s*. London: Phoenix.

Zakar R, Zakar MZ, Abbas S. 2016. "Domestic Violence against Rural Women in Pakistan: An Issue of Health and Human Rights." *Journal of Family Violence* 31(1): 15–25.

CHAPTER 2

# From "Mastership" to Active Management of Labor

## The Culture of Irish Obstetrics and Obstetricians

*Margaret Dunlea, Martina Hynan,*
*Jo Murphy-Lawless, Magdalena Ohaja,*
*Malgorzata Stach, and Jeannine Webster*

## Introduction: A Lengthy Tradition of Obstetric Authority

Sociologist Pat O'Connor (2000) has characterized Irish society as one where the "patriarchal dividend" continues to underpin a widespread cultural acceptance of male-oriented authority as entirely appropriate. Nowhere is this dominance more vividly to the fore than in relation to the institutions, policies, and practices surrounding childbirth in Ireland. So tightly configured are the operations of these elements that women are almost completely denied agency in pregnancy and birth, while midwives, who are generally present at births in Ireland, are consistently subordinated to obstetric protocols and denied professional autonomy (Kennedy 2002). The Irish state fully accepts obstetric authority, funding public maternity services with institutionally limited midwifery autonomy while allowing private obstetric care to flourish within the same complexes of the 19 publicly funded maternity units across the country. The 1953 Health Act marked the introduction of state financing for this two-tiered, exclusively hospital-based structure (Dunlea 2021), which also marked the ending of the existing domiciliary services (M. O'Connor 1995). Currently, while any woman in Ireland can access free antenatal, intrapartum, and postnatal care, including all hospital accommodation costs, there is no continuity of care for her and no guarantee that she will see the same midwife or doctor at each antenatal and post-natal visit, while intrapartum care will be dependent on the obstetric and midwifery team on duty.

Ireland has five hospitals exclusively for maternity care and gynecology—three in Dublin, one in Cork, one in Limerick, and an additional 14 maternity units in general hospitals. Midwife-led maternity services are few in number and extremely limited in scope. There are only two small alongside (next to or inside a hospital) midwifery-led units in the entire country. Eight of the 19 hospitals and units have birthing pools, but these can only be used with the obstetrician's consent. There is only one unit where women are able to birth their babies in the pool; the remaining seven "birth pools" are misnamed, as women can only use them for pain relief during labor. All midwifery-led initiatives are at risk of being closed down without warning and certainly without due oversight (Bowers 2020). The so-called "National Maternity Strategy" in 2016 arose from a highly critical review of Irish maternity services carried out by the Health Information and Quality Authority (HIQA)—the national safety and standards authority, following the high-profile death of Savita Halappanavar in Galway University Hospital in 2012 (HIQA 2013).[1] The 2016 Strategy—the first such national framework policy document—has continued obstetric control within its chosen risk framing, to the point of disallowing the very phrase "midwifery-led care" to be used on the grounds that it would be "professionally divisive" (Department of Health 2016). There are no concrete plans to add to the two existing alongside midwifery-led units in the Irish Republic (Angela Dunne, National Lead Midwife, quoted in Dunlea 2021: 56). The structure of care laid out in the 2016 National Maternity Strategy is one of retrograde obstetric control and "reflects the existing technocratic paradigm . . . viewing women's bodies in pregnancy as pathological" (Wood 2017:2). This Strategy puts women and midwives in Ireland well behind developments in Northern Ireland and Scotland in the last two decades.[2] There, under the UK National Health Service (NHS) and in line with UK maternity strategies, midwives and women have enjoyed far greater scope, including access to home birth through the public NHS (GAIN 2018). However, the NHS is now under considerable strain, reflected in growing concerns about its maternity services so that in 2022, the UK Royal College of Midwives drew attention as a matter of urgency to the multiple crises facing such services across the UK (see Royal College of Midwives 2022a, 2022b).

Here in the Irish Republic, the obstetric fraternity has long cultivated its private clientele on the basis that private practice secures the same obstetrician for a baby's birth whom the mother has seen in the private antenatal clinic. Behind this promise of continuity—the "conjuring of choice," as Marie O'Connor (2006) has termed it—lies the whispered promise of maximum safety in private obstetric-led care. In 1976, Comhairle na nOspidéal—the statutory body with the remit to deliver policy recommendations to the Minister for Health on the organization of all hospital services—published a report on maternity services that stated unequivocally that birth was safest in hospitals, and therefore all births should take place there. This conclusion, reached with no supporting evidence whatsoever, was accepted as an "an article of faith" (O'Connor 2006:111). It was implemented just before the publication of the first edition of the foundational Irish text *Active Management of Labour* (1980) by Kieran O'Driscoll and Declan Meagher of the National Maternity Hospital, Dublin. That text went through three more editions (O'Driscoll and Meagher 1986; O'Driscoll, Meagher and Boylan 1993; O'Driscoll, Meagher, and Robson 2003)[3] and cemented the international reputation of Irish obstetrics for strictly time-managed labor and birth according to a series of templates to be applied to each woman, along with recourse to augmentation with synthetic oxytocin, administered intravenously to any labor that deviated from the norms laid down by the templates.

These templates for active management were and are rigorously applied to first-time mothers in particular and are referred to in the textbook as "one of the fundamental truths in clinical obstetrics" (O'Driscoll and Meagher 1980:13). Thus, both the mantra about the only safe place for birth being a maternity hospital and the means to control a woman's body in labor according to obstetric dictates have produced a consistent pattern of obstetric control over practices, discourses, and crucially, allocations of public funding for these hospital structures throughout the last seven decades. Obstetric-led care has been reinforced during the same timespan when overwhelming evidence began to emerge about the safety of midwifery-led care and its implementation in other jurisdictions in Europe, including Northern Ireland (Murphy-Lawless 1998; Kennedy and Murphy-Lawless 1998; Mander and Murphy-Lawless 2013; Sandall et al. 2016; Stach 2020; Dunlea 2021). Yet Ireland's maternity services remain obstetric-led.

The long uninterrupted arc of the original 18th-century office of "Mastership" endures with its unquestioned status for the three major Dublin "lying-in hospitals," themselves historically laden with colonizing inferences of the subjugation of "poor" women. Mastership—a consultant obstetrician elected to a seven-year term of office as Master of a maternity hospital by fellow consultant obstetricians[4]—remains the favored form of governance; there is a call by consultant obstetricians, including Peter Boylan, former Master of the National Maternity Hospital, to extend this system to all other maternity units. According to Boylan:

> We wish to see the Mastership model of governance applied nationwide, with each unit having its own separate budget and governance structure. . . . This model has been in operation in the three Dublin maternity hospitals for more than 200 years. It is a tried and tested model that works. (Quoted in Mudiwa 2017)

This approach to governance—alongside the unreformed 1950s national Mother and Infant Scheme, which assigns care of the pregnant woman to the GP (general practitioner) and consultant obstetrician (Dunlea 2021), the rationales that produced *Active Management of Labour* (Murphy-Lawless 1998; O'Connor 2006), and finally the 2016 National Maternity Strategy, wherein a woman's "care pathway" is determined by obstetric risk criteria and must be approved in advance by the obstetrician—all carry the signs of continuing obstetric hegemony with adverse consequences for women, including poorer care (Edwards, Mander, and Murphy-Lawless 2018) and high rates of unnecessary interventions (Murphy and Fahey 2013). In 2019, of a total 59,352 births in the Irish Republic, the induction rate was 32.5% and the cesarean rate was 34.3% (National Women and Infants Health Programme Clinical Programme for Obstetrics and Gynaecology 2020). Studies have demonstrated how these high rates of intervention are "not fully accounted for by medical or obstetric risk differences" (Murphy and Fahey 2013:8); they are however associated with private practice, regardless of risk factors (Lutomski et al. 2014; Moran et al. 2020).

In this chapter, we examine the paradigms, power plays, and influences that sustain this unwieldy structure of care, to the benefit of obstetricians despite its clear detriments to childbearing women and to the midwifery profession. We examine how the strength and meanings of these obstetric discourses through texts, guidelines, policy documentation, and public testimony in front of our *Oireachtas* (Parliament) have proven difficult to subvert despite some three decades of activism, and conclude with strong suggestions about the need to take activism in more fruitful directions.

## Methods and Materials

We begin this section with a description of our respective areas of expertise. Margaret Dunlea and Magdalena Ohaja lecture in midwifery at

Trinity College Dublin and National University Galway, and along with Jeannine Webster are all registered midwives; Jo Murphy-Lawless and Malgorzata Stach are sociologists; Martina Hynan is an artist and a PhD researcher with the Centre for Irish Studies, NUI Galway. With a long history of activism around childbirth, all six of us work in collaboration to achieve definitive change for women and midwives in Ireland. The material for this chapter comes from our extensive literature reviews and from our multiple research undertakings and published works, many of which are cited in this chapter. Our most recent project, as part of what we named "The Elephant Collective" (because elephants surround the female elephant when she is calving to protect her), has been to create a new law mandating inquests for all maternal deaths in Ireland (Murphy-Lawless 2021). Before this law was passed, at best there was an internal hospital review of why the death had occurred and an inquest, if granted, frequently had to be fought for by a family's legal team.

## Obstetric Hegemony and Structural Violence in Irish Maternity Services

In the sciences, structures of formal language are classically employed to establish jurisdiction. They do so by seeking to delimit knowledges that strengthen any given field of power while excluding what they find troublesome or challenging. "What they sanction, what they exclude in order to function" (Foucault 1974:294) entails building a grammar that effectively becomes the sole legitimated mode of speaking. They also seek to secure that lodestone of seeming "objectivity" to underwrite their assertion of maintaining universal principles, but as Foucault observed, "the universality of our knowledge has been acquired at the cost of exclusions" (1974:294).

The language in *Active Management of Labour* is a useful starting point for understanding how Irish obstetric thinking has operationalized these exclusions in its determination to achieve the absolute primacy of the obstetrician in the delivery room. The authors of the successive editions of *Active Management of Labour* used their authority of speech and position to cement a control that was always there in any case, even while the authors asserted that their approach would transform labor and delivery. The tenets of *Active Management of Labour* meant that "the consultant obstetrician became actively involved in the conduct of labour on a regular basis as never before" (O'Driscoll and Meagher 1980:3). The implication was that the obstetrician was always present at birth. The reality was that midwives handled most births, without the obstetrician in attendance, albeit under the strict obstetric protocols laid out in *Active Management of Labour*, which, in O'Driscoll and Meagher's reading, meant that all births were under obstetric control; if the woman was a private patient, or if her labor was deemed high risk, the obstetrician would be expected to attend the birth in person.

In this influential text, there is an exclusion of the woman herself. Whatever she may have to say about her body, her pregnancy, or her labor is to be disregarded. The woman facing these iron laws of regulated labor should have not only no voice but her very conduct in the delivery room as laid down in all four editions of *Active Management* must be under obstetric direction and her actions censured when "needed." The woman should submit herself to the hospital prenatal education classes, which will show her precisely what is expected of her during labor and birth under active management "so as to learn the nature of their role and how best this may be fulfilled" (O'Driscoll and Meagher 1980:90). The woman who fails in this matter will be censured:

> [The] disruptive effect of one disorganized and frightened woman in a delivery unit extends far beyond her own safety and comfort . . . nurses are not expected to submit themselves to the sometimes outrageous conduct of perfectly healthy women who could not be persuaded . . . to learn how to behave with dignity and purpose during the most important event of their lives. Nor should nurses be held responsible for the degrading scenes that occasionally result from the failure of a woman to fulfil her part of the contract. (O'Driscoll and Meagher 1980:90–91)

The quotation above indicates the extent of the patriarchal hold on childbearing women. There is also an exclusion of the midwife, who is relegated to the offstage role of a "nurse-midwife" as companion, with her work being defined by obstetric rationales (1980:86). The midwife must fit into the obstetric authority then and now; hence the outright refusal to even incorporate the term "midwifery-led care"—a term that is fundamental to the organization of maternity services in all four of our neighboring jurisdictions. As Marie O'Connor (2006:112) has argued, this is the text that "institutionalised the domination of midwifery by obstetrics" in the modern era. *Active Management of Labor* sought to completely systematize women's births by application of its "truths," the focus being how to bring about "efficient uterine action" to successfully bring labor to an end:

The consultant, rather than remain off-stage waiting for a summons to perform an emergency operation on a belated attempt to retrieve a situation that could have been anticipated at a much earlier stage, now had to seek to prevent such emergencies arising in women who were normal when they first entered the hospital. (O'Driscoll and Meagher 1980:3)

In this firmly patriarchal society, these and similar efforts at controlling birth extend back to the origins of the Irish Mastership system in the 18th century (Murphy-Lawless 1998; Hynan 2018; Devane et al. 2020; Strong and Varley 2020). Patriarchy, paternalism, and the obstetric exercise of power within a rigid hierarchy are foundational for the three great Dublin "lying-in hospitals," which also date back to the 18th century. This weight of historical reputation has exercised a formidable influence, with the presumed universality of obstetric thinking extending to the local policies of every single maternity unit in Ireland since that time. Whereas midwives in Northern Ireland can train and work in NHS hospitals with a specific policy orientation of one-to-one woman-centered midwifery-led care, midwives in the Republic must continue to train and practice in systems entirely subordinated to obstetric rationales. Martina Hynan (2018) has shown how the "male obstetric gaze" has flourished from the 18th century onward, lying at the core of the Mastership system and imposing its "effective deletion of the mother's body" from a presumed scientific knowledge of how labor and birth occur, while simultaneously valorizing the technologies in the hands of the obstetricians that are supposedly used to make birth safe (Hynan 2018:126). This is what Melissa Cheyney and Robbie Davis-Floyd (2019:8) have called "the obstetric paradox": "intervene to keep birth safe, thereby causing harm." We can see a continuity dating from early efforts by Irish "men-midwives" to dilate the cervix mechanically (Murphy-Lawless 1989), through the policy of George Johnston, Master of the Rotunda Lying-in Hospital in the 1860s, to deliver unmarried women by forceps when they were as little as two-fifths dilated to preserve them from "remorse and fretting" due to their unmarried status (Murphy-Lawless 1988), to the overarching influence of *Active Management of Labour* and the complete exclusion of midwifery-led care as a national policy. Thus, Irish obstetrics reaches into normal pregnancies and births and legitimizes obstetricians' control of midwives' work, while rendering the role of the midwife as the guardian of physiologic birth superfluous.

The fact that there is no place for autonomous midwives in Irish obstetric thinking is evident in the response by consultant obstetrician

Peter Boylan, co-author of the 3rd edition of *Active Management of Labour* (O'Driscoll, Meagher, and Boylan 1993) and Chairperson of the Institute of Obstetricians and Gynaecologists, to the Oireachtas Committee on Health review of the National Maternity Strategy when he stated (with the inference that separate midwifery-led units such as those that prevail in the four jurisdictions of the UK are not optimum in his view): "We do not want to repeat the mistakes of separating out midwifery and obstetric care. They are both the same. All obstetricians are midwives and are proud to be midwives, but they are also looking after more complicated cases" (Boylan, quoted in House of the Oireachtas 2018). In this way, obstetric discourse obliterates midwives by coding obstetricians *as* midwives.

The perception that consultant-led, instead of midwife-led, hospital births are the safest option is entrenched in Irish obstetric thinking and is reinforced by obstetricians amongst other health professionals and politicians, as well as being accepted among the public generally, matched by a large uptake of private market health insurance to secure private care from a consultant obstetrician (Pope 2017). As Zygmunt Bauman (1989:142) succinctly put it, "the rationality of the ruled is always the weapon of the rulers." Margaret Dunlea (2021:256) has argued that senior Irish obstetricians continue to actively resist evidence that challenges their deeply held beliefs about hospital safety needing obstetric control, while also noting that any re-organization of the hospital space to accommodate midwifery-led units would disrupt obstetric surveillance. In Dunlea's ethnography, one participant—a senior obstetric advisor to the government on maternity care policy—commented:

> I do not buy this idea of . . . two separate labour wards, to me that's a non-starter because what you'll have is a situation where you'll have territorialism, you also have division and you also have, if you are very busy, an inability to run the service, so, what I argue for, okay, I said this to the HSE [Health Services Executive] . . . if you're building a labour ward, that every room in the labour ward should be capable of delivering every model of care, that no patient should be sent to another part of the hospital to access another level of care, you want your birthing pool, you want your resuscitaire [neonatal resuscitation unit] behind the wall, you want your bouncy ball . . . that if the low risk woman goes in there and she develops severe pre-eclampsia in labour that she does not move outside that room and that room then becomes a high risk room [that] midwives and obstetricians need to be able to work across. (Quoted in Dunlea 2021:256)

As for home birth, one Irish obstetrician expressed obstetric resistance to a homebirth policy in this rather euphemistic way: "Most obstetricians would not be philosophically well disposed to home birth" (quoted in Dunlea 2021:255). All contemporary evidence supporting midwifery-led services such as planned home birth or birth in an alongside or freestanding midwifery unit (see Birthplace in England Collaborative Group et al. 2011) is rejected out of hand by the members of this Stage 1, fundamentalist (see Chapter 1 in this volume) obstetric system.

## The Realities of Irish Maternity Services: An Economy of Violence

The universalizing discourses of obstetric power have created for women what the political philosopher Etienne Balibar (2015:104) terms "an economy of violence." Women come to this economy of violence largely unprepared for dealing with its multiple guises until it overtakes them in person. At its worst, women hear about this because of catastrophic outcomes. These include cases that portrayed instances of obstetric failure, such as:

- the Dunne case in the 1980s, in which inadequate monitoring of a twin pregnancy led to one stillborn twin, with the second twin sustaining massive brain damage and quadriplegia (Murphy-Lawless 1992);
- the 1999 inquest into the death of Mrs. Swarnili Basu following an elective cesarean to deal with placenta previa (Holland 1999);
- the revelations in 1998 about obstetrician Michael Neary, who performed at least 188 perioperative hysterectomies between 1974 and 1998 and was initially cleared of any charge of medical wrongdoing by his fellow consultant obstetricians before a concerted public campaign led to the revocation of his medical license (Matthews and Scott 2008);
- the needless baby deaths in the Portlaoise Hospital scandal, where five babies died through lack of care, but the actual accounts of these deaths did not come out until one of the mothers, Roisin Molloy, demanded an investigation on a national current affairs television program (Cullen 2015; Wall 2018); and
- the occasional reports on maternity hospitals in crisis due to understaffing, poor facilities, and so on (O'Regan 2007; Murphy-Lawless 2011).

In 2019, in its daily radio program *Liveline*, RTE—the national broadcaster—facilitated calls from more than 1,000 women over a two-week period to explain how they had felt abandoned, degraded, and damaged by their experiences in the maternity services (*The Journal* 2019). The then-Master of the National Maternity Hospital, Rhona Mahoney, the first female Master, contested the women's accounts, arguing: "It's just not comprehensive . . . while some of it might be deserved, if you paint a universally dismal picture, then that's genuinely at odds with my experience over 25 years" (quoted in O'Mahony 2019).

Yet the everyday experiences of pregnant women, starting with overcrowded facilities, are noted even by obstetricians: "We would have huge numbers, we would have traffic jams of people queueing up to try to get into the hospital, queueing up to get parking, and then queueing up to be seen by a consultant that may last five minutes" (quoted in Dunlea 2021:194). Inevitably this situation leads to neglect, small and large:

> people are kind of left behind and forgotten about a little bit and, um, I think that's, um, far from ideal, you know . . . You have doctors in such a rush to get people in and out of the room, they're far more likely to miss something because they're so intent in just getting those 120 patients through in two hours and you, kind of, just treat everybody the same and it's easy to just say, 'Come in, how are you doing? Fine. Here's your scan, off you pop.' And let's get the next patient in. (Obstetrician, quoted in Dunlea 2021:194).

Well may Marie O'Connor (2006:110) ask, "Why are Irish maternity services so unresponsive to women's wishes?"

## What Women Want

The commonplace experiences that pregnant and birthing women face in the obstetric wards run counter to their needs and desires, as evidenced in the 2014 Association for Improvement of Maternity Services in Ireland (AIMSI) survey: out of 2,836 women participants, 58.5% said they would opt for a freestanding birth center if available (AIMSI 2014). Malgorzata Stach's (2020) investigation into women's understandings of the uses of technology in childbirth revealed both ambiguity and conflict as women grapple with what the system lays out for them in pregnancy and birth. Stach has demonstrated how women must negotiate the issue of the technological promise of safety, endeavoring to make sense of it even as they try to come to terms with the discrepancies between their understandings and the discourses of technocratic biomedicine favored by Irish obstetricians. The ranges and uses of technologies within our maternity services offer at best a limited notion of care, yet such care is construed as clinically faultless when seen from obstetricians' perspectives. Women do often welcome the appropriate use of technology, but they want it underpinned by humane care that is genuinely enabling and addresses their needs. Women's voices as elicited by Stach (2020:233) challenge the persuasive strategies of biomedicine and expose its promises as deceptive, giving only the appearance of comprehensive maternity care:

> God, I think we have too much! We need to scale back on the interventions and just let women have their babies ... I think we should concentrate more on the person giving birth as an actual ... person—you're not just here to get this product out ... I suppose I would be thinking less about technology and machines and more about basic care. I think the basic care needs to improve. Like the ratio of midwives to labouring women, like breastfeeding support ... that should be provided ... So those kind of things I'd like to see, more than a particular technology. (Quoted in Stach 2020:227)

In 2020/21, the exigencies and constraints related to the COVID-19 pandemic led to the emergence of women's advocacy groups campaigning against the restrictions imposed on maternity care throughout the 19 maternity units. The restrictions were initially necessitated due to the unknown nature of SARS-CoV-2 and its impacts on pregnancy and newborns. Some obstetric units embraced innovative protective measures, such as increasing their midwifery clinics and introducing early transfer home; in contrast, one unit entirely banned partners from the labor ward. As the pandemic progressed, many restrictions proved to be contradictory to international evidence. As frustration grew, women began to speak out with, for example, heart-breaking accounts from those receiving the words "There's no heartbeat" alone, experiencing pregnancy loss alone, laboring alone, having major surgery alone, and parents unable to visit their newborns in the NICU for more than 15 minutes at a time, or sometimes not at all.

*In Our Shoes—Covid Pregnancy* is a social media movement that was founded in Ireland in September 2020 by two women who had given birth at the beginning of the coronavirus pandemic in spring 2020, when partners had overnight been removed from maternity units across the country.[5] They decided to help women take a stand, offering an invitation to parents to "tell us your story" on social media platforms. They describe what followed as a "bursting of the floodgates" that had held and hidden the grief and trauma of thousands of people who had been impacted by partner exclusions from labor and delivery rooms. The group allied itself with other advocacy groups in opening talks with the official state agency responsible for coordinating all health services—the Health Services Executive. Emma Carroll, the facilitator of the *In Our Shoes—Covid Pregnancy* website, argues that the body of experiences shared online should make clear that in order to provide good, person-centered care and to avoid the often-hidden traumas that so many women live with, radical systemic change is needed in the Irish maternity care system.

## Conclusion: Strengthening Midwifeship

The Midwives Association of Ireland (MAI), which had been formed as a radical campaigning voice for Irish midwives, issued a manifesto prior to the 2020 Irish General Election, held just before COVID-19 brought the country to lockdown. They expressed acute disappointment over the lack of progress relating to our troubled maternity services that so adversely affect women's pregnancy and childbirth experiences and outcomes. The broad issues were and remain the centralization and institutionalization of maternity services driven by obstetricians, as evidenced in the high rates of unnecessary interventions as described above. The hope was short-lived that even with the ill-configured 2016 National Maternity Strategy that sought to prioritize and retain obstetric control, there might be limited political space to establish outreach community midwifery services—which are vital for enhancing autonomous midwifery and returning birth to women. Cutbacks in funding and the lack of political will halted any concrete moves at that time (Cullen 2018). Again, currently there are only two alongside midwifery-led units (MLUs) within a hospital setting in the Republic of Ireland, while our neighbors Northern Ireland and Scotland have 8 and 17 MLUs respectively (GAIN 2018). In the absence of community midwifery services, the vast majority of women were being left with no alternative than to be forced into costly institutionalized, obstetric-led care. Sadly, women-centered care in hospitals remains a distant dream. Other critical concerns highlighted by the MAI included staff burnout, poor morale, and severe recruitment and retention challenges—all of which are a direct result of stressful working conditions that can put practitioners into what, in Chapter 1 of this volume, Davis-Floyd calls "Substage"—a condition of intense irritability, anxiety, and burnout, otherwise known as "losing it." In this condition, practitioners cannot feel empathy for others and may treat them with disrespect and even violence and abuse, especially those below them in the obstetric hierarchy, such as laboring women. Between 2007 and 2016, the State Claims Agency paid out €349 million to settle legal claims incurred as a result of poor obstetric outcomes ending in death or life-limiting conditions for women and babies (HSE Office of Legal Services 2016). These include the deaths of Savita Halappanavar and seven other women, for whom inquests were held only after families fought for them (Murphy-Lawless 2021). There are also persistent social inequalities in relation to access to care (MAI Midwives Manifesto 2020).

Of greatest concern is that most of the poor outcomes for women and babies could be avoided with appropriate care and good working conditions for midwives. However, a series of events has changed the parameters for midwifery and has taken these ongoing crises into the national political arena. In April 2022, a long-running argument broke into public discourse about the building in Dublin of a new National Maternity Hospital (the home of the book cited earlier, *Active Management of Labour*). At first this argument centered on this new hospital being located on a campus originally owned by a Catholic religious order, the Sisters of Charity, raising acute concern over the provision of full reproductive care, including procedures usually not carried out in Catholic hospitals, such as sterilizations. However, the resultant debate in the Dáil (the Irish Parliament), which was stormy (RTE 2022), expanded the reach of concerns. Not only were two government party parliamentary representatives (called Teachta Dála) suspended for their opposition to the new hospital (Bray and Burns 2022), but also the very structure of the maternity services was finally being questioned in strenuous public debates, in particular about the issue of publicly-funded subsidies to support private obstetric practices (Moore 2022). This was quickly followed by a national furor over the imposition of non-evidence-based restrictions on the provision of home birth for women in rural areas (Burns 2022), at the same time that the acute lack of midwifery staff also became a newsworthy story (Griffin 2022a). And then, in November 2022, a newly emerging umbrella group, the Birth Rights Alliance, held two protests, one in Cork about the homebirth restrictions, and one in Dublin about the deeply stressful working conditions for midwives (Griffin 2022b).

These developments have taken place against the backdrop of increasing rejection of and national discussion about the damages done to women's reproductive health care in a system that is now publicly acknowledged to be profoundly patriarchal and misogynistic (O'Connor 2022; O'Regan 2022). Vicky Phelan became a national figure as she campaigned for openness into the failures of a government cervical cancer screening program that led to her terminal illness and to the deaths of dozens of other women. Vicki's death in November, 2022 has placed the issue of dislodging paternalism from all aspects of women's reproductive care front and center in the national consciousness (O'Toole 2022).

There is urgent need for a thorough reconfiguration of Irish maternity services, increasing the numbers of midwives, the establishment of more midwifery-led units, and the development of community midwifery services across the country. We have the alternative knowledges—authoritative knowledges (Jordan 1997) grounded in women's and midwives' experiences—and a growing constituency for wide political action, drawing on a number of networks and resources, including the successful campaign to make all maternal deaths subject by statute to inquest. This campaign was initiated and carried through by midwives and by widowers who had lost their wives; together they fought to have inquests into maternity-related deaths made mandatory (Murphy-Lawless 2021). We *can* overturn archaic notions of Mastership and obstetric control. Our goal is a strengthened *Midwifeship*—that is, midwives enabled to practice to the full extent of their knowledge and skills.

**Margaret Dunlea** has served as a midwife for more than 30 years, having practiced in England, Saudi Arabia, and Ireland. She is also a feminist, academic, and childbirth activist. She has BSc in Anthropology, an MSc in Midwifery Education, and a PhD on Irish maternity care policies and practices. Currently she is an Assistant Professor in Midwifery at Trinity College Dublin. Her passion lies in supporting physiologic birth, childbearing women's empowerment, and midwives' autonomy. "To be a midwife is to be political."

**Martina Hynan** is a PhD researcher with the Centre for Irish Studies, National University of Ireland, Galway. She is an interdisciplinary artist, birth activist, and member of The Elephant Collective. Her practice-with-research PhD is an interdisciplinary and socially engaged project that explores the entanglement of birth with place. Her work sits at the intersection of reproductive justice and environmental humanities.

**Jo Murphy-Lawless** is a sociologist and social justice activist. Over many decades, she has written extensively on obstetrics and childbirth. She is one of the core coordinators of The Elephant Collective campaign, which in 2019 secured legislation for mandatory inquests for all maternal deaths. She is a Research Fellow in the Centre for Health Evaluation, Methodology Research and Evidence Synthesis, NUI Galway.

**Magdalena Ohaja** is a Nigerian and a midwife. She is currently a lecturer in midwifery at the School of Nursing and Midwifery, National University of Ireland Galway. She taught in the School of Nursing and Midwifery Trinity College Dublin for ten years, where she completed her PhD in 2015 on the concept of safe motherhood and its complexities as experienced and understood by women, midwives, and traditional birth attendants in southeast Nigeria. Her research interests include safety, risk, and normality in childbirth, women's/maternal health, women-led maternity care, culturally competent care, and socio-economic, cultural, and political determinants of maternal health.

**Malgorzata Stach** is a sociologist, an educator, and a feminist scholar. She holds a PhD from the School of Nursing and Midwifery, Trinity College Dublin, where she completed her research exploring women's conceptualizations of birth technology in the context of the Irish maternity services. Her research interests include women's reproductive health, maternity services, midwifery and obstetrics, appropriate use of technology, and provision of appropriate health care.

**Jeannine Webster** is a registered midwife, birth activist, campaigner for women's choice in health care, and lay advocate with the Irish College of Psychiatrists for improving Irish mental health services. She is a founding member of the Midwives Association of Ireland. She undertook her BSc in Midwifery as a mature student in 2007, fulfilling her long-held ambition to become a midwife. She completed her MSc studies in Health and Social Care at Glasgow Caledonian University in 2018. Her studies have focused on the views and experiences of midwives in screening for domestic violence during antenatal care in Ireland.

## Notes

1. Savita Halapannavar, who was a dentist by profession, died in Galway University Hospital on October 28, 2012, from septicemia following a catastrophic breakdown of care. She was 17 weeks pregnant with her first baby and had been admitted for an inevitable miscarriage. However, her request for a termination to deal with the miscarriage was denied by hospital staff, owing to overarching concerns about its legality, given Article 40.3.3 of the Irish Constitution—the so-called "right to life" Eighth Amendment inserted in 1983 after a campaign

heavily influenced and financed by American Catholic right-wing groups, who advocated an uncompromising pro-life position (Oaks 1999). The journalist Kitty Holland broke the story of Savita Halappanavar's death in the national press in November 2012, and then wrote the definitive account following the 2013 inquest into her death (Holland 2013). Savita's death brought about massive public protest, which precipitated a massive shift in the political climate in Ireland and laid the groundwork for the successful repeal of the Eighth Amendment by a 2 to 1 majority in 2018 and the subsequent legalizing of abortion in Ireland.

2. Northern Ireland's six counties comprise a separate jurisdiction that still belongs to Britain under the 1921 agreement between Britain and Ireland to establish an independent government for the other 26 counties of the island of Ireland, which became known as the Irish Free State from 1922 until 1948, when Ireland became a Republic.

3. It is not known why there have been no further editions. Lead author O'Driscoll died in 2007; he was in his 80s, but there has been no public statement as to why the book has not had a further updated edition.

4. A "consultant obstetrician" in British and Irish terms is one who has completed post-qualifying years after graduation with a four-year medical degree, first as a junior house doctor in hospital; then a senior house doctor in hospital; then enters an advanced training program, first as a junior registrar and then as a senior registrar.

5. "In Our Shoes – Covid Pregnancy." Facebook page. https://www.facebook.com/inourshoescovidpregnancy/

## References

Association for Improvement of Maternity Services in Ireland (AIMSI). 2014. "Survey: Maternity Care Choices in Ireland." *AIMS Ireland*. Retrieved 3 November 2022 from http://aimsireland.ie/care-choices/.

Balibar E. 2015. *Violence and Civility: On the Limits of Political Philosophy*. New York: Columbia University Press.

Bauman Z. 1989. *Modernity and the Holocaust*. Polity Press: Cambridge.

Birthplace in England Collaborative Group, Brocklehurst P, Hardy P, Hollowell J, et al. 2011. "Perinatal and Maternal Outcomes by Planned Place of Birth for Healthy Women with Low Risk Pregnancies: The Birthplace in England National Prospective Cohort Study." *British Medical Journal* 343: d7400.

Bowers S. 2020. "Call for the Protection of Midwifery-Led Maternity Units." *Irish Times*, 6 June.

Boylan P, quoted in Houses of the Oireachtas. 2018. "Joint Committee on Health Debate, Wednesday, 21 Feb 2018: Review of National Maternity Strategy 2016–2026; Discussion." *Houses of the Oireachtas*, 28 February. Retrieved 3 November 2022 from https://www.oireachtas.ie/en/debates/debate/joint_committee_on_health/2018-02-21/3/.

Bray J, Burns S. 2022. "National Maternity Hospital: Green Party Suspends Two TDs for Voting with the Opposition." *Irish Times*, 18 May.

Burns S. 2022. "HSE Proposal on Limiting Home Births 'Irresponsible and Dangerous'." *Irish Times*, 9 November.

Cheyney M, Davis-Floyd R. 2019. "Birth as Culturally Marked and Shaped." In *Birth in Eight Cultures*, eds. Davis-Floyd R, Cheyney M, 1–16. Long Grove IL: Waveland Press.

Comhairle na nOspidéal. 1976. *Development of Hospital Maternity Services: A Discussion Document*. Dublin: Stationery Office.

Cullen P. 2015. "HSE Report into Death of Baby Mark Molloy to Be Published: Case Spurred Inquiry into Fatalities at Portlaoise Hospital Which Led to Damning Report." *Irish Times*, 22 October.

———. 2018. "National Maternity Strategy: Funding for New Elements Halted." *Irish Times*, 1 April.

Department of Health. 2016. *Creating a Better Future Together: National Maternity Strategy 2016–2026*. Dublin: Department of Health.

Devane D, Webster J, Murphy-Lawless J, Hughes P. 2020. "COVID-19: Challenging Ireland to Move from Mastership to Midwifeship." *Medical Anthropology Quarterly Rapid Response Blog Series*. Retrieved 3 November 2022 from https://medanthroquarterly.org/rapid-response/2020/08/covid-19-challenging-ireland-to-move-from-mastership-to-midwifeship/.

Dunlea M. 2021. *Change and Entrenchment in Irish Maternity Care Policies and Antenatal Practices: An Institutional Ethnography*. PhD dissertation, School of Nursing and Midwifery, Trinity College, Dublin.

Edwards N, Mander R, Murphy-Lawless J. 2018. *Untangling the Maternity Crisis*. London: Routledge.

Foucault M. 1974. *The Order of Things: An Archaeology of the Human Sciences*. London: Tavistock Publications.

GAIN (Northern Ireland Guidelines and Audit Implementation Network). 2018. *Guideline for Admission to Midwife-Led Units in Northern Ireland*. Belfast: Regulation and Quality Improvement Authority, Northern Ireland.

Griffin N. 2022a. "Hundreds Attend Cork Protest in Support of Homebirth Access. *Irish Examiner*, 6 November.

———. 2022b. "Women and Babies 'at Risk' in Tipperary because of Staff Shortages, Warn Midwives." *Irish Examiner*, 3 November.

HIQA (Health Information and Quality Authority). 2013. *Investigation into the Safety, Quality and Standards of Services Provided by the Health Service Executive to Patients, Including Pregnant Women at Risk of Clinical Deterioration, Including Those Provided in University Hospital Galway, and as Reflected in the Care and Treatment Provided to Savita Halappanavar*. Dublin: HIQA.

Holland K. 1999. "Coroner Told How Woman Died after Childbirth." *Irish Times*, 6 October.

———. 2013. *Savita: The Tragedy that Shook a Nation*. Dublin: Transworld Ireland.

HSE (Health Service Executive) Office of Legal Services. 2016. "Response to Parliamentary Questions on the Funds Spent by the HSE on Legal Fees Concerning All Maternity Cases and Maternity Related Matters for Each of the Years 2007 to 2015." Written Response to Dáil Parliamentary Question 6417/16, submitted by Clare Daly TD.

Hynan M. 2018. "Hidden in Plain Sight: Mapping the Erasure of the Maternal Body from Visual Culture." In *Untangling the Maternity Crisis*, eds. Edwards N, Mander R, Murphy-Lawless J, 124–132. London: Routledge.

Jordan B. 1997. "Authoritative Knowledge and Its Construction." In *Childbirth and Authoritative Knowledge: Cross-Cultural Perspectives*, eds. Davis-Floyd R, Sargent C, 55–79. Berkeley: University of California Press.

Kennedy P. 2002. *Maternity in Ireland: A Woman-Centred Perspective*. Dublin: Liffey Press.

Kennedy P, Murphy-Lawless J. 1998. *Returning Birth to Women: Challenging Policies and Practices*. Dublin: Centre for Women's Studies, Trinity College Dublin and WERRC University College Dublin.

Lutomski J, Murphy M, Devane D, et al. 2014. "Private Health Care Coverage and Increased Risk of Obstetric Intervention." *BMC Pregnancy and Childbirth* 14(1): 1–9.

Mander R, Murphy-Lawless J. 2013. *The Politics of Maternity*. London: Routledge.

Matthews A, Scott A. 2008. "Perspectives on Midwifery Power: An Exploration of the Findings of the Inquiry into Peripartum Hysterectomy at Our Lady of Lourdes Hospital, Drogheda, Ireland." *Nursing Inquiry* 15: 127–134.

Midwives Manifesto (General Election). 2020. *Midwives Association of Ireland*. Retrieved 27 November 2022 from http://midwivesireland.ie/publications/.

Moore A. 2022. "Róisín Shortall: Questions over National Maternity Hospital and 'Murky' New Company's Role." *Irish Examiner*, 3 May.

Moran PS, Daly D, Wuytack F, et al. 2020. "Predictors of Choice of Public and Private Maternity Care among Nulliparous Women in Ireland, and Implications for Maternity Care and Birth." *Health Policy Experience* 124(5): 556–562.

Mudiwa L. 2017. "A Push for Mastership of Maternity Services." *Irish Medical Times*, 25 January. Retrieved 18 December 2021 from https://www.imt.ie/features-opinion/a-push-for-mastership-of-maternity-services-25-01-2017/.

Murphy D, Fahey T. 2013. "A Retrospective Cohort Study of Mode of Delivery among Public and Private Patients in an Integrated Maternity Hospital Setting." *BMJ Open* 3(11): e003865.

Murphy-Lawless J. 1988. "The Obstetric View of Feminine Identity: A Case History of the Use of Forceps on Unmarried Women in 19th Century Ireland." In *Gender & Discourse: The Power of Talk*, eds. Fisher S, Todd A, 177–198. Norwood NJ: Ablex Publishing.

———. 1989. "Male Texts and Female Bodies: The Colonisation of Childbirth by Men Midwives." In *Text and Talk as Social Practice*, ed. Torode B, 25–48. Amsterdam: Foris.

———. 1992. "Reading Birth and Death through Obstetric Practice: The Dunne Case." *Canadian Journal of Irish Studies: Women and Irish Politics* 18(1): 129–145.

———. 1998. *Reading Birth and Death: A History of Obstetric Thinking*. Cork, Ireland: Cork University Press.

———. 2021. "Holding the State to Account: 'Picking Up the Threads' for Women Who Have Died in Irish Maternity Services." *Éire-Ireland* 56(3–4): 51–79.

National Women and Infants Health Programme, Clinical Programme for Obstetrics and Gynaecology. 2020. *Irish Maternity Indicator System National Report 2019*. Dublin: HSE.

Oaks L. 1999. "Irish Trans/National Politics and Locating Fetuses." In *Fetal Subjects, Feminist Positions*, eds. Morgan LM, Michaels MW, 175–198. Philadelphia: Pennsylvania University Press.

O'Carroll C. 2022. "Vicky Phelan's Friend and Solicitor on Her Last Request: 'Tell them I asked for action, not praise.'" *Irish Independent*, 20 November.

O'Connor M. 1995. *Birth Tides: Turning towards Home Birth*. London: Harper Collins.

———. 2006. "Conjuring Choice While Subverting Autonomy: Medical Technocracy and Home Birth in Ireland." In *Risk and Choice in Maternity Care: An International Perspective*, ed. Andrew Symon, 109–122. London: Churchill Livingstone.

O'Connor P. 2000. "Ireland: A Man's World." *Economic and Social Review* 31(1): 81–102.

O'Driscoll K, Meagher D. 1980. *Active Management of Labour: The Dublin Experience*. St. Annes, Sussex: W.B. Saunders.

———. 1986. *Active Management of Labour, The Dublin Experience*, 2nd ed. London: Baillière Tindall.

O'Driscoll K, Meagher D, Boylan P. 1993. *Active Management of Labour: The Dublin Experience*, 3rd ed. Aylesbury, England: Mosby Year Book Europe Limited.

O'Driscoll K, Meagher D, Robson R. 2003. *Active Management of Labour: The Dublin Experience*, 4th ed. London: Mosby Elsevier.

O'Mahony C. 2019. "Baby Blues: Are Maternity Services Misogynistic?" *Irish Independent*, 20 April.

O'Regan E. 2007. "Stretched Services 'Put Lives of Mothers and Babies at Risk.'" *Irish Independent*, 12 December.

O'Regan E. 2022. "Dr Gabriel Scally Warns Cervical Check Change Must Come Not Just in Letter, but in Spirit. *Irish Independent*, 24 November.

O'Toole F. 2022. "Ireland Should Not Need Heroines Like Vicky Phelan." *Irish Times* 19 November.

Pope C. 2017. "Public or Private: What's the Best Way to Have a Baby?" *Irish Times*, 26 June.

Royal College of Midwives. 2022a. "NHS Maternity Staffing Crisis Puts Babies' Lives at Risk," Media release, 13 October. Retrieved 27 November 2022 from https://www.rcm.org.uk/media-releases/2022/october/nhs-maternity-staffing-crisis-putting-babies-lives-at-risk/#:~:text=The%20Royal%20College%20of%20Midwives,and%20babies'%20lives%20at%20risk.

———. 2022b. "Government Must Act Now to Reverse Rise in Maternal Deaths, Says RCM." Media release, 10 November. Retrieved 27 November 2022 from https://www.rcm.org.uk/media-releases/2022/october/government-must-act-now-to-reverse-rise-in-maternal-deaths-says-rcm/.

RTE. 2022. "Timeline: New National Maternity Hospital Saga." 17 May. Retrieved 27 November 2022 from https://www.rte.ie/news/ireland/2022/0517/1298418-maternity-hospital-timeline/

Sandall J, Soltani H, Gates S, Shennan A, Devane D. 2015. "Midwife-Led Continuity Models Versus Other Models of Care for Childbearing Women." *Cochrane Database of Systematic Reviews* 9: CD004667. https://doi.org/10.1002/14651858.CD004667.pub5

Stach M. 2020. *Deceptive Promises: Women's Understandings of Technology in Maternity Care*. PhD dissertation, School of Nursing and Midwifery, Trinity

College, Dublin. Retrieved 3 November 2022 from http://www.tara.tcd.ie/handle/2262/92447.

Strong, AE, Varley E. 2020. "COVID-19 and SRH/MNH: A Curated Online Collection for *Medical Anthropology Quarterly.*" *Medical Anthropology Quarterly Rapid Response Blog Series.* Retrieved 3 November 2022 from https://medanthroquarterly.org/rapid-response/2020/08/covid-19-and-srh-mnh-a-curated-online-collection-for/.

*The Journal.* 2019. "HSE Apologises to Women Callers to Joe Duffy's *Liveline* Who Shared Their Traumatic Childbirth Experiences." 20 April. Retrieved 27 November 2022 from https://www.thejournal.ie/childbirth-joe-duffy-4585612-Apr2019/.

Wall M. 2018. "Review of Portlaoise Baby Deaths Complete, Says HSE." *Irish Times,* 14 January.

Wood C. 2017. "A Review of the New Irish Maternity Strategy 2016–2026." *The Practising Midwife* 20(6): 1–3.

# CHAPTER 3

# Becoming an Obstetrician in Greece

## Medical Training, Informal Scripts, and the Routinization of Cesarean Birth

*Eugenia Georges*

In 2013, the UN Convention on the Elimination of Discrimination against Women (CEDAW 2013) declared Greece's cesarean birth (CB) rate to be "the highest in the world." Today, around 65–70% of births in Greece take place by cesarean—a rate double that of most of the rest of the EU nations (see Figure 3.1). However, the precise numbers are not known, because until recently, reporting of cesareans and other obstetric interventions to the Ministry of Health was on a voluntary basis only. As a result, the information available remains spotty and uneven. In addition to the obstacles this situation poses to researchers, who must rely on hospital records and the occasional survey to estimate rates, the absence of mandatory reporting has important consequences for attempts to monitor prevailing practices in hospitals and clinics, track changes over time, and devise and implement effective policies to reduce unnecessary interventions and improve the quality of maternity care. This lack of comprehensive and reliable information over time may also help to explain why, despite the public visibility of the issue, research on the factors promoting the normalization of cesarean birth in Greece remains sparse. The surveys that do exist, however, confirm my observations, those of the interlocutors, and reports in the press that CB rates have risen steadily over the last few decades.

In this chapter, I examine the often mutually reinforcing sociocultural, political-economic, and pedagogical processes that have led to the

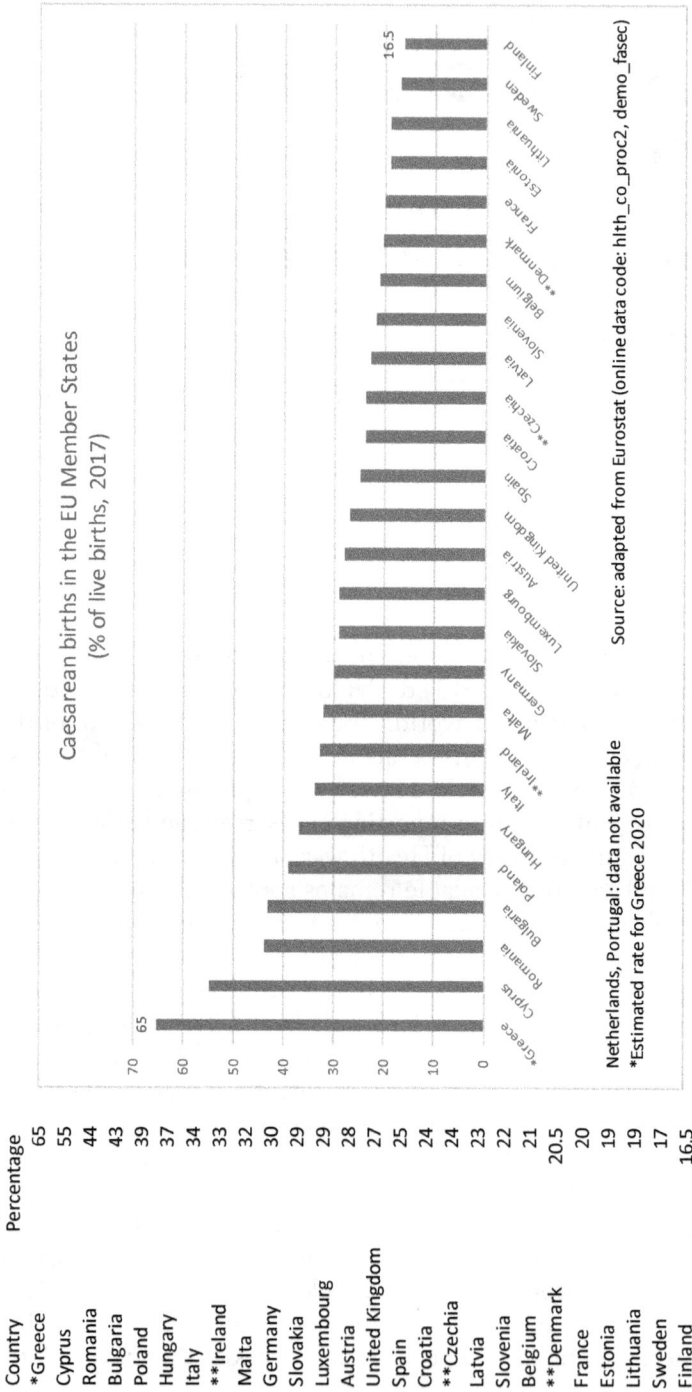

| Country | Percentage |
|---|---|
| *Greece | 65 |
| Cyprus | 55 |
| Romania | 44 |
| Bulgaria | 43 |
| Poland | 39 |
| Hungary | 37 |
| Italy | 34 |
| **Ireland | 33 |
| Malta | 32 |
| Germany | 30 |
| Slovakia | 29 |
| Luxembourg | 29 |
| Austria | 28 |
| United Kingdom | 27 |
| Spain | 25 |
| Croatia | 24 |
| **Czechia | 24 |
| Latvia | 23 |
| Slovenia | 22 |
| Belgium | 21 |
| **Denmark | 20.5 |
| France | 20 |
| Estonia | 19 |
| Lithuania | 19 |
| Sweden | 17 |
| Finland | 16.5 |

**Figure 3.1.** Cesarean Births in the Member States of the European Union. Adapted from Eurostat (online data code: hlth_co_proc2, demo_fasec).

mainstreaming of cesarean births in Greece. This mainstreaming has continued unabated despite heightened public awareness that many, if not most, cesareans are unnecessary. Across Greek society—from women and their families, the media, the Greek Parliament, and midwives to obstetricians themselves—there is widespread acknowledgment that the CB rate is excessively high. Indeed, over the course of my long-term ethnographic research on pregnancy and birth in Greece, I have often heard doctors lament the high cesarean rate. To date, however, there have been no qualitative studies that explore their points of view—a gap that this chapter is intended to fill.

## Methods and Materials

I have been conducting ethnographic research on reproduction-related issues in Greece since 1990, much of which is presented in my book *Bodies of Knowledge: The Medicalization of Reproduction in Greece* (Georges 2008), and in my more recent articles on the perspectives and experiences of pregnant women who had given birth vaginally and by cesarean (Georges 2010, 2013, 2022; Georges and Daellenbach 2019). This research took me to the maternity departments of three public hospitals—two in Athens and one in Rhodes—where I was able to observe pre- and postnatal visits, ultrasound exams, and births. Over the years and across these three field sites, I formally interviewed a total of 56 women, 26 obstetricians, and 12 midwives. In 2019, to gain a better sense of the historic role played by the United States in the transformation of Greek biomedicine after World War II, I researched the records of the American Mission of Aid to Greece (1945–1963) housed in the Tsakopoulos Hellenic Collection at California State University, Sacramento. I also conducted archival research in Athens and Lausanne, Switzerland, on the history and architectural design of Athens's first maternity hospital, completed in 1936.

In this chapter, I build and expand on this body of research to further examine Greece's high rate of cesarean births from the perspectives of obs (obstetricians) and obs-in-training. To plumb the "hidden curriculum" that may implicitly inform their understandings (Dixon, Smith-Oka, and El Kotni 2019), I interviewed an additional five mainstream obstetricians (with CB rates of 60–70%) as well as two humanistic/holistic obs who practice against the dominant grain (with CB rates of 15–17%). To understand the experiences and processes of biomedical training, I interviewed five medical students at three of Greece's seven medical schools, and one resident specializing in obstetrics. I also interviewed care providers who work alongside obstetricians, such as mid-wives and neonatologists, for the perspectives of those adjacent to but outside the specialty. With the exception of Dr. Louros (see below), all names used are pseudonyms.

## The Landscape of Maternity Care in Greece

The fundamental contours of contemporary maternity care in Greece diverge in a number of ways from those found in much of the rest of Europe. To make sense of the distinctive roles that cesareans have come to play in contemporary Greek obstetrics, this section provides a brief outline of the history of maternity care in Greece from the early decades of the last century to the present.

Throughout the first half of the 20th century, most women in Greece gave birth at home with the assistance of midwives. Obstetricians prac-ticed mainly in the largest cities, mostly serving an elite clientele. For models of the most advanced and modern medical practice and training, Greek doctors looked mainly to Germany and, to a lesser extent, France. For example, Dr. Nicolaos Louros (1898–1986), who served as Chair of Obstetrics and Gynecology at the University of Athens from 1936 to 1968, was educated in Germany, Austria, and Switzerland. An eminent professor, public figure, and obstetrician to the royal family, he exerted a powerful influence on the style and substance of Greek maternity care over the course of many decades (Manidaki et al. 2018). Dr. Lambrakis, a retired neonatologist who began his medical studies at the Univer-sity of Athens in time to witness Dr. Louros as a teacher, recalled his "authoritarian" pedagogical style, which Dr. Lambrakis attributed to the "Germanic mentality" that Dr. Louros, like others, had acquired while studying abroad. According to Dr. Lambrakis, Dr. Louros "would enter a patient's room lecturing to about 40 residents trailing behind him, and the ones in the back couldn't even hear what he was saying . . . It's not like that anymore, but in those days, there was only one maternity hospital, and all the obstetricians were his students, and they went on to teach the cohorts that followed that way for many years." As discussed below, traces of this top-down pedagogical approach can be discerned in Greek biomedical training to this day.

After World War II, the authority and prestige of European mod-els were gradually eclipsed by the influence of US-style biomedicine. In the immediate aftermath of this war and the Greek Civil War that followed (1946–1949), Greece began the process of rebuilding its dev-astated institutions. Greek national recovery took off in the context of the Cold War—a time when the United States was determined to contain the influence of the Soviet Union and to prevent the "dominos" of southeastern Europe from falling under Communist influence. Under the emergent policy of "soft power" inaugurated by the Truman Doctrine, Greece was identified as a frontline of Soviet containment. Massive amounts of non-military aid poured in to help rebuild the nation, and, at least partly as a result, by the early 1960s, the Greek economy had one of the highest growth rates in the world (Kalyvas 2015:105).

In the "American Era" that ensued, the United States exerted a strong cultural influence on the institutions being rebuilt as Greece recovered from the wars (Carpenter 2003). Biomedicine was no exception. Under the Truman Doctrine, doctors, nurses, and other healthcare professionals were given stipends to study in the United States with the proviso that they return to practice in Greece. Whereas before the wars, Greeks had looked to Europe for models of the most advanced and modern medical practice and training, by the 1960s and 1970s, many young Greek doctors, including both Directors of the Maternity Departments in which I conducted my earlier fieldwork, preferred to do their specialized training in the United States. Eventually, US influence on the development of Greek obstetric practice became decisive and remains so. Thus, in contrast to much of the rest of Europe, maternity care in Greece more closely resembles the technocratic model of US birth as classically described by Robbie Davis-Floyd in *Birth as an American Rite of Passage* ([1992] 2003, 2022). As in the United States, all births in Greece are generally understood to be pathological or potentially pathological events that should properly take place in hospitals under the surveillance of physicians and routinely subjected to a similar array of technological interventions.

Health care in Greece today consists of a mix of the public sector and a growing private sector. In 1983, Greece's social democratic government established the Ethniko Systema Ygeias (ESY) (National Health System) to provide universal and free access to health care to all Greek citizens. In 2016, refugees and asylees also formally gained the right to free care in the ESY system. However, because ESY hospitals are chronically underfunded—a condition exacerbated by the "debt crisis" that began in 2009 and continues to hobble the Greek economy today—facilities can be basic and hospital visits may involve long waiting times and other inconveniences. For these and other reasons, women who can afford to do so may opt to give birth in the comparatively more luxurious private clinics and hospitals where about half of all births now take place. Still, some ESY hospitals, including the three that I observed, enjoy strong reputations for good doctors and modern technology that attract a broad range of women, many of whom can afford private care. Greece as a whole boasts low rates of maternal (3.3/100,000) and infant (3.5/1,000) mortality that compare favorably with other member nations of the EU (Eurostat 2018; World Bank 2019), and these excellent outcomes are roughly the same across the two sectors. Most unusually from a cross-national perspective, CB rates are also roughly equivalent across both sectors.

One ostensible difference between the public and private sectors is the ability to chose one's physician. By law, most ESY doctors are prohited from seeing private patients. Pregnant women, however, regard the selection of their obstetrician as the most critically important decision they can make to ensure a good outcome. To finesse the restrictions on ESY doctors, and to ensure that they receive continuous care from the doctor of their choice, patients and their families resort to the widespread practice of informal payments, widely known as the *fakelaki*, literally, "little envelope" (Kaitalidou, Mladovsky et al. 2012; Souliotis et al. 2016). Currently running at about 1,000 EUR per birth, the *fakelaki* offers a powerful incentive for doctors to limit the access of others, such as midwives and residents, to "their" patients with whom they have established a quasi-private relationship. Ultimately, the existence of this deeply entrenched shadow economy of health care in which ethnic Greek women and their doctors are enmeshed effectively blurs the boundaries between private and public health care. This blurring, in turn, is reflected in the near uniformity in regimes of care, including the roughly equivalent CB rates in the public and private sectors.

Across Greece, all but a handful of births take place in hospitals and clinics. The country's only freestanding birth center closed a few years ago, and as a result, women's range of choice in childbirth today is essentially limited to deciding whether to go to a public or a private facility. Built into the design of Athens's oldest and largest public maternity hospitals is a stratified arrangement of space and care, in which rooms are divided into three tiers, called "Alpha," "Beta," and "Gamma." Ethnic Greek women typically pay an extra out-of-pocket fee to stay in a private suite or in an Alpha or Beta semi-private room. Immigrants, refugees, Roma, and poor ethnic Greek women, who overwhelmingly give birth in the public hospitals, are concentrated in the more basic Gamma rooms. These rooms may contain up to eight beds; due to Greece's very low fertility rate (1.3), only about half are occupied on any given day (Kaitelidou, Theodorou et al. 2013:28). Reflecting older medical beliefs in the therapeutic effects of light, air, and sun, the Gamma rooms in the hospitals I studied are relatively spacious, with high ceilings and tall windows—architectural design features that, along with the lack of crowding, help make them relatively pleasant spaces. Because Gamma patients are poor and often cultural "outsiders" who tend not participate in the informal economy, ESY obstetricians leave them mostly to the midwives. As a result, their CB rate is around half that of the better-off ethnic Greek women (Mossialos et al. 2005; Georges and Daellenbach 2019; Georges 2022).

Over the course of the 20th century, midwives have witnessed a steady reduction in the scope of their practice. In the decades following World War II, professional midwives attended births throughout the country. Rural women in particular relied almost exclusively on midwives, many of whom practiced in the countryside in fulfillment of the compulsory rural service that was part of their training and certification (*agrotiko*). By the 1970s, several trends combined to effectively end their stints of independent practice. Postwar migration to the nation's largest cities, particularly of young people, helped depopulate the countryside, diminishing the need and opportunities for rural service. At the same time, the supply of obstetricians began to expand rapidly as several new universities were built while Greece experienced unprecedented economic growth and social mobility.

During this period, five new faculties of biomedicine were founded throughout the nation, bringing the total up to seven. Doctors have long enjoyed status, prestige, and political influence in Greek society, and the biomedical profession attracted—and continues to attract—large numbers of the top students. Since 1990, for example, the number of medical school graduates has more than doubled. In the postwar years, obstetrics and gynecology became a particularly lucrative specialty, due in large part to the brisk demand for medical abortions as couples sought to limit their family size to two or three children (Georges 1996; Hionidou 2020:116). Technically illegal, though almost never prosecuted, safe medical abortion, almost always performed by ob/gyns, became a significant driver of the steep decrease in family size in the postwar period, when approximately 200,000–300,000 abortions were performed each year (Naziri 1988; Halkias 2004; Paxson 2004). At least in part in response to the financial opportunities created by this demand, the number of ob/gyns grew by a third—the greatest rate of increase of any biomedical specialization in Greece (Mossialos et al. 2005). However, as the birth rate plummeted to historic lows during this same period, the supply of obstetricians inevitably outstripped demand. By 2000, Greece's ratio of obstetricians to inhabitants was roughly double that found in the other countries of the EU, and Athens alone had four times the number of obstetricians per capita as London (Kaitelidou, Mladovsky et al. 2012). Inevitably, due to the considerable oversupply, competition between midwives and obstetricians, and among obstetricians themselves, intensified. Given the substantial political influence exerted by the organized biomedical profession in Greece (Nikolentzos and Mays 2016), competition for pregnant clients has also resulted in the near-total elimination of midwives as independent practitioners.

Midwives do play roles in contemporary Greek maternity care, but almost always as auxiliaries to a particular doctor—a dependent status clearly indexed by the fact that pregnant women and their families may refer to them as "the doctor's midwife." Midwives who work in hospitals are essentially restricted to teaching childbirth classes, attending most of the births in the Gamma rooms, providing doula-like support during labor and delivery (doulas are rare in Greece), and promoting breastfeeding among new mothers. As Dr. Kallopoulos—one of Greece's handful of holistic obstetricians and one of the very few who collaborates with homebirth midwives—put it: "Obstetricians believe that midwives are just chaperones." Their exclusion from active roles in the birth process belies the fact that Greek midwives are all highly educated professionals who undergo a rigorous four-year program of university coursework and clinical training. Upon completion, they become certified as direct-entry (non-nurse) midwives with the right to practice autonomously. Almost all, however, find work in hospitals or as part of an obstetrician's private practice. For example, in Athens—a city of over 3 million people—only three or four midwives practice autonomously, mainly serving a select clientele of well-educated ethnic Greek women, Greeks returned from the diaspora, expats, and a few celebrities who seek out a holistic birth experience, preferably a water birth. Not surprisingly, many midwives feel that the kind of work they typically perform does not make use of the extensive training and professional skills they acquired in midwifery school.

The erosion and de-skilling of midwives and the near-complete elimination of alternatives to biomedicalized birth were also abetted by the historical confluences of cultural and social developments rooted in the democratizing political climate of the mid-1970s. Before then, midwifery students were interned in schools associated with maternity clinics, where for four years they lived, attended classes given by professors of medicine, and worked their shifts. According to Dr. Dimou, a Professor of Midwifery, midwifery students and medical residents attended lectures side-by-side, and their diplomas, signed by the same professors, commanded more prestige and respect. Life for the interned midwifery students was highly regimented, closely surveilled, and the work was hard, but, as Dr. Dimou stated, "there was another sort of equality then" between doctors and midwives. Ironically, this equality was undermined by the democratizing reforms of the late 1970s that helped restructure and expand higher education: the residential midwifery schools were closed, and midwifery education was assigned to the newly created university tier entitled "Lower Technical Schools." As Dr. Dimou dryly observed: "The name says it all." At the same time, with the rapid expansion of biomedical schools throughout the country, the number of doctors quickly increased. In her opinion, these policies had a significant impact on the status of midwives; Dr. Dimou explained:

> Another important parameter was that [before the reforms] there were more midwives than doctors. Nowadays, we have more doctors, many more doctors than midwives. We have an oversupply, while then, we didn't have a lot of doctors; fewer studied medicine. And in general, there was respect for the midwives. Most women gave birth vaginally, and if a cesarean occurred, it was because it *had* to occur. There didn't exist the culture that exists today, where women feel safer with the ob than with the midwife. Then, they didn't feel safe with the doctor, because they didn't see him often. Rarely. The person they saw regularly was the midwife. When I did my rural practice in [a regional hospital in the 1990s], I encountered this situation with the old-school midwives (*i maes tis palies*). I saw that they were very dominant, these midwives, they weren't afraid of the doctors. The doctor was afraid of the midwife. If the midwife said [slapping her hand on the table for emphasis]: "This woman is going to give birth vaginally (*physiologika*)," how could the doctor say, "Ah no, I'm going to do a cesarean"?

Another significant factor that contributed to the erosion, devaluing, and de-skilling of professional midwives was the absence of organized oppositional or alternative social movements that seriously challenged the growing hegemony of obstetricians and the intensification of the interventionist protocols of hospital-based birth. In other high-resource countries, pressure from feminist activists has helped to protect, promote, and revive midwifery and push back against rising cesarean rates (Georges and Daellenbach 2019). The Greek feminist movement, which peaked in the 1980s and 1990s, was instrumental in effecting the profound cultural, social, and legal changes taking place throughout Greek society at the time (Papagaroufali 1990). However, much of the movement's energies coalesced around the urgent task of revoking Greece's repressively patriarchal family law (the now defunct "Family Code") that had effectively defined adult women as minors and enshrined their subordination to men in the judicial process. Issues in women's reproductive health, while also of concern, were not at the top of the feminist agenda. Ironically, the feminist currents of the time also contributed to the dismantling of the highly regimented (and sexist) model of interned midwifery education described above. Recently, a couple of activist midwives have founded organizations to contest current birth practices, but their members are few and their impacts are small.

I asked the two holistic obs I interviewed whether they saw any possibilities for change in the dominant model arising from consumers, the government, and activists from within or outside the biomedical profession. Dr. Kallopoulos, who has dedicated his career to practicing against the technocratic grain, responded with a sigh, "I think the answer is no." Dr. Broumas, who had trained with Michel Odent and other leading proponents of holistic birth practices, expressed similar resignation. With the dry humor that colored many of his responses to my questions, he offered this pragmatic evaluation of Greece's CB rate:

> The rate is way too high. At the same time, we have [among] the lowest rates of perinatal and infant mortality in the EU. That is to say, things can't be unambiguous. If today doctors were obligated to do vaginal birth only, the outcomes would be worse, because they haven't been trained to do them. Doctors are very good at doing CBs because they do so many. Look, it's the same with tonsillectomies and appendectomies: Greece's rates for both are the highest in the EU, but our outcomes are also the best—because we do so many!

Here Dr. Broumas also raises the critical issue of how obstetricians are taught and trained, to which I return below.

## The Dominant Model of Maternity Care in Greece

Due at least in part to the historical absence of organized opposition, the provision of maternity care throughout Greece is remarkably uniform. Whether Greek women give birth in a posh private facility or in a no-frills public hospital, they experience very similar protocols and procedures. When I began my research in Greece in 1990, pregnancy and birth were already thoroughly biomedicalized, and the traditional midwives who had long attended all Greek births had disappeared completely (Georges 2008). Since then, the use of technological interventions has steadily intensified, even as media reports of evidence-based critiques of conventional obstetric practices have proliferated.

In both ESY and private hospitals, vaginal births are routinely subjected to a similar array of technomedical procedures. Although women refer to them as "natural births" (*fisiologikos toketos*), they are in fact more accurately described as "operational deliveries." Episiotomies are nearly universal, and the women I interviewed were well aware that they would "cut either above or below" (as in many other countries, including almost all Latin American nations; see Diniz and Chacham 2004; Georges and Davis Floyd 2016; Davis-Floyd and Georges 2018, 2023). Women give birth almost exclusively lying flat on their backs in the lithotomy position (another legacy of postwar US influence). The use of electronic fetal monitors and IV drips is routine and universal, effectively immobilizing women during labor. Most have their contractions induced and augmented by rupturing the membranes (amniotomy) and by administering labor-enhancing drugs by the 39th week before their calculated due date. Almost no pregnancies are allowed to reach 40 weeks. Until recently, epidural analgesia was generally unavailable, and few anesthesiologists had acquired the training to administer it. Today, private hospitals offer epidurals, but they are still only sporadically available in public hospitals due to cost and a chronic shortage of anesthesiologists. Most doctors enter one of only seven specializations: obstetrics/gynecology, general surgery, cardiology, radiology, and neurology/psychiatry (which is considered to be a single specialty). Historically, anesthesiology has not been a popular choice (Kaitelidou, Mladovsky et al. 2012:726). Although nearly all these interventions intensify the pain of labor and birth, sometimes considerably, women who give birth in the public hospitals can only rely on getting substantial pain relief by undergoing a cesarean.

Unfortunately, the lack of national-level data on the rates of specific obstetric interventions makes it difficult to track changes over time and across sectors (Vlachidis, Iliodromiti et al. 2014). However, recent public health research on the increase in late preterm births over the last few decades provides valuable insight into the unremitting increase in CBs as well. Between 1991 and 2010, for example, the number of preterm births—live births at less than 37 weeks of gestation—increased 4.5-fold, leading researchers to label the "exponential" growth an "epidemic" (Vlachidis, Kornaru et al. 2013; see also Baroutis et al. 2013). As late as 1996, Greece had the lowest rate of preterm births in the European Union; by 2008 it had risen to second place (Vlachidis, Iliodromiti et al. 2014). By 2010, the 37th gestational week constituted almost half of preterm births and represented "the most important contributor to the overall incidence of preterm births" (2014: 1231). Most "worrying" for these researchers was the pronounced increase in births at 35–36 weeks—a practice not justified by the evidence and one that I intend to research further in the future. After taking into account the increasing numbers of older mothers and multiple births (IVF, which can result in multiple births, has become increasingly popular in Greece), they concluded that "changes in practice by Greek obstetricians have probably also played a major role in the decade's trend, particularly with regard to the late preterm birth increase" (Vlachidis, Kornaru et al. 2013:1231).

This educated guess is supported by Drs. Lambrakis and Kallopoulos, both of whom pointed to obstetricians routinely resorting to late preterm induction as a major factor in the high CB rate. Dr. Lambrakis, a neonatologist for whom science and evidence-based medicine were lodestars and who, although now retired, regularly keeps up with the medical journals in his field, described the typical sequence of events at the large public maternity hospital where he had worked as Department Head:

> So at 37 weeks and a bit, maybe a couple of days, it depends on if there's a holiday, or on Friday, typically on Fridays, the doctors say, "Let's start an induction." So they tell women to come in the morning, they put in the oxytocin [with exasperation] using *the same technique that was used when I returned* [from his Fellowship in the United States in the 1980s]—*it hasn't changed since then!* [His emphasis]. They start with this logic, then at noon and again in the afternoon, they check in on the woman, and then around 10–11:00 p.m., they start the CS [cesarean section]. Because if the cervix is not open, the baby can't be born. They start doing the CSs one after the other. It's like a CS party (*paniyiri*).
>
> Q: What do they say to the women?
>
> That the baby is stressed/in distress (*zoristike*). And that's the truth too, because *they stressed it* [his emphasis] with the oxytocin, so that's not a lie. And then the next birth will be a repeat CS. And they will do those early too.
>
> Q: Does that make more work for you?
>
> Sure, occasionally, if the baby needed help, a little oxygen maybe, they brought them in to our unit [NICU].
>
> Q: And if they had waited until 40 weeks . . .
>
> Forty!? Forty doesn't exist. If they had waited until 40 weeks, the babies would rightly (*canonika*) have been with their mothers.

In fact, however, Dr. Kallopoulos regularly goes up to 42 weeks; he said:

My induction rate is almost less than 5%. Why? Because I wait up until the time it is scientifically allowed for me to wait. [Q: Until?] Until 42 weeks. I go through completely 41 weeks; so, due date plus 7, plus 8—plus 10, I go for induction. By that time, most of the women have delivered. My experience working with diverse populations . . . because I studied in the UK, and I worked in Africa for about a year, having seen how patterns of labor progress—generally speaking, Greek women are very good in laboring. Once labor starts, the progression is quite quick and it's quite good. But . . . the problem is that generally here we don't allow them to labor properly. So you don't find difficulty in dealing with that [labor]; the difficulty is persuading the doctors to hold off until 41–42 weeks.

Q: I've been told that birth outcomes are as good as they are because women's health in general is good, do you agree with that?

Yes, we are a healthy population. Diet, exercise. Greek women are extremely privileged. They're not allowed to, but they labor extremely well. I am fascinated by how well they labor. Ok, we do have a higher rate of diabetes compared with other societies, but that is usually managed only with diet, and that's not an indication not to allow a woman to labor.

## So Why Is the Cesarean Birth Rate in Greece So High?

Despite widespread agreement that the cesarean rate is too high, explanations vary markedly across audiences. Popular opinion points to obstetricians' economic self-interest and to the convenience the operation affords them. Even women who've had CBs blame the doctors, although rarely their own, with whom they typically have forged a close and trusting relationship. The argument for profit most likely reflects the fact that cesareans used to cost more; however, this is no longer the case—or the difference is only marginal—and even the most critical of the interlocutors did not believe that profit is now a major driver of CB. The argument for convenience has gained traction through stories in the media that periodically report on research that finds that cesareans are more likely to be performed on Fridays and Saturdays in the ESY hospitals as doctors clear their schedules in preparation for their Sundays off (see, e.g., Mossialos et al. 2005)—findings echoed above by Dr. Lambrakis. Dr. Broumas, once again displaying the subtle sense of humor that colored many of his responses, added nuance to the ongoing debate. Supporting the position that "convenience" was the major reason that the CB rate is so high, he explained:

> Why is interventionist birth convenient? Because both the ob and the women know the when and the how [of the birth]. Previously, obs did interventionist births and CS because they got more money. This is no longer the case. Here, what is the case? "Time is money" [*in English*].
>
> Q: How so?
> Look, to know that I am going to do a CB on Wednesday, I can arrange my schedule. I don't lose my appointments, I don't lose my surgeries, I go out with my wife, with my children, everything. If I allow you to give birth, I am continuously left hanging, that is, I can't make a schedule. And consequently, [*he repeats, again in English and with emphasis*]: "Time *is* money and it's *a lot of money*."

Mainstream obstetricians, on the other hand, gave two principal reasons for the high CB rates: women's demands for the operation prompted by their fears of childbirth, and the fact that subsequent births will inevitably be by cesarean as well. Dr. Frangos, who directed the Maternity Department of a large public maternity hospital, put it thusly: "Greek women suffer from tokophobia"—a technical term derived from the Greek for "fear of birth" that began to circulate in the global biomedical literature in the 1990s—"and so they ask for or even demand the operation" to avoid the pain and trauma of vaginal birth. According to this logic, in responding to a woman's request, obstetricians are respecting her right to choose how she wants to give birth.

When I asked Marina, who had just begun her residency in obstetrics, why she thought the rate was so high, she offered her own complex perspective, which is simultaneously critical and empathetic:

> I've wondered this myself! I have asked my professors and discussed this with other obstetricians. In other countries, cost is more important. In Greece, I think, we don't have guidelines, everyone does what he wants. The Number One reason the obstetricians give is that it's what women want, they ask for it, it's their choice. That's why CB so high. But I think there are other considerations too. In Scandinavia and in the UK, for example, if something goes wrong with the birth, the state will provide funds to raise the child. In Greece we don't have this. The child might have a problem, we want to be safer. So, you do a CS to be a little safer.

Q: But why induce pre-term?
Lifestyle, because women want to program their lives. Also because of the increase in women's age—the risk goes up for complications [such as] preeclampsia, diabetes—for older women. [I probe her here to comment on whether there are advantages for the doctors.] In part, yes, I understand the doctor's nature, he also he wants to program his life a little bit. But also, the ob doesn't want the baby to be stressed, and because also the women may want it [CB]. And it's not done not super early—at 37 weeks, not at 35. And another reason is that in Greece almost all births are in the hands of obs, unlike other nations, where midwives play roles. So all births depend on the ob, he doesn't have help, and the system doesn't allow the midwives to do more. And so he says, "I may as well finish" (*as teliono*).

In this excerpt from our interview, Marina offers a thoughtful glimpse into mainstream obstetricians' points of view on many of the issues raised in this chapter.

Elsewhere, I have explored women's perceptions and experiences of cesarean birth in depth (Georges and Daellenbach 2019; Georges 2022). Here I briefly mention their points of view on some of the attitudes toward cesarean birth that doctors attribute to them. Most of the women I spoke with expressed a preference for vaginal birth. Nevertheless, their narratives typically revealed a mix of positive and negative perceptions of both vaginal and cesarean options. The most commonly mentioned undesirable aspects of the cesarean that women wished to avoid included postoperative pain. However, this concern was often outweighed by the aura of reduced risk for the baby that perceptually accrued to the operation. Doctors, women, and their families often described the process of labor as a "hardship" or "stress" for the baby, who has to navigate the birth canal, and it was commonly felt that the risk of injury or other harm only increased as the infant was "squeezed and stressed" as labor dragged on (*zorizete to moro*—the expression commonly used by both doctors and women to describe the experience of labor for the baby). The perception that CBs are a safer option is widespread in Greece, and even women who initially preferred to give birth vaginally accepted their obs' recommendations to undergo the operation once the suggestion of risk to the baby was introduced. Reflecting at least in part the intersection of a liberal discourse of "choice" with the maternal moral responsibility for their children's health, the cesarean has come to be seen by women (as well as their partners, mothers, and others) as one more among the many modern reproductive technologies that prudent women must consider to reduce potential risks and ensure an optimal outcome, in what I have called "the symbolic domination of modernity" (Georges 2008).

Reinforcing women's trust in their ob's recommendation to do a cesarean is the distinctively intimate nature of the doctor-patient relationship in Greek obstetrics that characterizes both private and public sectors. Dr. Frangos, who at the time was Director of a large ESY maternity department, had practiced in both the United States and Greece and compared his experiences in the two countries:

> My patients want an exclusive relationship with me [and thus, as he went on to explain, would not accept a group practice as his US patients had]. They are very tied to me, very dependent, even compulsive (*psichanangastikes*): they can call me 30 times, at my office or on my cell phone, at any hour, midnight even . . . That's the kind of relationship a Greek woman has with her doctor. It's very tiring, unbelievably tiring. I'm tied down, whereas in the US I had more free time. But if a doctor doesn't do these things for them, they don't stay, they will go elsewhere.

Dr. Broumas, whose practice is private and holistic, confirmed that his patients also had his cell number and called him "any old time." Although his tone did not convey the same sense of weariness as Dr. Frangos, he described the relationship in related terms:

> It's an erotic relationship, but it's not sexual. For example, I know everything about your family. I know if your husband has a lover and how you reacted, or if you have a lover, if your child uses narcotics, if he's doing well or not. But I believe that this is proper: doctors should be available to the women. And women don't abuse this [access]. If a doctor is a serious and humane person, it can be said that at this moment he is the last of the family doctors in Greece [where there is a serious shortage of family practitioners].

Elena, who was about to begin her residency in ob, got the message from both her teachers and fellow students in medical school that if she went on in her chosen field, "You won't have a life." At the same time, she favorably compared the close nature of the Greek ob-patient relationship with that experienced by her sister, who had just given birth in Canada. Following her sister's pregnancy long-distance, Elena grew concerned about some of the results of her lab tests and advised her to call the doctor to discuss them. She was dismayed when her sister responded that she couldn't do that; it was just not how things worked in Canada. Elena considered the accessibility and degree of support obstetricians provided to their patients to be a superior feature of Greek maternity care, one she valued and hoped to replicate when she practiced. However, the intimate nature of this relationship is double-edged. Once the bond of trust is in place, women and their families generally express confidence in their doctors' advice, including the "necessity" of undergoing a cesarean.

The second reason doctors gave for the high CB rate is that once a woman has a CB, subsequent births are all but guaranteed to be cesareans too, because mainstream obs do not know how to attend VBACs; they are not taught how during their clinical training. A handful of doctors in the private sector, like Dr. Kallopoulos, do attend VBACs, but as one ESY doctor lamented, "99.99% of women in the public hospitals do not get VBAC." Another ESY doctor, who learned how to attend VBACs in the UK, explained that "there are some doctors who have done some of their training abroad, especially in Europe, and over the last five years or so, some are performing more VBACs, but this is still in a transitional stage." In short, to learn how to attend a VBAC, Greek obstetricians must go abroad, and supposedly they must return to Greece to practice. However, as I further discuss below, there has been a massive exodus of doctors from Greece to Western Europe in recent years and thus, VBAC attendance in Greece is not occurring. I also note that in attributing the excessively high CB rate to women's demands (as well as to their age and weight), obstetricians also implicitly shift the blame to women for the multiplier effect set in motion by repeat cesareans, eliding the fact that because Greek obs lack the training, VBACs are unavailable to all but a few determined women.

Recently, three Greek obstetricians offered a novel argument in defense of Greece's high cesarean rate. In a letter to *The Lancet*, Georgios Pratilas, Alexandros Sotiridis, and Konstantinos Dinas (2019) proposed that because the budget cuts made after the 2009 financial crisis had compromised the quality of maternity care in public hospitals, cesareans were an essential strategy for maintaining the excellent maternal and perinatal outcomes that Greeks had come to expect. The authors concluded their letter with the provocative question: "Could the better-than-expected perinatal outcome in the context of the economic crisis in Greece be possible because of the *early* [my emphasis] recourse to CS?" Here these doctors appear to be defending not only routine CBs, but the routinization of preterm births as well. The letter is also revealing for their selective deployment of statistics in defending their position. Implicitly arguing against evidence-based medicine recommendations (for example, such as those of WHO [2015] for CB rates far lower than those in Greece), the authors cited their own statistical "evidence" in defense of Greek obstetricians' disregard for such guidelines.

## Becoming an Obstetrician in Greece: Biomedical Training

> *In Greece, we have the phenomenon that those who teach ob/gyn*
> *don't know how to do vaginal birth. So, when you don't know*
> *how to do vaginal birth, it's safer to do a CS. Consequently,*
> *the training of young doctors, and of young obs, needs to change,*
> *for them to be able to feel the confidence and security. But to do*
> *that, the old obs will have to change the way they do birth.*
> —Dr. Broumas

Many of the pedagogical issues that impede transformation in the entrenched technocratic obstetric model have been identified and critiqued by scholars of Greek biomedical education for more than four decades. The first critique of biomedical training appeared in 1975, when there were just two medical schools in Greece (Harrell 1975). Since then, as previously noted, five new schools have been built in different parts of the country. Because the biomedical curriculum has never been fully standardized, the new schools presented opportunities to rethink the organization of programs and pedagogical approaches. However, with the exception of the University of Crete, reform of biomedical education was not pursued or was lost sight of after being briefly piloted. Thus, most of the issues identified in the mid-1970s persist today (Cinoku, Zampeli, and Moustopoulos 2021).

In this section, I focus on the central issue raised by scholars of Greek biomedical education and the interlocutors alike: the compartmentalization of theory and practice and the resulting insufficiency of students' exposure to practical, hands-on experience, especially in their clinical years, when they are more often directed *what* to do and less often told the reasons *why*. I also discuss the implications of some informal aspects of training that introduce students to the spoken and unspoken norms of the profession that may also help to reproduce the high CB rate.

Getting into medical school in Greece is an arduous process. Only students who make top scores on the punishingly difficult national university entrance exams are admitted. Achieving such scores requires not only intensive studying during high school but also attending private "cram" classes after school. Consequently, students typically enter medical school with a strong science background. Elena, who had finished high school in Canada, told me that she struggled during her first year to keep up with her classmates, who arrived much better prepared than she was.

All higher education in Greece is free, yet housing and other living expenses are not included. A child's university education brings prestige to the entire family, and a distinctive feature of Greek society is the effort parents make to underwrite all aspects of their children's education (Georges 2008). Thus, in contrast to the United States, medical student debt is negligible and does not figure into the calculus of selecting a specialty. Elena, for example, described her family's reaction to her decision to go to medical school: "As soon as I told my parents, they said 'Yes!!' You know how parents are, they all want their kids to be a lawyer or a doctor." Indeed, the strong support provided by "the structure and ethos of the Greek family and society," including the (unremunerated) extra efforts of faculty, employees, and students, have been credited with maintaining the good quality of university education despite the steep budget cuts and hiring freezes in effect since 2009 (Kontos et al. 2015:610).

### Issues in the Formal Curriculum: Compartmentalization of Theory and Practice

The six years of medical education are divided equally into two distinct components: "theory" and "practice." The first three "preclinical" years are devoted exclusively to life science subjects and are taught by professors almost entirely through lectures. During these years, students may take up to ten courses per semester—all interlocutors considered that load too heavy, and repeating courses was not uncommon. Of necessity, students devoted themselves almost entirely to learning the massive amounts of scientific information required to pass their exams. Exposure to clinical practice during these years is absent or minimal (Moutsopoulos 2017; Moutsopoulos et al. 2017; Cinoku et al. 2021:289). Exceptionally motivated students, such as the interlocutors (as evidenced, among other things, by their willingness to take time from their over-scheduled lives to talk with me) try to participate in research or gain some practical hands-on experience outside the classroom during these years, but the burden is on them to find such opportunities and the faculty to advise and mentor them.

The three "clinical" years that follow take place in accredited departments or hospitals (Georgantopoulou 2009). There, students are exposed to clinical practice, usually for the first time. However, even then opportunities for hands-on training are often limited, especially in the busy hospitals of Athens and Thessaloniki. Learning in the hospital typically consists of teachers describing and explaining procedures to the students, who most often stand aside and observe (in a lingering echo of Dr. Louros's pedagogical style). The two major issues voiced by all the students I interviewed was the need for more hands-on patient treatment and experience during the clinical years, and more systematic integration of the theoretical and practical aspects of training across the curriculum.

On the whole, Elena appreciated her educational experience in Crete's reformed program, and compared it favorably to those of her friends who studied elsewhere in Greece. Still, she had this to say about her clinical years:

> To be honest, that [clinical training] is the gray area: the doctors work so hard, they have so much to do, that a lot of the time they don't really consider the educational part . . . you can get lost, because the doctors don't really take care of the [clinical] program, they're too busy. And I honestly understand, but at the same time, you're in a university hospital, and it's, like, your job.

Elena's experience can be generalized to the current state of clinical training across Greece. In the words of leading scholars of Greek biomedical education:

> During the . . . three years of clinical medical studies, in the majority of medical schools the clinical training is mostly theoretical . . . very limited "hands-on" patient training is enforced or performed. This results in young doctors with plenty of theoretical knowledge but a limited clinical experience . . . This has to change! (Cinoku at al. 2021:289)

However, because the number of students entering medical schools is not adjusted to accord with the nation's need for physicians, and because of budget cuts that place additional burdens on the time and energy of the faculty (as Elena sympathetically recognizes), changes in the prevailing model of clinical training are not likely to happen soon.

The same problem exists in the training of residents. I discussed the article cited above with Dr. Lambrakis, who knew one of the authors, and asked if he thought their critique was too harsh. Characteristically blunt, he responded by describing the training of residents in his hospital:

> No, the residents don't learn. They may know medicine theoretically. But when they are in front of the patient, they are lost. Here

the professor says, "Do this, do that. Run here, run there, we're going to do this." The resident can't learn if you treat him like an instrument, a tool. For instance, "Go do an X-ray" without explaining why. And what therapy will you use if there's a problem? But here they do tests without giving a reason, without an analysis—why do you do the exams? But most of them teach this way.

For Dr. Lambrakis, one of the most serious consequences of residents' inadequate practical experience was that:

> They *don't learn how to discern the serious from the light case*. For example, in pediatrics, how do you distinguish serious asthma in a baby? If the baby continues to drink the same amount of milk from the bottle, that means it's not serious. If it doesn't finish or drinks less, that means it gets tired, so it's a more difficult problem. (Emphasis mine)

Within this pedagogical context, it is difficult for students and residents to gain the self-confidence required to make such crucial distinctions, as Cinoku et al. (2021:289) pointed out. Without this confidence, they "can get lost," as both Elena and Dr. Lambrakis put it. This context also has implications for understanding why all pregnancies continue to be approached as though they are high-risk and why so many births end up as cesareans. Feeling lost, not knowing what to do, is an affective and embodied experience that, in the context of the clinic where much is at stake, can impel "even the most fluid of thinkers to shut down cognitively" and rely on Stage 1 rigid routines ("Our way is the only way"), as Robbie Davis-Floyd describes in Chapter 1 of this volume. As Dr. Lambrakis succinctly explained, students are not taught the sometimes-mundane technical skills (e.g., to observe how an infant drinks milk from a bottle) that would give them the confidence to differentiate the serious case. As a result, habitual practices are reproduced, and all births continue to be approached as "serious" and high-risk.

## Hidden Agendas: Informal Learning in Medical Schools

The students I spoke with were initially drawn to ob/gyn for many reasons—a fascination with birth, a desire to increase the representation of women in the field, and in one case, an early obsession with the television show *Grey's Anatomy*. Once in medical school, however, they were repeatedly exposed to discouraging stereotypes about obs from their classmates as well as from their professors that gave them pause. The one they faced most frequently was that obs are "in it for the money." This negative stereotype is so pervasive that when Elena was asked what she wanted to specialize in, she learned to preemptively defend herself:

> "So you want to be an ob? You're going to get rich" (*plousia tha gineis*). So now when they ask me, I say: "I want to be an ob, but not for the money." I say that automatically. That's why I started doing my MA, because I wanted to create that difference between me and the typical ob.

This stereotype, with which I was familiar from my previous fieldwork, may have its origins in the 1960s–1980s when many obs in fact did make a great deal of money from performing abortions.[1] Today, some, like a resident in psychiatry whom I met, point instead to the high CB rate to support the view that obs are "in it for the money." Medical students (like everyone else) know that some doctors in the public sector, especially those in surgical professions, accept or even elicit informal payments for their services. One student described glimpsing "behind the curtain" during his clinical training at the ways in which some of his professors differentially treated the patients that were "theirs"—that is, from whom they would be getting "the little envelope" after the birth. All the students I spoke with told me that they did not want to accept informal payments, but they also understood why the temptation would exist. Niko, for example, hopes that he won't take money, but also said that this was a "gray area" for him. Citing the low salaries, hard work, and long hours, he confessed that, "In all honesty, I'm not sure what I will do in the future."

More surprising for me was the stereotype, perhaps related to the assumption that money was their main motivator, that obs were not as smart or as knowledgeable as other doctors. For example, one of Alexandra's professors, an ob/gyn himself, told her she was "too bright" to be an ob! Disappointed with ob/gyn for her own reasons, Alexandra later decided to switch to ophthalmology. Elena was also very familiar with the negative views held by her colleagues: "The stereotype is that they are considered bad doctors, doctors that only want the money. And I contemplated within myself, do I want to have that label within the medical community—the bad doctor that's not as knowledgeable and stuff? And then you decide to become the good doctor to prove them wrong." But for others, the widely circulating negative images were sufficiently discouraging that ultimately, they decided to switch to another specialty.

# The Brain Drain

Medical students like the interlocutors, with the passion and desire to acquire knowledge and practical skills, actively try to participate in patient care during their clinical rotations. Some seek out mentors in their "free" time to help out in those mentors' practices; others get involved in research projects or enroll in Master's programs. However, as Ilir Cinoku, Evangelia Zampeli, and Haralampos Moutsopoulos (2021) also found in their review of the current state of medical education in Greece, these highly motivated young doctors usually find ways to continue their education in hospitals in other EU countries or in the United States. Professors may even advise their best students to leave. Alexandra, for example, was encouraged to start prepping for the USMLE (United States Medical Licensing Examination) early in her medical school career.

Given the serious doctor shortage in the rest of the EU, especially in the UK, Greek medical school graduates seeking residencies abroad are readily "scooped up," as Dr. Broumas put it. Many, if not most, who leave will not return, resulting in a massive brain drain for Greece. A recent survey of Greek medical students found that 86% were considering emigration to continue their studies abroad (Labiris et al. 2014). The medical associations of Athens and Thessaloniki estimated that between 2009 and 2013, some 7,500 doctors emigrated from these two cities alone (Chatziprodromidou et al. 2017:289).

Another factor pushing students to go abroad is the notoriously long wait time for obtaining a residency in Greece. The combination of an oversupply of medical school graduates and deep cutbacks in the public health sector has created a serious bottleneck in the pipeline from graduation to residency. The wait for an opening can last four to six years or even longer. The current wait time for a residency in endocrinology, for example, is around ten years. Elena, who wants to specialize in reproductive endocrinology, told me that if she could find an opening in Greece without having to wait, she probably wouldn't go abroad. But four of the five obstetric students I interviewed planned to leave to do their residency (and the fifth was undecided). Those who go abroad must usually devote additional time, energy, and money to mastering a foreign language. Alexandra, for example, is taking advanced English classes to do her residency in the UK. Elena, who lived for many years in Canada and switched effortlessly between Greek and English during our conversations, had also considered the UK. However, citing the decline of the NHS (the UK's National Health System), she is now looking to

Switzerland, considered the best place in the EU for her chosen specialty; she is currently studying French. Both are uncertain as to whether they will return to Greece to practice medicine once they complete their studies.

While the loss of economic and human capital represented by the Greek medical brain drain has attracted considerable attention from researchers (see, e.g., Ifanti et al. 2014; Labrianidis and Pratsinakis 2014; Moris, Karachaliou, and Kontos 2017), a hidden dimension of particular relevance to this chapter is the loss of young doctors who have been trained abroad in more evidence-based approaches and/or exposed to holistic or humanistic alternatives to the prevailing Greek technocratic model of birth. Drs. Kallopoulos and Broumas are two exceptional holistic obs who prove the rule. When they trained in the UK, both learned how to attend VBACs and water births and how to work collaboratively with midwives. Like the holistic obs whom Robbie and I studied in Brazil (Georges and Davis-Floyd 2016; Davis-Floyd and Georges 2018; see also our chapter in Volume III of this series, Davis-Floyd and Georges 2023), these doctors were motivated by deeply held ethical commitments, left-political for the one, religious-spiritual for the other. Their humanistic values also impelled them to return to practice holistically in Greece and sustained them when their colleagues mocked them for doing so. But, again, most of the doctors who go abroad will not return. Coupled with the fact that mandatory continuing medical education (CME) is nonexistent in Greece, their loss most likely will help to ensure the reproduction of the dominant technocratic model of maternity care for years to come.

## Conclusions: The Distinctively Greek Adaptations of the Technocratic Model

As I have shown in this chapter, reaching a CB rate that is "the highest in the world" is the outcome of multiple trends, some global, and some specific to Greece. I have described the historical development of Greek obstetrics and the distinctive features of Greek obstetric training to understand the processes that have impelled the seemingly unstoppable momentum driving up the cesarean rate over the past three decades. As I have shown, the foundations of the distinctively Greek technocratic approach to childbirth were laid during the Cold War when the United States attempted to influence the direction of Greece's postwar recovery. The promotion of US "soft power" under the Truman Doctrine succeeded in redirecting Greek biomedicine toward North America in the postwar period, instead of toward Western Europe, where the elite doctors of the first half of the 20th century had studied. In the ensuing years, the technocratic model was reinforced, reproduced, and intensified within a complex constellation of political, social, and cultural factors that constituted the distinctively Greek adaptations of the technocratic model. These include not only Greece's extremely high CB rate, but also among the highest rates of scheduled deliveries of pre-term babies in the EU.[2] Other distinctively Greek adaptations of the technocratic model include using general anesthesia for CBs; the informal payments given to their obs by "their" patients; and the close relationships established between obstetricians and patients—very few US obs would be willing to be available to their patients 24/7, and those are the 50 or so US obs (out of a total of around 35,000) who attend home births (Davis-Floyd 2022).

As the Greek biomedical profession came to occupy a powerful position in the context of a relatively weak state, regulations, constraints, and oversight of doctors were relatively loose, porous, or nonexistent (for examples, no obligatory continuing medical education, no board certification). The political power wielded by the biomedical profession also worked to eliminate competition from midwives, first by promoting the passage of laws that barred them from performing abortions (Hionidou 2020) and later, as the number of doctors began to multiply exponentially, by effectively restricting midwives' scope of professional practice to the role of doctors' assistants. Over time, the midwifery option was foreclosed for most Greek women. Unlike in many other places, in Greece, as previously noted, feminist activism around reproductive health was never an important force, even in the 1970s and 1980s when the feminist movement was organized and was achieving success in the dismantling of longstanding patriarchal laws. The lack of attention paid to reproductive issues is perhaps due to the fact that the technical illegality of abortion during these years did not prevent women from accessing safe medical abortions. In any case, organized demands for alternatives to the prevailing model of birth, which in other places have helped to restrain excessive cesareans and other interventions, have not formed a significant part of the agenda of healthcare activists in Greece.

This broader historical, political, and social context is critical to understanding the question at the heart of this chapter: why is the Greek CB rate so high? Yet it is also essential to look at the education and training of obstetricians-to-be, as I have done, to more fully understand how the routinization of cesarean birth has become as encompassing as it is today. As discussed in this chapter, students acquire a vast store of life science knowledge in medical school, but at least since the 1970s when the first critique of Greek biomedical education appeared in print, far less practical experience and hands-on clinical training. Across the board, this was the chief complaint of all interlocutors. Insufficient exposure to practical experience has several implications for understanding the reproduction and intensification of cesarean births. First, as a result, to quote both Elena and the most prominent critics of Greek biomedical education, students "can get lost." As previously noted, feeling lost, not knowing what to do, is an affective and embodied experience that, in the context of the clinic where much is at stake, can impel "even the most fluid of thinkers to shut down cognitively" and rely on Stage 1 rigid routines ("Our way is the only way"; see Chapter 1, this volume). As Dr. Lambrakis succinctly explained, students are not taught the some-times-mundane technical skills (e.g., to observe how an infant drinks milk from a bottle) that would give them the confidence to differentiate the serious case from one that is not. As a result, all births continue to be approached as "serious" and high-risk. Additionally, the top-down ped-agogical approach that consists of telling students *what* to do, but not encouraging them to understand the practical and theoretical logics of *why*, has obvious implications for reproducing conventional protocols.

In this chapter, I have suggested that this approach to biomedical training may be a vestige of the European training experienced in the last century by the influential pioneers in Greek obstetrics. However, further research would help to clarify why, given that many doctors since then were trained in the United States and elsewhere under differ-ent pedagogical approaches, the top-down Greek model remains robust. Finally, and not least, the progressive de-skilling of obstetricians that has resulted from the reduced number of vaginal births they attend also contributes to the reproduction of routine cesareans. As Dr. Broumas put it, obstetricians are very skilled practitioners of the operation "be-cause they do so many." Less skilled at attending non-interventionist births, they teach their students only what they know.

Another current in the confluence of factors intensifying recourse to cesareans that needs to be considered is the Greek perception that cesareans mitigate risk and are thus safer. This perception is shared by Greek women, their families, and their obstetricians. Although most women I have interviewed told me that they preferred to give birth vaginally, they accepted their doctors' advice to undergo cesarean at any hint of risk to the baby. The distinctively close nature of the doctor-patient relationship in the Greek cultural context helps to reassure most women that the operation was necessary and in the best interest of their babies.

Two final factors that encourage the reproduction and impede the transformation of the current model are the massive brain drain that usually permanently removes from the Greek healthcare system doctors trained "otherwise" while abroad, and the negative stereotypes that typecast obstetricians as greedier and less intelligent than other doctors. Those students who find these stereotypes sufficiently discouraging—presumably those who are motivated by a different set of values—may switch to another specialty, and thereby their potential to transform obstetric practice may also be lost. In short, the recourse to cesarean birth at its currently spectacularly high levels has been impelled by a disparate yet powerful assortment of trends, all working in the same direction. Although I would prefer to end this chapter on a more hopeful note, the fact is that up to the present, there are no countervailing currents to dissipate these trends.

## Acknowledgments

I am grateful to the Tsakolopoulos Hellenic Foundation for a generous Fellowship that enabled me to conduct archival research in the Tsakolopoulos Hellenic Collection at the California State University, Sacramento in the summer of 2019, and to the support and assistance offered to me by the Curator of the Collection, George Paganelis. My profound thanks to Robbie Davis-Floyd for suggesting the topic of this chapter, which led me to conduct additional research in Greece in 2021–2022, and for her care-full editing. I also gratefully acknowledge the invaluable help that my research assistant, Anastasia Zanetoulis, provided in recruiting interlocutors for this project as well as for her insights into the process of biomedical education. Not least, I am deeply grateful to the interlocutors for their time and for their support of this project.

**Eugenia Georges** is Professor of Anthropology at Rice University and former long-term Chair of the Department of Anthropology. She has conducted research on medicalization and reproduction in Greece, the movement to humanize childbirth in Brazil, and Dominican transnational migrants in the Dominican Republic and New York City. She is the author of multiple articles and of *The Making of a Transnational Community: Migration, Development and Cultural Change in the Dominican Republic* (1990) and *Bodies of Knowledge: The Medicalization of Reproduction in Greece* (2008).

## Notes

1. The number of abortions has decreased considerably among married couples due to more consistent use of contraception. In recent years, however, the number has been rising among Greek teens, due in part to a lack of sex education in the schools.
2. In the United States, in most circumstances, labors are not induced and CBs are not scheduled until 39 weeks, in compliance with the guidelines set out by the American College of Obstetricians and Gynecologists (ACOG 2021), which are specifically designed to avoid unnecessary preterm births.

## References

American College of Obstetricians and Gynecologists (ACOG). 2021. "Committee Opinion No. 831: Medically Indicated Late-Preterm and Early-Term Deliveries." *Obstetrics & Gynecology* 138: e35–39.

Baroutis G, Mousiolis A, Mesogitis S, et al. 2013. "Preterm Birth Trends in Greece: A Rising Concern." *Acta Obstetricia et Gynecologica Scandinavica* 92: 575–582.

Carpenter M. 2003. "On the Edge: The Fate of Progressive Modernization in Greek Health Policy." *International Political Science Review* 24(2): 257–272.

CEDAW. 2013. "Concluding Observations on the Seventh Periodic Report of Greece Adopted by the Committee at its 54th Session." www2.ohchr.org/english/bodies/cedaw/docs/co/CEDAW.C.GRC.CO.7.doc.

Chatziprodromidou I, Emmanouilides C, Yfanti F, et al. 2017. "Brain Drain: The Greek Phenomenon." *International Research Journal of Public and Environmental Health* 4(11): 289–293.

Cinoku I, Zampeli E, Moutsopoulos H. 2021. "Medical Education in Greece: Necessary Reforms Need to Be Reconsidered." *Medical Teacher* 43(3): 287–292.

Davis-Floyd, R. 2003 [1992]. *Birth as an American Rite of Passage*, 2nd ed. Berkeley: University of California Press.

———. 2022. *Birth as an American Rite of Passage*, 3rd ed. Abingdon, Oxon: Routledge.

Davis-Floyd R, Georges E. 2018. "The Paradigm Shift of Humanistic and Holistic Obstetricians: The 'Good Guys and Girls' of Brazil." In *Ways of Knowing about Birth: Mothers, Midwives, Medicine, and Birth Activism*, Davis-Floyd R and Colleagues, 141–161. Long Grove IL: Waveland Press.

Davis-Floyd R, Georges E. 2023. "The Paradigm Shifts of Humanistic and Holistic Obstetricians: The 'Good Guys and Girls' of Brazil." In *Obstetric Violence and Systemic Disparities: Can Obstetrics Be Humanized and Decolonized?* eds. Davis-Floyd R, Premkumar A, Chapter 9. New York: Berghahn Books.

Diniz S, Chacham AS. 2004. "'The Cut Above' and 'the Cut Below': The Abuse of Cesareans and Episiotomy in Sao Paulo, Brazil." *Reproductive Health Matters* 12(23): 100–110.

Dixon LZ, Smith-Oka V, El Kotni M. 2019. "Teaching about Childbirth in Mexico: Working across Birth Models." In *Birth in Eight Cultures*, eds. Davis-Floyd R, Cheyney M, 17–48. Long Grove IL: Waveland Press.

Eurostat. 2018. Infant Mortality Rate Halved between 1998 and 2018. https://ec.europa.eu/eurostat/web/products-eurostat-news/-/ddn-20200309-1

Georgantopoulou C. 2009. "Medical Education in Greece." *Medical Teacher* 31(1): 13–17.
Georges, E. 1996. "Abortion Policy and Practice in Greece." *Social Science and Medicine* 42(4): 509–519.
———. 2008. *Bodies of Knowledge: The Medicalization of Reproduction in Greece.* Nashville TN: Vanderbilt University Press.
———. 2013. "'An Intervention Just Like Any Other': Changing Meanings of the Caesarean in Contemporary Greece." In *Motherhood in the Forefront: Recent Research in Greek Ethnography,* ed. Kantsa V, 143–155. Athens: Alexandra Press.
———. 2010. "Guiding Pregnancy: Expert Advice and the Modern Greek Mother." *Journal of Mediterranean Studies* 18(2): 387–412.
———. 2022. "Making Ethnographic Sense of Caesarean Rates in Greek Public Hospitals: Immigrants, Midwives, and Stratified Maternity Care." In *The Work of Hospitals: Global Medicine in Local Culture,* eds. Olsen W, Sargent C, 232–244. New Brunswick NJ: Rutgers University Press.
Georges E, Daellenbach R. 2019. "Divergent Meanings and Practices of Childbirth in Greece and New Zealand." In *Birth in Eight Cultures,* eds. Davis-Floyd R, Cheyney M, 129–164. Long Grove IL: Waveland Press.
Georges, E and Davis-Floyd R. 2016. "Humanistic Obstetric Care in Brazil." In *The Routledge Handbook of Medical Anthropology,* eds. Manderson L, Cartwright L, Hardon A, 340–350. New York: Routledge.
Halkias A. 2004. *The Empty Cradle of Democracy: Sex, Abortion, and Nationalism in Modern Greece.* Durham NC: Duke University Press.
Harrell G. 1975. "Medical Education in Greece." *Annals of Internal Medicine* 82(2): 278–279.
Hionidou V. 2020. *Abortion and Contraception in Modern Greece: 1830–1967.* Cham, Switzerland: Palgrave.
Ifanti A, Argyriou A, Kalofonou F, et al. 2014. "Physicians' Brain Drain in Greece: A Perspective on the Reasons and How to Address It." *Health Policy* 117: 210–215.
Kaitelidou D, Mladovsky P, Leone T, et al. 2012. "Understanding the Oversupply of Physicians in Greece: The Role of Human Resources Planning, Financing Policy, and Physician Power." *International Journal of Health Services* 42(4): 719–738.
Kaitelidou D, Theodorou M, Sourtzi P, et al. 2013. "Informal Payments for Maternity Health Services in Public Hospitals in Greece." *Health Policy* 109: 23–30.
Kalyvas S. 2015. *Modern Greece: What Everyone Needs to Know.* New York: Oxford University Press.
Kontos M, Demetrios M, Zoografos M, Liakakos T. 2015. "The Greek Financial Crisis: Maintaining Medical Education, Against the Odds." *Postgraduate Medical Journal* 91(1081): 609–611.
Labiris G, Vamvakerou V, Tsolakaki O, et al. 2014. "Perceptions of Greek Medical Students Regarding Medical Profession and the Specialty Selection Process during the Economic Crisis Years." *Health Policy* 117(2): 203–209.
Labrianidis, L Pratsinakis M. 2014. "Outward Migration from Greece during the Crisis, Final Report." Project funded by the National Bank of Greece through the London School of Economics Hellenic Observatory. Retrieved 10 February 2022 from https://www.lse.ac.uk/Hellenic-Observatory/Assets/Documents/

Research/External-Research-Projects/Final-Report-Outward-migration-from-Greece-during-the-crisis-revised-on-1-6-2016.pdf.

Manidaki A, Tsiligianni I, Trompoukis C. 2018. "Nikolaos Louros (1898–1986): The Reformer of Greek Obstetrics and Gynecology of the 20th Century." *Acta Medico-Historica Adriatica* 16(2): 253–266.

Moris D, Karachaliou G-S, Kontos M. 2017. "Residency Training in Greece: Job Dissatisfaction Paves the Way to Brain Drain." *Annals of Transactional Medicine* 5(5): 123–124.

Mossialos E, Allin S, Karras K, Davaki K. 2005. "An Investigation of Ceasarean Sections in Three Greek Hospitals." *European Journal of Public Health* 15(3): 288–295.

Moutsopoulos H. 2017. "Παθολόγος στην Ελλάδα—αλλά με τιεκπαίδευση" [Internist in Greece—But with What Education?]. In *Ανθρωπολογία της παρακμής* [Anthropology of Decadence], 2nd edn., ed. Moutsopoulos H, 48–54. Athens: Medusa Publishers.

Moutsopoulos H, Vlachoyannopoulos P, Samarkos M. 2017. "Αναμόρφωση των υπηρεσιών υγείας στη σύγχρονη Ελλάδα" [Reformation of Health System Services in Modern Greece]. In *Ανθρωπολογία της παρακμής* [Anthropology of Decadence], 2nd edn., ed. Moutsopoulos H, 56–71. Athens: Medusa Publishers.

Naziri D. 1988. *La Femme Grecque et L'avortement: Étude Clinique du Recours Répétitif L'avortement* [*The Greek Woman and Abortion: A Clinical Study of Repeated Recourse to Abortion*]. PhD dissertation, University of Paris.

Nikolentzos A, Mays N. 2016. "Explaining the Persistent Dominance of the Greek Medical Profession Across Successive Health Care System Reforms from 1983 to the Present." *Health Systems & Reform* 2(2): 135–146.

Papagaroufali E. 1990. *Greek Women in Politics: Gender Ideology and Practice in Neighborhood Groups and the Family*. PhD dissertation, Columbia University.

Paxson, H. 2004. *Making Modern Mothers: Ethics and Family Planning in Urban Greece*. Berkeley: University of California Press.

Pratilas G, Sotiridis A, Dinas K. 2019. "Is High Use of Cesarean Section Sometimes Justified?" *Lancet* 10192: 25–26.

Souliotis K, Golna C, Tountas Y, et al. 2016. "Informal Payments in the Greek Health Sector amid the Financial Crisis: Old Habits Die Hard." *European Journal of Health Economics* 17(2): 159–170.

Vlachidis N, Kornaru E, Ketenas E. 2013. "The Preterm Birth Epidemic in Greece." *Acta Obstetricia et Gynecologica Scandinavica* 92: 1231–1235.

Vlachidis N, Iliodromiti Z, Creatsas G, Vrachnis N. 2014. "Preterm Birth Time Trends in Europe: The Worrying Case of Greece." *BJOG: An International Journal of Obstetrics and Gynecology* 121(3): 372–373. World Bank 2019. Maternal Mortality Ratio (Modeled Estimate Based on 100,000 Live Births, European Union. Retrieved 27 November 2022 from: https://data.worldbank.org/indicator/SH.STA.MMRT?locations=EU&name_desc=true

World Health Organization. 2015. *WHO Statement on Cesarean Section Rates*. Geneva: Department of Reproductive Health and Research, World Health Organization. Retrieved 27 November 2022 from http://apps.who.int/iris/bitstream/handle/10665/161442/WHO_RHR_15.02_eng.pdf;jsessionid=6DD7FE73BFF95ACC729E60C2BF047D77?sequence=1.

# CHAPTER 4

# "Physiologic Birth Implies Economic Damage"

## Financial Incentives for the Performance of Cesareans in Chile

*Michelle Sadler and Gonzalo Leiva*

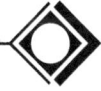

## Introduction: Childbirth in Chile

Chile is a country of 19 million inhabitants, located in the extreme South of the Americas. Despite being one of the countries with the fastest economic growth in recent decades, and being categorized as a high-income country (Lange, Wodon, and Carey 2018), Chile is currently the second most unequal country among those in the Organization for Economic Cooperation and Development (OECD 2021). The income of the richest 20% of the population is ten times higher than that of the poorest quintile, surprisingly higher than the average for OECD countries (Mieres 2020). Since October 2019, in the context of an unprecedented social upheaval in the country, a profound reform process has been underway, facing central questions about governance, the economic model, and the social contract. (A "social contract" is an implicit agreement among the members of a society to cooperate for social benefits, for example by sacrificing some individual freedom for state protection.) And, as we will discuss throughout this chapter, the inequities in childbirth care are faithful reflections of the structural inequalities of Chilean society.

Since the 1990s, more than 99% of births have occurred, and still occur, in biomedical healthcare facilities—public and private—and are attended by trained biomedical personnel (Koch et al. 2012), with no insured or regulated out-of-hospital alternatives (Sadler, Leiva, and Gómez 2021). Since then, there have been enormous reductions in maternal and infant mortality rates. In 2017, Chile's IMR (infant mortality ratio; infant deaths/1000 live births) was 6/1000 (UNICEF 2018) and its MMR (maternal mortality ratio, maternal deaths/100,000 live births) was 13/100,000 (WHO 2019). Although these are excellent indicators for the country, they hide the problems of an excessively biomedicalized childbirth system and huge gaps in access and quality of health care among the different modes of health insurance. The standards of childbirth care are very far from national and international guidelines (MINSAL 2008; WHO 2018; Lalonde et al. 2019). And although the excessive rates of routine obstetric interventions are similar in private and public healthcare facilities (with the exception of cesareans), the mistreatment of women by biomedical personnel is much higher in public hospitals. An online survey with a sample of 5,697 births that took place in Chile between 2014 and 2017 reported that verbal and physical abuse toward birthing women was more than triple in the public sector compared to the private (OVO Chile 2018), in a context in which the public healthcare system has important deficiencies such as hospital infrastructure deficits, low privacy in patient care, and a low level of wages for practitioners (Goic 2015). The causes of these deficiencies date back to the 1970s, when a neoliberal healthcare system was introduced by the Pinochet regime (1973–1990), creating a private healthcare system that has led to inequality of access and has created a structural disadvantage for several segments of the population, including women (Rotarou and Sakellariou 2017).

The privatization of childbirth has been steadily rising in Chile, from less than 20% in 2000 to 35% in 2016 (Sadler et al. 2018; De Elejalde and Giolito 2019a), and has translated into a steep rise in cesarean births (CBs), which accounted for 59% of births in the country in 2021 (DEIS 2022). These numbers are consistent with the rising trend in this intervention in Latin America and the Caribbean, which led to a CB rate for this region of 44.3% in 2015 (Boerma et al 2018). The WHO Statement on Cesarean Section Rates of 2015 expressed concern about the increase in the number of these surgeries and the possible negative consequences for maternal and child health. This document is emphatic in stating that cesareans are effective in saving the lives of mothers and newborns only when they are truly needed (WHO 2015). In addition to the adverse health effects of CBs, concerns have been raised regarding the inequities in their use—between and within countries—and the excessive costs that CBs impose on healthcare systems (Villar, Valladares, and Wojdyla 2006; Betrán, Ye et al. 2016).

As A. P. Betrán, M. R. Torloni and colleagues (2016:667) argue, the reasons that may explain the rise in CBs "are not fully understood but emerge as a complex multifactorial labyrinth involving health systems, healthcare providers, women, societies, and even fashion and media." Changes in maternal characteristics (older age of pregnant women; increase in assisted reproduction; increase in weight issues, obesity, and diabetes, among others) play a role, but cannot account for the dramatic increase in the CB rates. Attention should be paid to the "non-medical" factors influencing the trend; these factors relate to sociocultural, organizational, and economic dynamics. These are evident in the case of Chile, given that cesareans in private health care are more than double those of the public sector.

As previously noted, Chile's healthcare system is organized into two insurance systems: public and private. In 2016, 78% of the country's population was insured by the public National Health Fund (FONASA), 18% by private institutions called ISAPRES (the acronym for Instituciones de Salud Previsional), and the remaining 4% by an armed forces insurance plan (OECD 2017). In private health care, there are several ISAPRES plans to choose from; these offer multiple healthcare plans with different kinds of health coverage. These private entities receive and administer the mandatory health contribution of 7% of the taxable remuneration, or more, depending on the health plan and coverage chosen, whereas in public health, all insured members join FONASA and are assigned to different groups according to their income brackets. Individuals with no income are assigned to Group A, and those who contribute 7% of their taxable salary monthly are assigned to Groups B, C, and D, according to their incremental incomes. FONASA Group A can only access the public network, while Groups B, C, and D can also access the private network of affiliated institutions through a diagnosis-related payment system called PAD (*Pago Asociado a Diagnóstico*). This system includes childbirth, and for women to be eligible for PAD Birth, their pregnancies have to be singleton, categorized as "low risk," and past 37 weeks of gestation. In 2021, the PAD Births' standardized cost was 1,180,000 CLP (Chilean pesos) (1,430 USD, exchange rate of November 2021), of which 75% is financed by FONASA and 25% by the childbearer, independent of the mode of birth (FONASA 2021).

In 2017, the latest year for which we have breakdown data, the cesarean rate in the public sector—FONASA—reached 28%; in the private sector—ISAPRES—62%, and in the public-private scheme of PAD Birth, 72%. Of these subsystems, the public and private sector's rates have remained stable over recent decades, while the PAD has experienced a steep rise (Subsecretaría de Salud Pública 2018). Women giving birth under the PAD scheme with healthy full-term pregnancies should present the lowest rates of cesareans in the country, but the opposite is occurring: they have 2.5 more chances of having a CB than those of the public sector, considering that the public sector concentrates the poorest women and most of the "high-risk" pregnancies.

Recent national studies carried out by economists confirm that the PAD Birth insurance program increases CB rates. Ramiro de Elejalde and Eugenio Giolito (2019a, 2019b) show that, since the co-payment that women must contribute was reduced from 60% (in 2001–2002) to 25% of the total price of the PAD Birth in 2003, births in the private sector increased significantly. In the first quarter of 2003, 10% of the births recorded for women insured under FONASA (Groups B, C, and D) were financed under the PAD Birth program. The rate had increased to 45% in the first quarter of 2008. Between 2003 (when the cost was reduced) and 2005, the rate of cesareans for women in these three Groups of FONASA increased from 30% to 40% (but the rate did not increase for women belonging to FONASA Group A or ISAPRES). From 2008 onward, a quarter of births nationwide have been financed under the PAD program (De Elejalde and Giolito 2019a, 2019b). Florencia Borrescio-Higa and Nieves Valdés (2019) have shown that by 2014, births financed through this insurance program contributed 52% to the overall weighted cesarean rate in the country.

In addition to understanding the insurance systems for childbirth, it is important to describe the organization of care in the different subsystems. In the public sector, professional midwives (called *matronas*) are the main caregivers for low-risk pregnancies and births, and are supervised by on-duty obstetricians who manage high-risk cases, instrumental deliveries (such as forceps), and cesareans. In the private sector, including the PAD Birth, although *matronas* are present throughout labor and birth, obstetricians are the primary care providers. The payment system operates per client, which means that shorter labors and elective cesareans increase the providers' and the hospitals' profits (Murray 2000; Sadler and Leiva 2016). As private care and CBs have been increasing, the number of births attended by midwives has been decreasing: in 2000, *matronas* were in charge of 52% of all births, while in 2015 that figure had dropped to approximately 38% (Leiva 2016).

Until now (early 2022), the national recommendations for humanistic childbirth that have been promoted since 2008 (ChCC 2015; MINSAL 2008) have not been effective (Binfa et al. 2016; OVO Chile 2018), because the problem has been approached mainly as one of the low quality of services resulting from the difficult working conditions of the health personnel, or from their lack of ethical training (Castro

2014), or as an issue of women's lack of autonomy or empowerment (Sadler 2021), without paying attention to the structural and organizational components of this problem (Sadler, Santos et al. 2016).

Having described the context of childbirth in Chile, in the rest of this chapter we delve into the perceptions of Chilean obstetricians about the high rates of cesareans, focusing especially on the differences between health subsystems and insurance systems. Given obstetricians' power in childbirth, their explanations about what influences their clinical practice are critical to understanding the problem.

## Materials and Methods

This chapter is built on documental examinations of various sources (press, national birth policies, and public information on hospital fees, among others), and on qualitative interviews and discussion groups carried out with ob/gyns during 2014–2016 and 2020–2021. From 2014–2016, we carried out a research project centered on understanding the non-medical factors influencing the rise in cesareans in Chile. The project was funded by the Chilean National Fund for Research and Development in Health (FONIS project SA13I20259) and was approved by the ethics committees of two health services of the Metropolitan Region (North and Southeast). It was a mixed methods study, of which we will refer herein to only part of its qualitative component, consisting of 14 in-depth interviews with obstetricians. In public health care, we chose three major public hospitals of the Metropolitan Region to carry out fieldwork, in order to attend to different territories presenting different rates of CBs (the highest and the lowest within the region, and a rate similar to the national average). Hospital authorities facilitated our fieldwork, asking their staff to collaborate with us and giving us access to their databases. In private health care, we privileged snowball sampling, starting from an initial list of contacts because private hospitals were not open to facilitating fieldwork. We used an opportunistic maximum variation sampling, selecting obstetricians of different ages with different approaches toward childbirth, from technocratic to humanistic (Davis-Floyd 2018, 2022; see also the Introduction to this volume), who worked in the private and/or public sector and in a range of institutions.

During 2021, we expanded the sample to deepen our previous findings and to include new voices in the obstetric field. Via snowball sampling, we contacted ob/gyns from several maternity facilities, and included young female ob/gyn members of a new professional association, Ginecólogas Chile. Their inclusion is important because, although only

26% of the total number of ob/gyns in the country are women, those under 40 years of age amount to 74.5% (Venegas 2020). A new research protocol was approved by the Ethics Committee of Eloísa Díaz I. Hospital—La Florida. We carried out four in-depth interviews and two discussion groups with obstetricians (with four and six participants each).

In sum, this chapter is based on 18 in-depth interviews and two discussion groups with obstetricians, with 28 participants overall. Of these, seven were Chiefs of maternity departments at the time of the interviews: 12 were women and 16 were men. All but six were working in public and private health care at the time of the interviews, of which three were only working in the public sector and three only in the private sector. The interviews and discussion groups were recorded and transcribed verbatim from the audio tracks. The material was coded through narrative content analysis, with a priori categories derived from the topics covered in the encounters and emerging categories developed from the data.

Please note that throughout this chapter, we use the letter "I" followed by the number of the interview (from 1 to 18) when we quote interviews, and "G" when referring to discussion groups, followed by the correspondent number of the group (1 or 2), and by the number of the participant, after a comma. For example: (E8) corresponds to interview number 8 and G2,3 corresponds to Group 2, participant number 3.)

## Why So Many Cesareans in Chile?

All but one of the obstetricians interviewed were extremely critical of the excessive biomedicalization of childbirth in the country, characterized by the routine practice of obstetric interventions, especially cesareans. However, most of them—even those who adhere more explicitly to a humanistic model—performed many more cesareans than recommended. Thus what we found is an "evidence-discourse-practice gap" (Kramer 2002)—the discursive recognition of updated scientific evidence, which, however, is not translated into practice.

When asking ob/gyns about the non-medical factors contributing to the high rates of cesareans in the country, almost all framed the problem in the context of an extremely biomedicalized birth culture that is difficult to change, and that is installed in the imaginaries and practices of biomedical teams and in the population as a whole. As true as this can be, and with ob/gyn curricula having a strong technocratic approach and the popular culture being blanketed with media images of the risks and complications of childbirth (Sadler 2021), it does not explain the differences among the cesarean rates of the three insurance systems. In addition, most of the ob/gyn interlocutors referred to the "judicialization" of obstetrics (which we will discuss critically later on) and to clinicians' "practice styles" as driving forces for the performance of cesareans. But again, these factors are common to both public and private health care. When we delve into the enormous differences among health subsystems, the factors mostly mentioned are maternal request and economic/convenience benefits for ob/gyns and hospitals.

These factors behave differently, depending on each obstetrician's approach to childbirth: those more closely aligned with a technocratic view of birth put more weight on causes that are somehow considered "external" to their own practices, such as maternal request and the judicialization of obstetrics, and are less critical of their own influences on the trend of rising CB rates. On the other hand, those who ascribe more fully to a humanistic approach to birth place greater weight on economic incentives and ob/gyns' personal approaches to childbirth. We will engage critically in the discussions of these dimensions in the following sections.

## Women's or Obstetricians' Preferences?

We begin by questioning the weight of some of these categories. A great deal of responsibility in the private system is put on women who request a CB in the absence of clear medical indications. This was mentioned in all interviews, and some ob/gyn interlocutors noted it as the single most influencing factor for the rise in cesareans (especially those who work solely or primarily in the private healthcare sector). This idea is reproduced in medical literature and in the press. For examples, an article written by two Chilean ob/gyns in 2012 stated that among the non-medical factors most likely to influence the rise in cesareans was maternal request (Farías and Oyarzún 2012); and a headline of a major Chilean newspaper in 2014 said that "Women with private health insurance prefer cesarean sections" (Fernández and Sandoval 2014). Nonetheless, several studies in the country show that in both the private and the public healthcare sectors, most women prefer vaginal birth in the absence of medical complications. These studies report a strong preference for vaginal birth: 78% in A. Angeja and colleagues's (2006) study with pregnant women (with 13% declaring to be undecided); 89% in two studies with university students who wished to have children in the future (Bravo and Cox 2015; Weeks, Sadler, and Stoll 2020), and 80% in a sample of women who had all experienced cesareans in the past (Sadler, Leiva et al. 2018). In this latter study, only 6.6% of women who had undergone at least one cesarean during the previous ten years declared having requested the procedure.

These numbers are consistent with studies around the world, which show that only a minority of women in a wide variety of countries and situations prefer cesareans (Mazzoni et al. 2011; Betrán, Temmerman et al. 2018). A review of studies published from 2003–2016 on women's right to request a cesarean (Loke, Davies, and Mak 2019) concluded that in countries with well-developed private healthcare systems, a higher percentage of stakeholders—particularly obstetricians—support cesarean by maternal request, compared to countries with stronger public healthcare systems, where stakeholders fear that cesareans will impose a greater burden on such systems. In their critique of literature on women's requests for cesareans, Jenny Gamble and Debra Creedy (2000) concluded that such requests have a minimal influence on the overall rates of cesareans, and highlighted that there is an over-estimated use of "women's request for cesarean" as a reason to perform the surgeries. This was discussed by two young women ob/gyns in one of our discussion groups:

> Deep down, we have to recognize that from many ob/gyns' point of view, anything qualifies as maternal request . . . we could say that every woman who at some point during pregnancy and birth mentioned "cesarean" can qualify! (G2,1)

> The easiest thing to say is that cesarean was the mother's request, but in most of the cases, it was the doctor's convenience. I once heard a doctor saying he could get a woman to accept a cesarean with a thousand arguments. (G2,2)

Thus, we see the importance of asking how the categories of "preference for mode of birth" and "maternal request" are constructed. As several authors have pointed out, much of the research claiming to demonstrate women's birth preferences has failed to explore the information that women are given before making birth choices and has also failed to acknowledge obstetricians' influences during clinical encounters (Gamble and Creedy 2000; Weaver, Statham, and Richards 2007; Mazzoni et al. 2011). Along these lines, several of the ob/gyn interlocutors recognized their power to manipulate information in ways that align with their own preferences:

> One can relativize the truth and tell the patient a half-truth . . . and given the asymmetry in the relationship, since there is a person who knows more about the subject, if you tell the patient a half-truth,

she may believe that a normal birth and a cesarean pose the same risks. (E6)

If one wants cesareans, one makes cesareans. If the best option for one is a cesarean, it is terribly easy; one can search among thousands of arguments that will convince the patient. (E11)

[The obstetrician] decides the mode of birth, not the woman. (E14)

These obstetricians recognize that the power asymmetry that characterizes the doctor-patient relationship is often used to "relativize the truth" and make the woman ascribe to the medical teams' interests. So, even though they discursively express the benefits of vaginal birth, they acknowledge that they can perform cesareans very easily if it is in their best interests to do so. And, in contexts where obstetricians feel pressure to justify high cesarean rates, providing the indication "maternal request" is a way of shifting their own responsibility toward women (Gamble and Creedy 2000; Sadler 2021). In the context of the strong women's preference for vaginal birth that studies in the country have shown, the above ob/gyns' quotations make a strong case for arguing that women's requests are not driving the country's high rates of cesarean, and that obstetricians' views on childbirth and the decision-making power they hold play much more relevant roles. In 2007, McCourt and colleagues argued that obstetricians' own personal preferences were emerging as important factors in decision-making related to mode of birth, which was confirmed in a more recent systematic review that identified ob/gyns' personal beliefs as major factors influencing the performance of cesareans (Panda, Begley and Daly 2018). This in turn confirms Robbie Davis-Floyd's ([1992] 2003, 2018, 2022) long-standing insistence that the paradigm of the practitioner, not the desires of the birthing person, is the primary determinant of the mode of birth (see also Hodnett 2002a, 2002b).

## "Perverse Financial Incentives"

A 2015 article in *The Economist* stated that "The global rise of cesarean sections is being driven not by medical necessity but by growing wealth and perverse financial incentives for doctors." A year later, a commentary in the *British Journal of Obstetrics and Gynaecology* about rising cesarean rates worldwide noted that "Where rates are high, the real reason is money" (Geirsson 2016). This is certainly true for Chile, and we will argue that money is in fact the primary element influencing the rise in cesarean births. As we briefly described in the Introduction to this chapter, how childbirth care is organized in the three available insurance schemes enables or hinders the emergence of certain incentives that we will call "perverse," since they allow the agendas and personal interests of individual or institutional healthcare providers to go well beyond the medical needs of pregnant women.

## Payment Systems: Shifts versus Procedures

A great difference between the public and private healthcare sectors relates to the ways in which obstetricians are paid. In public maternity care, the salary is determined by hierarchy and by hours/shifts of work, independently of the number of births attended. In private maternity care, the bulk of the salary is obtained from consulting hours and births that are charged "per procedure." Thus, the more procedures obstetricians perform, the greater is their income.

In public health care, FONASA assigns the same value for childbirth throughout the country. In contrast, in the private sector, each institution and healthcare team charges different figures, with large price variations. These values are not public knowledge; therefore, we requested them during 2015 in all private hospitals in the city of Santiago. Of a total of 14 hospitals in the city, 12 gave us budgets. Of these, only five turned in the total budgets—including institutional and practitioner fees—and the remaining eight disclosed only the institutional fees, but not those of the practitioners. The average value of vaginal birth (without practitioner fees) among the 12 hospitals was 11 times higher, and of cesarean 15 times higher, than FONASA's valuation of birth, with fluctuations for vaginal births of 463% between the lowest and highest value, and of 570% for CBs. In 2017, a survey carried out by the national newspaper *La Tercera* showed similar results, exposing differences of up to 375% among a dozen private hospitals (Leiva and González 2017) without considering the practitioners' fees: the average fee per birth for obstetricians in the five hospitals that disclosed the information for our study was 826,000 CLP (around 1,000 USD)), considering that the top-range hospitals did not provide this information. The hospitals that didn't turn in the full budgets argued that practitioner fees were only disclosed to patients. The secrecy and lack of regulation regarding transparency in the private sector have led to obstetric collusion, as happened in 2015 in the Region of Ñuble, where 25 ob/gyns were convicted by the Chilean Competition Tribunal because they had colluded to establish minimum fees for consultations and births, raising by 69% the cost of private childbirth (Excma. Corte Suprema 2016).

The difference in practitioner fees among the health sectors is stunning. One of the obstetricians interviewed, who works only in the public sector, expressed the huge ethical dilemma that this situation causes:

> Let's put it in numbers. I am Head of shift, and I earn 3.5 million CLP a month [4,235 USD]. I live well, I don't need anything else. But it is not enough for them; many colleagues want to make seven, ten, 15 million or more per month. They cannot do that in public health, they need to go to private [ISAPRES], and/or to PAD Births, where they work by volume. But if you work by volume, you cannot have humanized births, because they can last 24–48 hours . . . When I worked in private health, I was the only one willing to spend 12 hours in the clinic, and since I was not willing to do more cesareans, I stopped doing private, and I dedicated myself only to public medicine. (E8)

This obstetrician's monthly salary would be reached by a private ob/gyn doing only four cesareans on women insured by ISAPRES (using the average fee we got from the clinics). This is why, as we put into the title of our chapter, one of the interviewed ob/gyns stated that "physiologic birth implies economic damage," going on to clarify that: "It is different to schedule a cesarean at an appropriate and suitable time that will not interrupt your patients' appointments than physiologic labor, which begins at any time and constitutes significant economic damage" (E3).

## "Once You Have Tasted the Apple, You Cannot Stop Eating Apples!"

Describing vaginal birth as causing economic damage, this obstetrician talked about the extent to which a commercial logic has permeated childbirth care. It is in this context that we talk about "perverse" incentives, because they don't only allow, but also encourage births to be scheduled to accommodate ob/gyns' agendas and to increase their incomes. Such scheduling means pharmacologically accelerating labor (artificial induction, artificial rupture of membranes, oxytocic acceleration) and also performing an excess of cesareans that are not due to medical reasons. These factors help to explain why cesareans are almost double in private compared to public health care, despite the fact that that the population served in the private sector is healthier than that from the public. Susan Murray, who studied the relation between private insurance and cesareans in Chile, had reached this conclusion two decades ago:

Obstetricians do private work to increase their income. Conflicting demands arise from complex peripatetic work schedules and the need to provide personalized care for private patients. These are resolved by liberal use of caesarean section, which permits maximum efficiency in use of time. The prevailing business ethos in health care encourages such pragmatism among those doctors who do not have a moral objection to nonmedical caesarean section. (Murray 2000:1504)

These finding were confirmed by the obstetricians interviewed:

The high rate of cesareans has to do with the private system, with obstetricians working in many places, and organizing their agendas. (E7)

It is much easier to program a cesarean, because what we get paid for vaginal birth or cesarean is the same; therefore, I optimize my time. (E16)

If we talk about costs, how much it means, how much is [paid for] a normal birth . . . it is extremely cost-inefficient . . . it is very exhausting and not adequately valued. (E2)

The commodification of medicine is the most relevant factor; my colleagues, rather than looking for the wellbeing of the patient, are basically looking to improve their incomes. (E18)

The main factor is monetary, without a doubt; no matter how much evidence and protocols you may have, once you have tasted the apple—as many politicians well know—you cannot stop eating apples! (G2,1)

Even a former Minister of Health, Dr. Jaime Mañalich, declared that: "As there is a very great economic incentive for doctors to perform cesareans, we have one of the highest numbers in the world in the private sector" (INDH 2016). Susan Murray's study (2000) was carried out before the PAD Birth was implemented, so we can see that this scenario has only worsened as the privatization of childbirth care has risen.

## PAD Birth

As we described earlier, the PAD Birth scheme can be accessed by women with low-risk pregnancies and beyond 37 weeks of gestation, insured in Groups B, C, and D of FONASA, who pay a fixed amount of money to be transferred to private health care. Although women who access the PAD have healthy full-term pregnancies, they have the highest cesarean rates of all insurance schemes—72% in 2017. This is 10% higher than women insured in the "full" private system of ISAPRES (Subsecretaría de Salud Pública 2018). But, if in both of these systems, births are attended in private health care, why such differences? Moreover, we must take into account that the PAD Birth was designed to *lower* the cesarean rate. When it was implemented, the economic incentive for the medical team (obstetrician-midwife) was higher for vaginal than for cesarean birth. However, the income difference was small and could not match the economic benefit derived from the volume of interventions that the scheduling of cesareans allowed. Thus, the PAD system now provides the same medical fees for vaginal or cesarean birth—as in ISAPRES—but with a much lower economic return.

The total price of the PAD in 2021 was 1,180,000 CLP (1,430 USD) (FONASA 2021). This amount is divided between practitioner fees for the entire team and fees for the hospital:

> The full PAD bonus is paid to the institution, and then distributed: they pay the ob/gyn, the midwife, the neonatologist and the anesthetist, the supplies, hospital ward costs, and in case of a cesarean, two extra nurses. So the institution is left with very little . . . it falls short. That is why they privilege everything to be done quickly; it becomes an issue of volume. (O.E9)

In this logic, it is only by volume of births—or, to be more precise, of cesareans—that those clinicians and institutions can economically "compensate" for the low returns of the PAD Birth procedures. One interlocutor stated, "Looking at it coldly, it is the equation of time/money that counts. Sadly, in the PAD, it is very difficult to tell a doctor 'Try to go for a vaginal birth in eight hours, and earn 200,000 CLP [242 USD],' when he can earn the same in less than an hour [by doing a cesarean]" (G1,2). Another ob/gyn interlocutor stated that "The answer you will get from most colleagues is: 'I will not run the risk of a vaginal birth for 200 *lucas* [200,000 CLP/242 USD]'" (G1,3). There are even reports of institutions that establish conditions for paying the practitioner fees under the PAD scheme:

> To access the PAD, the woman has to have a healthy term pregnancy, without pathology, because those are cases that will most likely not develop complications. In other words, for the PAD to be a business for the institution, it has to be cheap, meaning that mother and baby are discharged after two days, they don't use extra supplies, they

don't require extra tests, drugs or treatments. In this hospital, in order to get paid the medical fees of a PAD Birth, the birth has to take place within the first 12 hours since the woman was admitted.

Q. Why?

So that she can be discharged in two days. If more than 12 hours have passed since admission, it implies an extra bed/day that she will stay, and that the hospital loses. And with cesareans it is the same—the days of hospitalization are the same for vaginal or cesarean birth. And if discharge is postponed for more than three days because of any complication, they apply the same criteria; they no longer pay the doctors' fees. This contaminates the whole birthing process, and most colleagues choose to operate earlier on patients with a very high chance of a vaginal birth. (E11)

This situation becomes critical in a healthcare system that only regulates the public sector. For private births, there is no data available, apart from some very broad indicators, as an ob/gyn interlocutor pointed out:

It is ridiculous that the cesarean rate is used as an indicator of quality of care when it is only applied to the public system. It is the public system that has to make efforts and keep the cesareans low, but the private sector can do whatever! A hospital can have 80 or 90% cesarean births, an ob/gyn can cross the street from a public to a private maternity and triple his cesarean rates, and they don't care, because nobody is looking at them. (G1,2)

Moreover, this is a system that transfers exorbitant amounts of resources from the public to the private sector. In 2017, FONASA financed 56,000 births through the PAD, which meant an expense of approximately 60 billlion CLP (75 million USD) and made up to 51% of the total expenses through the PAD system of the public system in that year. (The PAD system includes a total of 55 conditions/diseases [Subsecretaría de Salud Pública 2018].) As one ob/gyn stated: "A lot of FONASA's resources are being spent that should be invested in strengthening public births" (E8).

## Cross-Cutting Factors: The Judicialization of Birth and Obstetricians' Lack of Skills in Attending Physiologic Births

We have discussed how ob/gyns can influence patient demand to suit their own interests, and how economic/convenience incentives play a large role in the rising numbers of cesareans in the country. These factors apply mainly to private health care. And although the main focus of this chapter is to understand the differences in cesarean rates among the Chilean health insurance systems, there are some cross-cutting factors that we consider important to discuss.

The "judicialization" of obstetrics was mentioned by most of the obstetricians interviewed, referring to the performance of cesareans in the absence of medical indication as "defensive medicine" driven by the fear of litigation:

> There is this extreme judicialization of medicine, and particularly of obstetrics, which makes our colleagues act with fear and think that a safe way to do things is to practice mostly cesareans. (E4)

> Why would you take the risk of a vaginal birth or of a forceps if you could end up being prosecuted? The judges are going to crucify you in case of a bad outcome. We have entered a vicious cycle—no efforts are done [for vaginal birth], no teaching is done, it is all judicialized, therefore it is comfortable and practical to do a cesarean. (E15)

> Gynecologists are among the most persecuted specialists, which I think has prompted many people to avoid lawsuits by handling everything with a cesarean that is often incorrectly indicated. (G2,4)

Although in Chile, there was a strong increase in lawsuits against doctors during the first decade of this century, between 2008 and 2018 they stabilized, with an average of 310 per year, and the last four years of this period were below the average (FALMED 2019). What *have* been increasing year by year over the last two decades are mediations (FALMED 2019). In 2015, 278 trials for malpractice were closed, with general medicine (20.5%), ob/gyn (20.1%), and surgery (19.8%) taking the lead of specialties involved (Bravo et al. 2019). In 2018, there were 257 lawsuits and 578 mediations (we do not have the breakdown of specialties for this year). As an exercise, if 30% of lawsuits and mediations in 2018 were related only to childbirth—which is a big exaggeration—and with 223,000 births in the country during that year, there would be a 0.1% chance that each birth ended up in a lawsuit or a mediation. It is thus correct that ob/gyn is one of the most litigated medical specialties, but we can question the excessive weight attributed to this phenomenon. It is therefore possible that the expressed fear of judicialization does not correlate with the actual number of cases, but that it is exaggerated to justify the high rates of cesareans as a user-driven trend—that is, as a kind of "external" factor driven by the intolerance of "patients" for negative birth outcomes, as one ob/gyn expressed:

> An important factor [for the rise in cesareans] is the judicialization of medicine, which implies that faith and trust were lost; now we are not friends, we are enemies. Years ago, the doctor was like the village priest, like the mayor, like the president of the bank—they were demigods. If a problem occurred, the patient would say: "Don't worry, it was God's will, thank you very much, you did what you could." But now, instead, everything is negligence. And we say: "You know what? We'd better do cesareans and avoid all these problems." (E1)

But why was "trust" lost? Can the doctor-patient relationship be brought to justice in a context in which many women feel cheated by the system and report not receiving evidence-based information on biomedical practices and procedures? The fact that women report an association between feeling informed and feeling confident is a consistent finding internationally (O'Brien, Butler, and Casey 2021). The reversal of the trend toward judicialization and defensive medicine is only possible if clinicians stop creating distance from women and invest in humanizing their relationships. This would be practicing in accordance with the international recommendations for humanistic childbirth (WHO 2018; Lalonde et al. 2019).

Another relevant factor mentioned for the increase in cesareans is obstetrician's lack of skills for attending physiologic births. Although this factor had far fewer mentions than the ones previously described, it was proposed by the obstetricians most aligned with the humanistic approach:

> And there is a second factor [after economic incentives], which I think is very important and relevant, and needs to be highlighted, and which makes me feel ashamed as an obstetrician. After really trying to answer this question for a long time, I have come to realize that as obstetricians, we are really not prepared for vaginal births. This is super-shocking to say out loud—it involves looking at yourself in the mirror and being able to say something that will sound ugly and unexpected. But we are completely unprepared for vaginal birth, we know very little about physiologic obstetrics. (G2,5)
>
> [Obstetricians are ignorant and have a] lack of skills regarding vaginal birth. . . I work in a public hospital in Santiago that has a very

high rate of cesareans. They are done out of fear, ignorance of how physiologic birth progresses. (G2,4)

## Vaginal Birth as Economic Damage: Winds of Change?

In Chile, women who birth in the public system, FONASA, have a relatively low (28%) rate of cesareans (for the local standards). Regarding the reasons for these cesareans, Chilean ob/gyns identify the prevailing heavily medicalized obstetric (technocratic) model and the fear of litigation as the main non-medical contributing factors. These factors are common to private health care, where the rate of cesareans increases to 62% in the private insurance, ISAPRES, and to 72% in the PAD Birth system—public insurance until the 37th week of gestation followed by transfer to the private system. As we have shown, this situation can only be explained by certain incentives that the private sector facilitates. The private ISAPRES insurance system, which pays per birth, provides high practitioner fees and institutional revenues. As cesareans allow ob/gyns to schedule their time efficiently, the more cesareans, the more money, to the extreme of vaginal birth being described as "economic damage." In the PAD Birth, which pays much lower practitioner fees and institutional revenues, because there is a lack of price incentives, "hospitals use cesareans to smooth out demand over time to optimize the use of their resources" (De Elejalde and Giolito 2019a:1). Defenders of the PAD Birth system argue that it promotes equity by giving access to private health care to women from public insurance. But is that really the road to equity? As we have seen, it is a system that: (1) excludes the poorest women in society, who are insured via FONASA; (2) it "cesareanizes" the healthiest women from the public sector; and (3) it transfers an exorbitant amount of resources from the public to the private sector, which could be otherwise invested to provide better public health care. Clearly, this is very far from an equitable system.

The convenience of performing cesareans for institutions and ob/gyns has a much stronger weight than women's desires and more weight than the evidence on what is best for women's and newborns' health. The power these obstetricians hold allows them to manipulate information to align their clinical practices with those interests. Instead of the TMTS (too much too soon [Miller et al. 2016]) over-performance of interventions, including cesareans, the care that should be given— RARTRW care (the right amount at the right time in the right way [Cheyney and Davis-Floyd 2020])—is being jeopardized, and obstetrics' *lex artis* is being profoundly compromised. This Latin concept, mainly used in the legal domain, refers to the set of rules that professionals should honor when exercising their skill or art, to the true guarantee of good medical practice (Arimany-Manso 2012). "Let us continue practicing obstetrics as art, without forgetting it as science," was a warning given in 1949 by Dr. Avendaño, a Chilean ob/gyn who was concerned about the development of the discipline. The dimensions of care that need to be recovered in Chilean birth—indeed, in birth everywhere—are the art of the skills of facilitating physiologic births and the recovering of humanistic values in childbirth care. The recognition of where obstetrics has come was expressed by a young woman ob/gyn:

> I am really ashamed of my guild, plain and simple. What we do goes beyond the limits of professional and moral ethics in all its aspects. We have a tremendously great power, and we are using it so badly, we are abusing it so much. Instead of making all of this available to women and pregnant bodies, we are using it for our personal benefit. We are robbing the person of a life experience that is so important! I include myself because at some point, like everyone else here, I learned and practiced the same kind of obstetrics. But one can deconstruct and start doing it differently. (G2,5)

This powerful testimony illustrates the winds of change we are beginning to witness in the country (Sadler, Leiva, and Gómez 2021). The field of obstetric practice is being placed in tension by various concurrent factors: an increasingly organized civil society demanding changes; a bill advancing in Parliament that consecrates childbirth rights; the rise in home births (even though they are not insured) and an association of homebirth midwives called *Maternas Chile*; the experiences of hospital maternity wards that are implementing midwifery units with great success (Leiva et al. 2021); the updating of clinical guidelines for physiologic birth; and a growing public problematization of cesareans with the recent publication of a guideline for their monitoring and surveillance (MINSAL 2021). Finally, and very importantly, a new association of feminist midwives—ASOMAT—the Asociación Nacional de Matronas y Matrones (National Association of Midwives of Chile) and feminist women ob/gyns, Ginecólogas Chile—are pushing the agenda for humanized childbirth and piercing the traditional patriarchal dynamics of maternity care.

A paradigmatic shift is no small thing, and complex problems need complex solutions. Only a set of measures that address the cultural imaginaries of childbirth and the incentives that are driving the extreme medicalization and technocratization of birth can lead us to a "deep humanism" (Davis-Floyd 2018, 2022; see also the Introduction to this volume) that includes: comprehensive sexual education from early childhood; educational curricula in schools and universities that thoroughly integrate the psychosocial dimensions of health; training, updating, and re-socializing practicing clinicians; childbirth education programs for pregnant families; and stronger regulations to implement the humanistic model of childbirth (described in the Introduction to this volume). And although some studies have shown that regulatory legislative interventions have reduced cesarean rates (but with low certainty of evidence) (see Opiyo et al. 2020), in Chile we have witnessed the reluctance of technocratic obstetricians to change their practices after more than a decade of programmatic efforts by birth activists, humanistic ob/gyns, the national government, and others. Recognizing ob/gyns' insufficient training in physiologic birth, we should advance in models based on autonomous midwifery for physiologic birth such as midwifery-led birthing units (Long et al. 2016; Sandall et al. 2016). Promising models for private health care are those that reduce the scheduling/economic incentives, such as a collaborative midwifery-obstetrician program based on care provided primarily by midwives, with 24-hour backup from an obstetrician who provides in-house labor and birth coverage without other competing clinical duties (Rosenstein et al. 2015) (called a "hospitalist" or "laborist" in the United States).

We know that childbirth matters, and that there is strong evidence to support the facts that physiologic birth is related to the wellbeing of mother and baby in the short-, middle-, and long-terms and is more sustainable for healthcare systems and for societies as a whole. It is time to use biomedical power for the benefit of humankind by providing the best birth experiences that we can, in line with the *lexis artis* and with the art of caring.

## Acknowledgments

We deeply thank all ob/gyns who shared their views on childbirth with us. This publication is based on research funded by FONIS (Chilean National Fund for Research and Development in Health) project SA13I20259. The participation of Michelle Sadler was also supported by the Israeli Science Foundation (Grant No. 328/19). We thank both FONIS and the Israeli Science Foundation for their support.

**Michelle Sadler** is a Chilean anthropologist with a PhD in Medical Anthropology. She is an Adjunct Researcher in the Faculty of Liberal Arts, Universidad Adolfo Ibáñez, Chile; and a Postdoctoral Researcher at the Women's and Gender Graduate Studies Program, University of Haifa, Israel. She also serves as the Director of the Chilean Observatory of Obstetric Violence. Michelle has 20 years of experience researching childbirth models in Chile and abroad, has assessed policies toward respectful maternity care, and has led civil society organizations that seek to promote change in maternity related issues.

**Gonzalo Leiva** is a Chilean father and midwife with a Master's in Health Administration. He taught in midwifery programs for more than a decade. For five years, he served as Chief of the Safe Model of Personalized Childbirth Unit at the Dra. Eloísa Díaz Hospital-La Florida—a unit that has recently joined the *International Childbirth Initiative (ICI): 12 Steps to Safe and Respectful MotherBaby-Family Maternity Care* and is recognized as a pillar and example of respectful care within the country. Leiva has also served as Founder and Director of the Chilean Observatory of Obstetric Violence, and as Director of the National Association of Midwives of Chile (ASOMAT), a trade association that works to strengthen midwifery and that advocates for sexual and reproductive rights. He currently works as Comprehensive Care Manager at the Dra. Eloísa Diaz-La Florida Hospital in Santiago, Chile.

## References

Angeja A, Washington A, Vargas J, et al. 2006. "Chilean Women's Preferences Regarding Mode of Delivery: Which Do They Prefer and Why?" *British Journal of Obstetrics and Gynaecology* 113(11): 1253–1258.

Arimany-Manso J. 2012. "Professional Liability in Cardiology." *Revista Española de Cardiología* 65(9): 788–790.

Avendaño O. 1949. "La Pelvis de la Mujer: Estudio Morfológico y Clínico." Tesis para optar al título de Profesor Extraordinario de Clínica Obstétrica de la Facultad de Biología y Ciencias Médicas. Santiago, Chile: Universidad de Chile.

Betrán A, Temmerman M, Kingdon C, et al. 2018. "Interventions to Reduce Unnecessary Caesarean Sections in Healthy Women and Babies." *Lancet* 392: 1358–1368.

Betrán A, Ye J, Moller A, et al. 2016. "The Increasing Trend in Caesarean Section Rates: Global, Regional and National Estimates: 1990–2014." *PLoS ONE* 11: e0148343.

Betrán A, Torloni M, Zhang J, et al. 2016. "WHO Statement on Caesarean Section Rates." *BJOG* 123(5): 667–670.

Binfa L, Pantoja L, Ortiz J, et al. 2016. "Assessment of the Implementation of the Model of Integrated and Humanised Midwifery Health Services in Chile." *Midwifery* 35: 53–61.

Boerma T, Ronsmans C, Melesse D, et al. 2018. "Global Epidemiology of Use and Disparities in Caesarean Sections." *Lancet* 392(10155): 1341–1348.

Borrescio-Higa F, Valdés N. 2019. "Publicly Insured Caesarean Sections in Private Hospitals: A Repeated Cross-Sectional Analysis in Chile." *BMJ Open* 9(4): e024241.

Bravo P, Cox M. 2015. "Percepciones sobre el parto de estudiantes de la Pontificia Universidad Católica de Chile." Taller de Titulación I, Instituto de Sociología, Facultad de Ciencias Sociales, Universidad Católica de Chile.

Bravo R, Lidia A, Lagos T, et al. 2019. "Responsabilidad Médica en Chile: Fallos de la Corte Suprema de Justicia 2017." *International Journal of Odontostomatology* 13(3): 367–373.

Castro R. 2014. "Génesis y Práctica del Habitus Médico Autoritario en México." *Revista Mexicana de Sociología* 76(2): 167–197.

Cheyney M, Davis-Floyd R. 2020. "Birth and the Big Bad Wolf: A Biocultural, Co-Evolutionary Perspective, Part 2." *International Journal of Childbirth* 10(2): 66–78.

ChCC, Chile Crece Contigo. 2015. *¿Qué es Chile Crece Contigo?* Ministerio de Desarrollo Social, Gobierno de Chile. http://www.crececontigo.gob.cl/wp-content/uploads/2015/11/que-es-Chile-Crece-2015.pdf.

Davis-Floyd R. (1992) 2003. *Birth as an American Rite of Passage*, 2nd edn. Berkeley: University of California Press.

———. 2018. "The Technocratic, Humanistic, and Holistic Models of Birth and Health Care." In *Ways of Knowing about Birth: Mothers, Midwives, Medicine, and Birth Activism*, Davis-Floyd R and Colleagues, 3–44. Long Grove IL: Waveland Press.

———. 2022. *Birth as an American Rite of Passage*, 3rd edn. Abingdon, Oxon: Routledge.

De Elejalde R, Giolito E. 2019a. *More Hospital Choices, More C-Sections: Evidence from Chile.* IZA Institute of Labor Economics DP No. 12297.

———. 2019b. "Altas Tasas de Cesáreas en Clínicas Privadas ¿Una Relación Causal?" *Revista Observatorio Económico* 135.

DEIS Departamento de Estadísticas e Información en Salud, Ministerio de Salud de Chile. 2022. Request of transparency to Subsecretaría de Salud Pública N° AO001T0018394.

Excma. Corte Suprema. 2016 [January 7]. *Sentencia Rol N° 5609–2015.* Excma Corte Suprema, Poder Judicial. Chile.

Farías M, Oyarzún E. 2012. "Cesárea Electiva Versus Parto Vaginal." *Medwave* 12(3): e5335.

Fernández O, Sandoval G. 2014. "Mujeres con Seguro de Salud Privado Prefieren la Cesárea." *Diario La Tercera*, 22 November.

FONASA. 2021. *Bonos PAD, Parto.* Retrieved 8 November 2022 from https://www.fonasa.cl/sites/fonasa/parto.

FALMED (Fundación de Asistencia Legal del Colegio Médico de Chile). 2019. *Cuenta Pública FALMED.* Retrieved 30 November from https://www.falmed.cl/falmed/nosotros/cuenta-publica-2019.

Gamble J, Creedy D. 2000. "Women's Request for a Cesarean Section: A Critique of the Literature." *Birth* 27: 256–263.

Geirsson R. 2016. "From Half to a Third: A Step Towards Reducing Unnecessary Caesarean Sections." *British Journal of Obstetrics and Gynaecology* 123(10): 1628.

Goic A. 2015. "El Sistema de Salud de Chile: Una Tarea Pendiente." *Revista Médica de Chile* 143(6): 774–786.

Hodnett ED. 2002a. "Caregiver Support for Women During Childbirth." *Cochrane Database of Systematic Reviews* 2: CDC000199. Doi: 10.1003/14651858. CD000199.

———. 2002b. "Pain and Women's Satisfaction with the Experience of Childbirth: A Systematic Review." *American Journal of Obstetrics and Gynecology* 186(5): S160-S172.

INDH (Instituto Nacional de Derechos Humanos). 2016. *Informe Anual Situación de los Derechos Humanos en Chile 2016*. Santiago, Chile.

Koch E, Thorp J, Bravo M, et al. 2012. "Women's Education Level, Maternal Health Facilities, Abortion Legislation and Maternal Deaths: A Natural Experiment in Chile from 1957 to 2007." *PLoS ONE* 7(5): e36613.

Kramer K. 2002. Unpublished class paper for a course taught by Robbie Davis-Floyd at Southern Methodist University, Dallas, Texas.

Lalonde A, Herschderfer K, Pascali-Bonaro D, et al. 2019. "The International Childbirth Initiative: 12 Steps to Safe and Respectful MotherBaby–Family Maternity Care." *International Journal of Gynecology and Obstetrics* 146(1): 65–73.

Lange G, Wodon Q, Carey K. 2018. *The Changing Wealth of Nations 2018: Building a Sustainable Future*. Washington, DC: World Bank.

Leiva G. 2016. "La Formación de la Matrona y su Contribución a la Atención a la Maternidad en Chile." In *La Atención a la Maternidad en Diferentes Países la Contribución de la Comadrona*, 32–35. Catalunya: Consell de Collegis d'Infermeres i Infermers de Catalunya.

Leiva L, González K. 2017. *Costo Base de un Parto en Clínicas Fluctúa Entre $1 Millón y $7 Millones*. La Tercera, 8 May. Retrieved 8 November 2022 from https://www .latercera.com/noticia/costo-base-parto-clinicas-fluctua-1-millon-7-millones/.

Leiva G, Sadler M, López C, et al. 2021. "Protecting Women's and Newborns' Rights in a Public Maternity Unit during the COVID-19 Outbreak: The Case of Dra. Eloísa Díaz—La Florida Hospital in Santiago, Chile." *Frontiers in Sociology* 6: 614021.

Loke A, Davies L, Mak Y. 2019. "Is it the Decision of Women to Choose a Cesarean Section as the Mode of Birth? A Review of Literature on the Views of Stakeholders." *BMC Pregnancy and Childbirth* 19(1): 286.

Long Q, Allanson ER, Pontre J., et al. 2016. "Onsite Midwife-Led Birth Units (OMBUs) for Care around the Time of Childbirth: A Systematic Review." *BMJ Global Health* 1: e000096.

Mazzoni A, Althabe F, Liu N, et al. 2011. "Women's Preference for Caesarean Section: A Systematic Review and Meta-Analysis of Observational Studies." *BJOG* 118(4): 391–399.

McCourt C, Weaver J, Statham H, et al. 2007. "Elective Cesarean Section and Decision Making: A Critical Review of the Literature." *Birth* 34(1): 65–79.

Mieres M. 2020. "La Dinámica de la Desigualdad en Chile: Una Mirada Regional." *Revista de Análisis Económico* 35(2): 91–133.

Miller S, Abalos E, Chamillard M, et al. 2016. "Beyond Too Little, Too Late and Too Much, Too Soon: A Pathway Towards Evidence-Based, Respectful Maternity Care Worldwide." *Lancet* 388(10056): 2176–2192.

MINSAL, Ministerio de Salud. 2008. *Manual de Atención Personalizada en el Proceso Reproductivo*. Ministerio de Salud, Gobierno de Chile.

———. 2021. *Norma Técnica y Administrativa Monitoreo y Vigilancia de la Indicación Cesárea*. Ministerio de Salud, Gobierno de Chile.

Murray S. 2000. "Relation between Private Health Insurance and High Rates of Caesarean Section in Chile: Qualitative and Quantitative Study." *BMJ* 321(7275): 1501–1505.

O'Brien D, Butler MM, Casey M. 2021. "The Importance of Nurturing Trusting Relationships to Embed Shared Decision-Making during Pregnancy and Childbirth." *Midwifery* 98: 102987.

OECD (Organisation for Economic Cooperation and Development). 2017. *Reviews of Public Health: Chile, a Healthier Tomorrow*. Paris: OECD Publishing.

———. 2021. "Income Inequality (Indicator)." *OECD Data*. Retrieved 8 November 2022 from https://data.oecd.org/inequality/income-inequality.htm.

Opiyo N, Young C, Requejo J, et al. 2020. "Reducing Unnecessary Caesarean Sections: Scoping Review of Financial and Regulatory Interventions." *Reproductive Health* 17(1): 133.

OVO Chile (Chilean Obstetric Violence Observatory). 2018. *Resultados Primera Encuesta Sobre el Nacimiento en Chile*. Santiago: Observatorio de Violencia Obstétrica. https://www.researchgate.net/publication/325933924_OVO_Chile_2018_Resultados_Primera_Encuesta_sobre_el_Nacimiento_en_Chile.

Panda S, Begley C, Daly D. 2018. "Clinicians' Views of Factors Influencing Decision-making for Caesarean Section: A Systematic Review and Metasynthesis of Qualitative, Quantitative and Mixed Methods Studies." *PLoS ONE* 13(7): e0200941.

Rosenstein MG, Nijagal M, Nakagawa S, et al. 2015. "The Association of Expanded Access to a Collaborative Midwifery and Laborist Model with Cesarean Delivery Rates." *Obstetrics and Gynecology* 126(4): 716–723.

Rotarou ES, Sakellariou D. 2017. "Neoliberal Reforms in Health Systems and the Construction of Long-Lasting Inequalities in Health Care: A Case Study from Chile." *Health Policy* 121(5): 495–503.

Sadler M. 2021. "La Tecnocracia Biomédica Vestida de Humanismo. La Atención del Parto Institucional en el Chile Contemporáneo." PhD dissertation, Tarragona, Spain: University of Rovira i Virgili.

Sadler M, Leiva G. 2016. "Nacer en el Chile del Siglo XXI: El Sistema de Salud como un Determinante Social Crítico por Cabieses, Bernales, Obach, Pedrero." In *Vulnerabilidad Social y su Efecto en Salud en Chile*, 61–77. Santiago, Chile: Universidad del Desarrollo.

Sadler M, Leiva G, Gómez R. 2021. "Childbirth in Chile: Winds of Change." In *Sustainable Birth in Disruptive Times*, eds. Gutschow K, Davis-Floyd R, Daviss BA, 131–144. Switzerland: Springer.

Sadler M, Leiva G, Perello A, Schorr J. 2018. "Preferencia por Vía de Parto y Razones de la Operación Cesárea en Mujeres de la Región Metropolitana de Chile." *Revista del Instituto de Salud Pública de Chile* 2(1): 24–29.

Sadler M, Santos M, Ruiz-Berdún D, et al. 2016. "Moving beyond Disrespect and Abuse: Addressing the Structural Dimensions of Obstetric Violence." *Reproductive Health Matters* 24: 47–55.

Sandall J, Soltani H, Gates S., et al. 2016. "Midwife-Led Continuity Models Versus Other Models of Care for Childbearing Women." *Cochrane Database of Systematic Reviews* 4, CD004667.

Subsecretaría de Salud Pública, MINSAL, Gobierno de Chile. 2018. *Identificación Clínico Sanitaria de las Intervenciones en los Partos Naturales y los por Cesárea.* (Licitación Pública ID 757-120-L118 DIPLAS 02661).

*The Economist.* 2015. "Caesar's Legion." *The Economist*, 15 August. https://www.economist.com/international/2015/08/15/caesars-legions.

UNICEF. 2018. *Levels and Trends in Child Mortality, Report 2018: Estimates by the United Nations Inter-Agency Group for Child Mortality Estimates.* New York: UNICEF.

Venegas M. 2020. "Género y Medicina." Charla Especialidad de Ginecología y Obstetricia, y en Violencia Obstétrica. Comité de Cultura, Sociedad y Bienestar (CSB) y Comité de Consejería Académica (CCA), Centro de Estudiantes de Medicina (CEM) UNAB Santiago.

Villar J, Valladares E, Wojdyla D. 2006. "Caesarean Delivery Rates and Pregnancy Outcomes: The 2005 WHO Global Survey on Maternal and Perinatal Health in Latin America." *Lancet* 367: 1819–1829.

Weaver J, Statham H, Richards M. 2007. "Are There 'Unnecessary' Caesarean Sections? Perceptions of Women and Obstetricians about Caesarean Sections for Nonclinical Indications." *Birth* 34: 32–41.

Weeks F, Sadler M, Stoll K. 2020. "Preference for Caesarean Attitudes toward Birth in a Chilean Sample of Young Adults." *Women and Birth* 33(2): e159–e165.

WHO. 2015. *WHO Statement on Caesarean Section Rates.* Geneva: World Health Organization.

———. 2018. *WHO Recommendations: Intrapartum Care for a Positive Childbirth Experience.* Geneva: World Health Organization.

———. 2019. *Trends in Maternal Mortality 2000 to 2017: Estimates by WHO, UNICEF, UNFPA.* Geneva: World Health Organization.

# CHAPTER 5

# The Introduction of the "Gentle Cesarean" in Swiss Hospitals

## A Conversation with One of Its Pioneers

*Caroline Chautems, Irene Maffi, and Alexandre Farin*

## Introduction

In Switzerland, as in most high-resource countries, labor and delivery are conceived of as risky and unpredictable events that can only be considered "normal" in retrospect (see, e.g., Maffi 2012; Scamell and Alaszewski 2012; Maffi and Gouilhers 2019). Anticipation regarding what could go wrong is not limited to birth but is already present throughout the course of pregnancy. Risk surveillance during pregnancy includes a range of tests to assess the mother's and the fetus's health, along with various recommendations regarding optimal behaviors to maximize the future child's health (Manaï, Burton-Jeangros, and Elger 2010). Such continuous medical surveillance reveals a risk-oriented comprehension of birth that healthcare professionals and society share. The ongoing debates in many countries of the Global North about the safety of home birth or birth in a freestanding birth center versus birth in biomedical settings further reflect the prevalent preoccupations about risks. These discussions occur within a context in which maternal and infant mortality and morbidity are at their lowest levels ever worldwide, while residual risks (serious complications and deaths associated with birth) are deemed socially and medically intolerable (Lupton 1993; Burton-Jeangros, Cavalli et al. 2013; Burton-Jeangros, Hammer 2014). The focus on risk in managing pregnancy and childbirth reflects the broader cultural context of Euro-American societies in which the discourse of risk orients public institutions' policies and private behaviors (Lupton 1993; Beck 2003).

In 2017, 98.3% of all births in Switzerland took place in hospitals, and almost one-third (32.3%) of all children were born via cesarean (OFS 2019a). Half of these cesarean births (CBs) were planned, while the other half were emergency cesareans. The Swiss CB rate decreased by 1.4% between 2014 and 2019 (OFS 2019b). However, in comparison with other European countries, the cesarean rate in Switzerland remains among the highest (Euro-Peristat Project 2018), behind Cyprus (56.9%), Romania (46.9%), Bulgaria (43%), Hungary (39%) and Italy (35.4%). For comparison, the European countries with the lowest rates include France (19.7%), Sweden (16.6%), Finland (16.5%), the Netherlands (16.2%), and Norway (16%) (OECD Indicators 2019). Furthermore, important variations exist across the Swiss cantons—Jura's rate is below 20%, while Glaris's reaches 40%—and healthcare infrastructures, with 45.6% of CBs for women with (semi)private insurance versus 30.7% for those with standard health insurance (OFS 2019a). Variations also occur in accordance with women's sociodemographic features: cesarean rates are higher among older women (OFS 2019a) and among women of non-Swiss origins—for example, those from South America, Africa, or Italy (Hanselmann and Von Greyerz 2013). Depending on the specific birth circumstances, certain women are also more likely to undergo a cesarean birth: in Switzerland, 79.9% of multiple births and 94% of the births of babies in the breech position take place via cesarean.

In 2014, the Swiss Society of Gynecology and Obstetrics (SGGG 2014) took a stance in favor of vaginal birth, asserting that it should be the default procedure for a normal, low-risk pregnancy, while "planned C-section should be the exception." However, the cesarean rate remains a relatively neglected topic in the Swiss biomedical literature (Hohlfeld 2002; Morales et al. 2004; Roth-Kleiner 2007; Bonzon et al. 2017; Horsch et al. 2017; Baud et al. 2020). Current Swiss CB rates contradict the growing international movement promoting "normal childbirth" (Downe 2008), which emphasizes how biomedical practices have become too interventionist, resulting in over-screening, over-diagnosis, and over-treatment (Cassel and Guest 2012; Moynihan et al. 2012; Miller et al. 2016). In practice, healthcare professionals appear to face difficulties in inversing the cesarean trend, and those working in obstetrics are well aware of the adverse consequences of cesarean overuse. In addition, most parents want to limit technical and biomedical interventions because they consider pregnancy and birth to be important and intimate familial events (Maffi 2012; Chautems 2022). Although maternal requests for cesareans are often evoked as a factor exacerbating the increase in cesarean rates, the literature suggests that these play only a marginal role (see Moffat et al. 2007; Potter et al. 2008; Tully and Ball 2013; ACOG 2019).

Despite the high rate of cesareans in Switzerland, the current social context promotes "natural" physiologic birth. The dominant social representations, which most healthcare professionals also share, conceive of a normal birth as a vaginal one. Hence, CBs may foster a sense of failure for women who had planned a "natural" childbirth (Fenwick et al. 2009; Chautems 2022; Davis-Floyd 2022). In this context, "gentle" cesareans have appeared as attempts to reconcile the natural childbirth ideal with the cesarean birth. (A photo of a gentle cesarean birth, taken by photographer Elsa Mesot, appears on the cover of this volume. After this photo was taken, the newborn was passed directly to the mother.) The British obstetrician N. M. Fisk and his team (Smith, Plaat, and Fisk 2008) created the "gentle cesarean" technique, which aimed at mimicking a vaginal delivery. This technique stands out from the classic cesarean, as it allows newborns to be placed immediately on their mothers' chests for their first skin-to-skin contact, the mothers to play a more active role, and the environments and hospital staff to be more respectful of the event. Considering that early skin-to-skin contact can increase the rate and duration of breastfeeding (Rowe-Murray and Fisher 2002; Moore et al. 2016), as part of the 10 Steps of the Baby-Friendly Hospital Initiative (WHO 2018), this practice is currently standardized throughout Swiss maternity wards after a vaginal birth. Early skin-to-skin contact can also favor the bonding process between mother and child (Moore et al. 2016). A gentle cesarean is also intended to be inclusive of parents, allowing them to see their baby when extracted, and/or offering the father or other parent the opportunity to cut the umbilical cord (Smith, Plaat, and Fisk 2008). Yet despite the intention to enhance parents' participation, gentle cesarean, like any surgery, is still defined by normative expectations regarding "the appropriate behaviors in the operating theatre" (Maffi 2013:6). The hospital staff's requirements and the operating room's constraints thus frame the parents' participation. Few studies have explored parents' expectations and experiences regarding this technique.[1]

## Our Collaboration

The collaboration among the three authors of this chapter started in early 2020 when Caroline and Irene decided to prepare a research project on parents' experiences of cesareans in Switzerland,[2] and asked Alexandre whether he and his colleagues working in the maternity ward of the Hospital Riviera-Chablais (HRC)—a medium-sized public hospital located in the French part of Switzerland—would be interested in becoming partners in this project. Alexandre and most of his colleagues accepted our proposition with enthusiasm. One of the aspects that facilitated our collaboration was our common interest in "gentle cesarean," which has become a routine practice at HRC. This technique, which Alexandre and his colleague Christian Valla, the former head of the maternity department at HRC, introduced to Switzerland in late 2019, is particularly interesting for all of us, although not exactly for the same reasons. The quality of care and the clinical results are central from a biomedical point of view, whereas from a social science perspective, it is important to investigate whether and how this technique transforms parents' experiences of surgical birth. We decided to write this chapter in the form of an interview because we wanted to give voice to an obstetrician who has made a reflexive journey transforming him "from doctor to healer" (Davis-Floyd and St. John 1998)—meaning that he transformed several aspects of his training and previous clinical practices in accordance with a humanized conception of surgical birth and his moral concern for parents' and newborns' experiences of childbirth.

In what follows, we trace Alexandre's professional trajectory from medical school to his present position at HRC. We believe that his journey is significant because it uncovers some important characteristics of the two national systems in which it took place (France and Switzerland), of obstetric training (or the lack thereof) in biomedical schools, of hospital cultures, and of professional attitudes toward childbirth and the actors involved in it. The interview took place in French, and the other authors translated it to English.

## The Interview with Alexandre

*Irene: Could you tell us about your medical training and how you arrived in Switzerland?*
*Alexandre*: I grew up in Lyon,[3] where I attended medical school. At the end of my last year, I didn't want to choose a specialty, and hence I decided to train in general medicine [three years]. In the French system, you can choose the service and the hospital according to your ranking. I was not among the best students and thus had little choice. The first semester I was in a pneumology department; in the second semester, without having chosen it, I landed in an obstetrics and gynecology department. I initially hated gynecology and obstetrics because I had done

an internship in a department of the Hospital Hôtel Dieu in Lyon during my studies and had not liked it at all [in France, internships are done during the third year of medical school]. There, I had seen a female doctor perform a cesarean, and the sight of a woman opening another woman' s belly struck me. At the end of this internship, I had to pass an exam that consisted of inserting a speculum. I did it on a young girl, and it was my first time. I remember it as a very unpleasant experience.

Thus, during my second semester of specialization in general medicine, when I was sent to a gynecology and obstetrics department in the Hospital of Montélimart [a small-sized peripheral hospital], I was not very motivated. Unexpectedly, it was a good experience that changed my professional life. I was the first resident there who was not doing his specialization in gynecology and obstetrics. As the attending doctors [an attending physician has completed residency] weren't certain about what they could get me to do, I had a lot of freedom. There was only one thing I didn't like: the operation theater. I had asked the Head of the department not to attend operations. However, he made me understand that I had to attend at least some surgeries. At the end of the day, I had a blast during this residency. Although I performed cesareans and ultrasounds, I was very inexperienced and was often in awkward situations. I realized that when you know little, you are not experienced, you make mistakes and missteps. I remember one time when a couple asked me when children's teeth grow and I answered "at the age of four or five"! I also realized that obstetricians/gynecologists are trained to pay attention to pathology rather than physiology. After that semester, I decided I wanted to change and specialize in obstetrics and gynecology, but I learned it wasn't possible. I had to finish general medicine first, work for two years as a general practitioner, and then take the specialty exam for gynecology and obstetrics. At that time, I thought about doing my specialization in Belgium or Switzerland because they are also francophone countries. Considering that in Belgium, it was quite complicated to be admitted as a resident doctor, I opted for Switzerland where, at that time [2003], to specialize in gynecology and obstetrics, all you had to do was visit the Head of the department and be accepted by them. After finishing my specialty in general medicine in France, I started my residency in 2006 at the Hospital Le Samaritain in Vevey.[4]

It was difficult to adapt to the Swiss system because, for example, the names of medications were different. In France, we tend to use the names of the medications' active ingredients. In Switzerland, health professionals use the names given by the pharmaceutical manufacturers. I was familiar with the French names but not with the Swiss ones. Once, a nurse asked me what she could give to a woman with a headache, and

I said the name of the medication we use in France, and she didn't understand. I felt quite overwhelmed at first.

I spent two years at the Hospital Le Samaritain, one year at the University Hospital of Canton of Vaud (CHUV), and a year and a half at the Hospital of Morges.[5] At the Hospital Le Samaritain, it was just like a party: I had a very nice colleague with whom it was very good to work. I had a great deal of autonomy, and I liked that. I had never done surgeries [with the exception of cesareans], whereas my colleague was more of a surgeon. Therefore, we had very different attitudes toward the situations to be treated: I was very conservative, leaving surgery as a last resort, while my colleague was very interventionist, always putting surgery first. It's still like that today. I believe that I am much less interventionist than my colleagues at HRC are, even in the case of certain uterine ruptures where I do not want to intervene because I know they heal very well without surgery. My colleague at Le Samaritain always had the scalpel in his hand and operated on everything that came along.

*Irene: Could you tell us how and why you developed a different attitude toward childbirth compared to many of your colleagues?*
*Alexandre*: My conservative attitude is probably related to my experience as a general practitioner. During my internship in France, I took part-time responsibility for the office of a general practitioner in Saint Marcel d'Ardèche, a small town located south of Lyon. I learned a lot working as a general practitioner because I had to rely mostly on the clinic and evaluate which patients to send to the hospital to access medicine that was more high-tech. I had to develop a holistic approach to patients by assessing their family and social situations in making medical decisions.

In Switzerland, you have to do two years of surgery experience before becoming an obstetrician/gynecologist. This is at the origin of a very interventionist culture in this specialty. To obtain the FMH (Swiss Medical Association) diploma in obstetrics and gynecology, there is a list of surgical interventions you must perform. However, obstetrics is the poor relative of gynecology: We do not train obstetricians, but we do train gynecologists (surgeons). Therefore, resident physicians fight to go to the operating room. In France in the early 2000s, there was no operating catalogue. What counted was to have practiced five years of obstetrics/gynecology—the number of years rather than the number of surgical acts performed was important. For example, a friend of mine finished her specialization in France after performing three hysterectomies, while in Switzerland I had to perform 25. One colleague I met during my internship in Morges also told me that "obstetrics is for fags!" [Note from Caroline: This was a homophobic comment meant to discredit obstetricians, who only perform routine surgeries like cesareans or other birth emergency procedures, compared to gynecologists, who are trained to perform more challenging and varied surgeries including treatment of pathologies not necessarily related to childbirth.] I believe that in obstetrics, technical acts are few and rather banal: forceps, vacuum, cesarean. I am convinced that other aspects are more important: the psychosocial environment, parents' experiences, etc. These are not technical procedures. In obstetrics, we are not in the process of extracting a tumor.

For me, a cesarean is easy to do. I used to feel bothered when performing it a lot, so I was almost happy when there were complications because it became more interesting. The cesarean easily solves all the problems, and it is not very complicated to do, which is why it is so easily performed. In my opinion, in Switzerland, there are few gynecologists/obstetricians practicing only obstetrics. I would say that in obstetrics, most of my colleagues are like drivers of a car, but have never put their hands in the engine. I am a driver in gynecology, but I know how the engine works in obstetrics. For example, when I did my internship, most of my attendings preferred to do more cesareans rather than try maneuvers that were more complicated. They argued that the Swiss population was not ready for anything else. More generally, I think that the Swiss world of gynecology and obstetrics is rather closed to other European countries' influence: most Heads of maternity wards in Switzerland have been trained in Switzerland and are rather locked into their local culture.

When I was working at Le Samaritain, I was a young attending and the only full-time, in-hospital physician: at the beginning I had few outpatients, and hence, I had a lot of time to read. I also participated in several European congresses and saw that the practices that seemed indisputable in Switzerland were not at all the same elsewhere. For example, in some hospitals where I did my internship, it was mandatory to give the woman five international units (IU) of oxytocin after the child's shoulder came out, while Portuguese obstetricians gave ten IU after the expulsion of the placenta. I discovered that what seemed so true in Switzerland was not true in some other European countries. I sometimes think that many of my colleagues have lost their sense of what childbirth involves because the interventions they perform disrupt the process. In many hospitals, you find what I would call a "cold obstetrics." I think many things we do are useless or even deleterious. I will give you some examples.

Let's talk about continuous fetal monitoring. We know that, compared with intermittent auscultation, under continuous fetal monitoring, fewer newborns would have convulsions at birth, but we do not know what the consequences of these are on the children in the long term. We know there is no difference for NICU admission, acidosis, fetal death, or neurological injuries. On the contrary, we do know that continuous fetal monitoring increases the risk of fetal extraction by vacuum, forceps, or cesarean. Nonetheless, habit and medico-legal issues lead to the use of continuous fetal monitoring for all woman in our delivery rooms. We don't dare to change that, despite the mentioned consequences on our patients. Over the years, I have come to trust the women and their bodies much more. A woman gives birth. I wonder why in our hospital we have 30% of inductions of labor, 25% of cesareans and 12% of forceps/vacuum, whereas women who give birth know how to give birth.

Another experience that helped me to develop a critical perspective on my practice was the advanced course on ultrasound taught by Israel Nisand, who is a very well-known French obstetrician. Nisand explained that ultrasounds are practically useless, except for a few pathologies, such as certain cardiac malformations that require an intervention immediately after birth. For the rest, there is nothing to do, even if things are detected.[6] For instance, trisomy 18 and 13 cause the fetus's death in utero or shortly after birth. However, except for interrupting the pregnancy once you discover it, you cannot change the situation. I believe that ultrasounds are a source of stress for many future parents and can even harm them. Despite my opinion, I still perform ultrasounds to see the fetus because it has become routine and also for medico-legal reasons.

Finally, I believe that I learned a lot in the field when I was doing my internship in the delivery ward. I started thinking about the situations I observed and became interested first in the quality of care and the clinical aspects. I had the opportunity to attend a special training in patient safety coordination and another one in quality of care. I then realized that healthcare professionals are the third most important cause of death for patients. When I was a resident at CHUV, I was on the team in charge of setting up the procedure for reporting adverse events. I was also the one who created the written protocol of the delivery ward, which did not exist before. At that time, I started to think that it was important to discuss couples' wishes and the possibility of birth attendants being less paternalistic. When you start this kind of reflection, you open your eyes to many things. You realize that science is not everything. In sum, I started to think from a clinical point of view, but I later switched to consider the patients' point of view.

*Caroline: What about cesarean birth and gentle cesareans?*
*Alexandre*: I was very bored doing cesarean births because it was always the same procedure. When it comes to gentle cesareans, the idea came

from Christian Valla, the former Head of the department at the hospital Le Samaritain in Vevey. One day, he told me about a technique that we could introduce in our service. He proposed: "What if we had gentle (*douce*)—as it is usually called in French—cesareans?" I wanted to laugh at him, but I said to myself, "Go see what this is first." I read the article from 2008 [Smith, Plaat, and Fisk 2008]. It's far from everything you are taught during your training. You have to rethink your convictions and be open to change. For example, I learned that when you find the fetal head, you should immediately pull it out. People get excited, doing it very quickly. You also have to be careful that everything is perfectly sterile. On the paternalistic side, parents should not see anything because the father could faint. You should never lower the sterile drape separating the upper part of the mother's body from her abdomen.

Therefore, you have to get past everything you learned during your training. The pediatricians want the baby right away, to stimulate her or him. The anesthetists say that if it is a high-risk surgery, you need strong light everywhere. They are afraid of bleeding. If you want to do gentle cesareans, you must fight against all of that, all these beliefs. Even if it's not just beliefs, because there *are* situations where things can go wrong. You have to show that it is entirely possible, and that even if there is a problem, you can always make up for it. The gentle cesarean technique highlights that this event is a birth, not a surgery. The patients are there to give birth, not have a surgery. They want to give birth to their child. We must not forget that.

*Caroline: How did you manage to implement gentle cesareans in your service? It must have been challenging.*
*Alexandre*: Before the move to Hospital Riviera-Chablais, we started introducing it in Vevey with Dr. Valla and the midwives. We gradually tested small parts of the gentle cesarean protocol: slowly taking out the child's head, then dimming the lights, then lowering the surgical drape. We realized that everything was fine and that the women were delighted. During this transition stage, we had to convince medical staff from different disciplines, both pediatricians and anesthetists. At first, we were walking on eggshells. I was asking questions, and I negotiated with the teams to get them accustomed to it slowly. The midwives and pediatricians joined first. It was more difficult to convince the anesthetists, but it depended on the teams and individuals.

When we moved from Vevey to Hospital Riviera-Chablais, we had the opportunity to institutionalize gentle cesareans; therefore, they became the default protocol. Attending pediatricians were immediately on board with gentle cesareans. On the other hand, resident pediatricians were not informed of the protocol change; thus, they still wanted to take the babies right after birth, to clear them, to put them on the examination table. It was hard for them. There was little or incomplete training from attending pediatricians. Now, we are training resident obstetricians to perform gentle cesareans. I try to explain to residents that even though the woman has an epidural during the surgery, we pull and push on her stomach, and she can feel everything, even if there is no pain. Regarding extracting the child, we have to be gentle; this is not a Kinder Surprise Egg![7]

Now gentle cesareans are well established in the hospital, even if there are variations among the staff, and not everyone performs them the same way. Some colleagues are not entirely at ease with the technique, and they don't integrate all its components. It is also probably easier now that I am the Head of the obstetric unit. I have more influence than before [at Vevey]. Members of the medical staff from hospitals located in French-speaking Switzerland often contact me about gentle cesareans. They attend gentle cesareans births to perform them in their institutions. The other day, one physician asked me, "Why have I never done this before?" However, when I present the gentle cesarean protocol at national medical conferences, there is still a lot of reluctance, in particular from physicians working in university hospitals—for example, anesthetists or neonatologists. They are often quite condescending with our team because we are based in a regional hospital. They tell me that it would not be possible for them to perform gentle cesareans because they attend premature births. But in fact, they have few preterm births compared with full-term ones. I think that a relatively small percentage of premature births is not an acceptable reason for refusing to perform gentle cesareans. Indeed, there is *no* acceptable reason! It is even possible to perform a gentle cesarean in cases of emergency situations.

I hope that what we are doing at the HRC can help to grow a new generation of obstetricians. Although my colleagues at CHUV do not perform gentle cesareans, we are collaborating on other important aspects to improve work conditions in maternity wards. For example, with my colleague David Desseauve [associate physician and Head of the laboratory at CHUV], we have been able to introduce some hours of the TeamSTEPPS training in the Swiss French-speaking medical school, and we are also training some attending physicians. [The TeamSTEPPS training is an international program promoting strategies and tools to improve patient safety and the reliability of collaborations and teamwork to avoid adverse events.] We hope that this can improve things on both sides by addressing the issue during training and with attending physicians: to make teamwork more reliable, to adequately coordinate and avoid adverse medical events.

*Irene: Do you think that gentle cesareans also have an impact on the medical staff and on the atmosphere in the operating room?*
*Alexandre*: As I already said, I was bored during cesarean sections. You rarely get a surprise. When I started doing gentle cesareans, what I saw touched me. Parents' reactions, the expressions on their faces affected me. This is what made it possible to transform the cesarean section into childbirth. Furthermore, this is contagious—you can see it when you attend this kind of birth—everybody is happy! Gentle cesareans are also different for the medical team. For cesarean sections to become child-births requires a shift in the team culture—that is, [to see birth as] an important event and not a technical routine. It brings humanity to the operating room, because otherwise, it is technical. It is surgery: we are cutting meat. And, based on my experiences, I can say that the human-ization of the operating room has a positive impact on the morbidity rate and the patients' recovery.

I wonder if it affects [other] surgeries. There are changes occurring. Some anesthetists use hypnosis. They speak to patients; they prepare them. Before gentle cesareans, few anesthetists were interested in ob-stetric patients' experiences. Now they all look at them and interact with them during surgery. They are more present in general. One sur-geon told me that gentle cesareans have changed his approach to other surgeries under epidural anesthesia. He wants to lower the surgical drape to keep eye contact with the patients. I believe that gentle cesareans can help build a new culture of the relationships between the medical team and patients.

*Irene: During prenatal consultations, I observed that some women asked to be informed at each step of the cesarean procedure during the surgery. How do you address these demands?*
*Alexandre*: I think they do not actually want to be informed step by step, but just to be reassured . . . If I told them, "I cut the skin, I move apart the abdominals," and so forth, I do not think it would be helpful nor reassuring. I just give them general information, not the details of the technical actions performed. The tone of your voice is very important.

*Caroline: There are different elements constituting gentle cesareans. What is important in your opinion?*
*Alexandre*: I believe that gentle cesareans are primarily based on respect for the child's birth: it is a newborn, a little human who comes to life,

and we must respect this moment. It is a matter of humanity—or rather humanism. It is also a question of respect toward parents, for whom this birth is an extremely important moment. There is an inconsistency between the way we consider the baby before birth as an extractable fetus and what it eventually becomes—a lovely baby. For example, sometimes when you use forceps, you have to pull very hard, and you apply this pressure on a little baby. Whereas once babies are in the cradle, you hardly dare to touch them anymore. Many doctors who handle them rather roughly at birth are uncomfortable taking babies in their arms when they are in their bassinets. There is a sort of disconnection. The same disconnection happens in surgery. There are times when you must take a medical rather than a human posture. We are in the action, and we do not think about what we are doing. We turn into technicians. There is a disconnection also in obstetrics: we do not realize, and we do not want to realize. However, this disconnection has to stop at a certain point; we have to return to this child's birth. We must respect her or him, going at her or his pace. Gentle cesareans contribute to restoring this connection.

*Caroline: I was wondering, what do you think of the proposition made to women that they push to deliver their baby in the gentle cesarean protocol? Is it helpful for obstetricians?*
*Alexandre*: From a medical point of view, there is no point. It is useless. It is symbolic. At the beginning, it was part of the gentle cesarean procedure, so I did it. I wanted to observe if pushing was effective, and I asked several patients to do it. I realized that it has little effect on the baby's presentation. However, I had positive feedback from several patients who said, "Thank you for letting me push!" They told me it was super important for them. So, I keep doing it.

*Irene: Regarding the postpartum period, did you observe some changes in parents' experiences and recoveries since the introduction of gentle cesareans?*
*Alexandre*: I have the feeling that yes, there is a change. Before, no one ever wanted to return home the day after surgery. I feel that the parents' experience is different compared to when I was doing standard cesareans. Some patients thank me and tell me, "You healed me from my previous delivery." They also said, "It's so great to have my baby skin-to-skin right after birth!" I know that for them, seeing the birth or having their baby immediately, skin-to-skin, are fundamental elements. I have much more positive feedback with gentle compared to standard cesareans.

## Discussion

Biomedical training tends to encourage future physicians to distance themselves from their feelings and to avoid dealing with patients' emotions (Davis-Floyd 1987; Davis-Floyd and St John 1998; Davis-Floyd 2018a). Breaking from "cold obstetrics," which Robbie Davis-Floyd (2018b) would call "technocratic obstetrics," the gentle cesarean procedure as Alexandre and his colleagues perform it acknowledges the importance of emotions in obstetrics—those of the patients and those of the staff. From this perspective, gentle cesareans and the humanization of the operating room can potentially reconfigure the relationships among health professionals, parents, and child. They partly disrupt the technocratic hierarchy and the subordination of the individual to the institution and to the practitioners representing it (see Davis-Floyd 2022). Gentle cesareans also produce better health outcomes, as women's recoveries can be easier or at least better experienced. This could explain why parents who have experienced gentle cesareans often leave the hospital only one day after the operation, according to the data collected at HRC. The empowerment they feel from their gentle cesarean births may make them less dependent on hospital recovery care. However, as each practitioner reinterprets the procedures of gentle cesareans in their own way, there are significant variations in the ways they are performed, and normative behaviors that comply with the operating room requirements and protocols are still expected from parents (Maffi 2013).

Gentle cesarean proponents generally emphasize the parents' perspectives; the procedure is presented as a "woman-centered technique" (Smith et al. 2008). Our volume lead editor Robbie Davis-Floyd adds a personal note here:

> When my 26-hour labor with my first child, during which I felt completely embodied, ended in a cesarean, I was beyond shocked at the sudden and total mind-body separation I experienced when the epidural took effect. This separation was also visual: I could not even *see* the body that I could not feel. Being "awake and aware," I asked the obstetrician to *please* place the curtain blocking my view above my head, so that I could bear witness to the birth of my daughter, but this was in 1979—a time when such a concept was "beyond conception." I would have given anything to have a gentle cesarean like the ones described in this chapter!

Interestingly, Alexandre also insists on the importance of newborns' experiences. Indeed, gentle cesareans include a set of procedures aimed at easing the baby's birth experience in line with the child-centered approach that the French pediatrician Frédérick Leboyer developed more than 40 years ago, in 1974. This approach includes dimming the lights, allowing babies time to establish respiration while still connected to the placenta—a process that J. Smith, F. Plaat, and N. M. Fisk (2008) called "autoresuscitation"—and placing babies on their mothers' chests as soon as possible, thereby enabling them to initiate breastfeeding in the operating room.

As Alexandre stated, in contemporary obstetric culture, physicians are usually alienated from their patients, both women and babies (see also Davis-Floyd 2018b, 2022). The ways in which obstetricians consider and handle babies at the time of birth contrast with their attitude toward them once they are dressed and lying in their bassinets—in other words, once they appear as members of the society rather than as naked, not-yet-socialized bodies. Before the inscription of the baby's body into the social environment of the hospital, "newborns are considered in many cultural contexts to be unripe, unformed, ungendered, and not fully human" (Kaufman and Morgan 2005:317). This is also true in Swiss maternity hospitals where, as Line Rochat (2017) has shown, an important part of nurses' work in the neonatology intensive care unit (NICU) consists of helping the parents to bond with their premature or sick child.

Although the socialization process and the humanization of the care of sick or premature babies may be extreme cases, they nevertheless very well show the work usually performed in ordinary postpartum care. This work—generally entrusted to nurses and midwives—consists of helping to create a strong affective and physical bond between the mother, the father/partner, and the baby. Mothers must devote themselves entirely to their babies to abide by the norms of the "good mother" and to avoid being criticized or even pathologized by healthcare providers. In the Swiss NICU where Line Rochat conducted her doctoral research (2019), mothers had to spend days, sometimes months, at the sides of the incubators in which their babies were struggling to survive. They regularly had to pump their milk, touch their babies, speak to them—in short, to forget their personal lives and wellbeing, and even their other older children and partners, to build the bond considered necessary to adequately care for the hospitalized child. No other family members, not even the fathers, were exposed to this social and biomedical pressure because they were not seen as playing primary roles. Although in the mentioned NICU, the often dramatic health conditions of the babies emphasized mothers' sacrificial roles, this norm was clearly also present in the regular post-partum department of the same hospital (Rochat 2019; Chautems and Maffi 2021).

The attitudes of medical staff toward women during standard cesar-eans reveal a deep disconnection that is both symbolized and reinforced by the surgical drape. The woman's head, representing her social per-sonhood, is visually and physically separated from her abdomen, which becomes a "piece of meat" that the obstetrician can dissect. This discon-nection allows the staff to discuss personal and often insignificant sub-jects during the cesarean, completely ignoring the woman's personhood and feelings, and that the cesarean is the birth of a child and a most significant event for the parents, as Alexandre described. Removing the surgical drape and making eye contact between the staff and the woman during gentle cesareans completely transforms their relationships: at-tention to the parents, respect for the importance of the moment, and the space in the operating theater all reinforce the importance of the parents'—and especially the mothers'—emotions.

## Conclusion: Spreading Gentle Cesareans

On a broader scope, Alexandre's professional trajectory sheds light on some specific features of Swiss obstetric training. For example, unlike the French training, the Swiss training includes a list of mandatory surgical procedures—an "operating catalogue"—with a determined number of qualifying surgical acts that must be performed before graduating. This requirement both reflects and reinforces a technocratic and interven-tionist obstetric culture in which relational aspects and parents' expe-riences are secondary. Alexandre's reflexive account of his journey and his commitment to a humanistic approach to obstetric care challenges Swiss dominant obstetric culture. Alexandre's and other obstetricians' adoptions of gentle cesareans contribute to reinforcing this practice, which is now spreading locally in French-speaking Switzerland and is also being adopted in other parts of the world as other obstetricians and parents become aware of its value.

**Caroline Chautems** is a social and medical anthropologist and a Swiss National Science Foundation Research Fellow at the University of Laus-anne, Switzerland. Her research interests focus on human reproduction, the body and parenthood, and gender issues underlying these themes.

She is the author of *Negotiated Breastfeeding: Holistic Postpartum Care and Embodied Parenting* (2022).

**Irene Maffi** is Professor of Cultural and Social Anthropology at the University of Lausanne. She has conducted ethnographic research in Jordan, Tunisia, and Switzerland in two primary domains: political anthropology and the anthropology of sexuality and reproduction. She is the author of *Women, Health and the State in the Middle East: The Politics and Culture of Childbirth in Jordan* (2012) and of *Abortion in Post-Revolutionary Tunisia: Medicine, Politics and Morality* (2020).

**Alexandre Farin** is the Head of the Obstetrics Unit at the Riviera-Chablais Hospital, Rennaz, Switzerland.

## Notes

1. Jolien Onsea and colleagues's (2018) comparative study of experiences with "standard" and "gentle" cesareans is one rare exception. The authors concluded that gentle cesareans may improve parents' satisfaction.
2. The project's title is "Parents' Experiences of Surgical Birth: A Socio-Anthropological Study of Cesarean Culture in Switzerland" and is funded by the Swiss National Science Foundation (project number 10001A_197393) for four years (2020–2024). Two hospitals are partners of the project: the University Hospital of the Canton of Vaud and the Hospital Riviera-Chablais.
3. Lyon is one of the largest cities in France and is located in the central-eastern part of the country.
4. Alexandre here mentions the Hospital Le Samaritain, which used to be located in Vevey. In 2019, following a large merger involving five regional hospitals, Le Samaritain and another small-sized hospital closed and their teams were displaced to a new site. Alexandre Farin has been the Head of the obstetric unit since the opening of this new interregional institution Hospital Riviera–Chablais in Rennaz in 2019.
5. Vevey and Morges are two small cities located on the shores of the lake of Geneva. Two of the hospitals where Alexandre did his internship are peripheral hospitals serving a small population.
6. Fetal therapy for issues like alloimmunization and certain congenital anomalies, such as fetal myelomeningocele (in which a portion of the baby's spinal cord and surrounding nerves protrude through an opening in the spine into an exposed, flat disc or sac that is visible on the back. This exposes the baby's spinal cord to the amniotic fluid in the mother's womb and can be harmful to fetal development) have risen over the past 50 years and are commonplace within high-risk obstetrical practice. Here, ultrasound remains critical for detection and counseling (see, e.g., Bianchi et al. 2010).
7. The Kinder Surprise Egg is a hollow chocolate egg that contains a plastic capsule with a small toy inside.

# References

ACOG. 2019. "Cesarean Delivery on Maternal Request." ACOG Committee Opinion No. 761. *Obstetrics & Gynecology* 133(1): e73–e77.

Baud D, Sichitiu J, Lombardi V, et al. 2020. "Pelvic Floor Dysfunction 6 Years after Uncomplicated Vaginal Versus Elective Cesarean Deliveries: A Cross-Sectional Study." *Scientific Reports* 10: 21509.

Beck U. 2003. *La Société du Risque: Sur la Voie d'une Autre Modernité.* Paris: Flammarion.

Bianchi DW, Crombleholme TM, D'Alton ME, Malone FD. 2010. *Fetology. Diagnosis and Management of the Foetal Patient,* 2nd ed. New York: McGraw Hill.

Bonzon M, Mechthild M, Karch A, Grylka-Baeschlin S. 2017. "Deciding on the Mode of Birth after a Previous Cesarean Section—An Online Survey Investigating Women's Preferences in Western Switzerland." *Midwifery* 50: 219–227.

Burton-Jeangros C, Cavalli S, Gouilhers S, Hammer R. 2013. "Between Tolerable Uncertainty and Unacceptable Risks: How Health Professionals and Pregnant Women Think about the Probabilities Generated by Prenatal Screening." *Health, Risk & Society* 15(2): 144–161.

Burton-Jeangros C, Hammer R, Maffi I. 2014. *Accompagner la Naissance: Terrains Socio-Anthropologiques en Suisse Romande.* Lausanne: BSN Press.

Cassel CK, Guest JA. 2012. "Choosing Wisely: Helping Physicians and Patients Make Smart Decisions about Their Care." *Journal of the American Medical Association* 307(17): 1801–2.

Chautems C. 2022. *Negotiated Breastfeeding: Holistic Postpartum Care and Embodied Parenting.* Abingdon, Oxon: Routledge.

Chautems C, Maffi I. 2021. "Mères et Pères face à l'Allaitement: Savoirs Experts et Rapports de Genre à l'Hôpital et à Domicile en Suisse." *Nouvelles Questions Féministes* 40(1): 35–41.

Davis-Floyd R. 1987. "Obstetric Training as a Rite of Passage." *Medical Anthropology Quarterly* 1(3): 288–318.

———. 2018a. "Medical Training as Technocratic Initiation." In *Ways of Knowing about Birth: Mothers, Midwives, Medicine, and Birth Activism,* Davis-Floyd R and Colleagues, 107–140. Long Grove IL: Waveland Press.

———. 2018b. "The Technocratic, Humanistic, and Holistic Paradigms of Birth and Health Care." In *Ways of Knowing about Birth: Mothers, Midwives, Medicine, and Birth Activism,* Davis-Floyd R and Colleagues, 3–44. Long Grove IL: Waveland Press.

———. 2022. *Birth as an American Rite of Passage,* 3rd ed. Abingdon, Oxon: Routledge.

Davis-Floyd R, St. John G. 1998. *From Doctor to Healer. The Transformative Journey.* New Brunswick: Rutgers University Press.

Downe S., ed. 2008. *Normal Childbirth: Evidence and Debate,* 2nd Edition. Edinburg: Elsevier.

Euro-Peristat Project. 2018. *European Perinatal Health Report: Core Indicators of the Health and Care of Pregnant Women and Babies in Europe in 2015.* Paris: Euro-Peristat. Retrieved 28 January 2022 from https://www.europeristat.com/images/EPHR2015_web_hyperlinked_Euro-Peristat.pdf.

Fenwick S, Holloway I, Alexander J. 2009. "Achieving Normality: The Key to Status Passage to Motherhood after a Cesarean Section." *Midwifery* 25(5): 554–563.
Hanselmann V, Von Greyertz S. 2013. *Accouchements par Césarienne en Suisse: Rapport en Réponse au Postulat Maury Pasquier (08.3935).* Berne: Office Fédéral de la Santé Publique (OFSP).
Hohlfeld P. 2002. "Cesarean Section on Request: A Case for Common Sense." *Gynäkol Geburtshilfliche Rundsch* 42: 19–21.
Horsch A, Vial Y, Favrod C, et al. 2017. "Reducing Intrusive Traumatic Memories after Emergency Cesarean Section: A Proof-of-Principle Randomized Controlled Study." *Behaviour Research and Therapy* 94: 36–47.
Kaufman SR, Morgan LM. 2005. "The Anthropology of the Beginning and Ends of Life." *Annual Review of Anthropology* 34: 317–341.
Leboyer F. 1974. *Pour une Naissance sans Violence.* Paris: Seuil.
Lupton D. 1993. "Risk as Moral Danger: The Social and Political Functions of Risk Discourse in Public Health." *International Journal of Health Services: Planning, Administration, Evaluation* 23(3): 425435.
Maffi I. 2012. "L'Accouchement Est-il un Événement? Regards Croisés sur les Définitions Médicales et les Expériences Intimes des Femmes en Jordanie et en Suisse." *Mondes Contemporains* 2: 53–80.
Maffi I. 2013. "Can Cesarean Section be 'Natural'? The Hybrid Nature of the Nature-Culture Dichotomy in Mainstream Obstetric Culture." *Journal for Research in Sickness and Society* 10(19): 5–26.
Maffi I, Gouilhers S. 2019. "Conceiving of Risk in Childbirth: Obstetric Discourses, Medical Management and Cultural Expectations in Switzerland and Jordan." *Health, Risk and Society* 21(3–4): 185–206.
Manaï D, Burton-Jeangros C, Elger B, eds. 2010. *Risques et Informations dans le Suivi de la Grossesse: Droit et Pratiques Sociales.* Berne: Stämpfli.
Miller S, Abalos E, Chamillard M, et al. 2016. "Beyond Too Little, Too Late and Too Much, Too Soon: A Pathway Towards Evidence-Based, Respectful Maternity Care Worldwide." *The Lancet* 388(10056): 2176–2192.
Moffat M, Bell J, Porter M, et al. 2007. "Decision Making about Mode of Delivery among Pregnant Women Who Have Previously Had a Cesarean Section: A Qualitative Study." *British Journal of Obstetrics and Gynaecology* 114(1): 86–93.
Moore ER, Bergman N, Anderson GC, Medley N. 2016. "Early Skin-to-Skin Contact for Mothers and Their Healthy Newborn Infants." *Cochrane Database of Systematic Reviews* 11. CD003519.
Morales M, Ceysens G, Jastrow N, et al. 2004. "Spontaneous Delivery or Manual Removal of the Placenta During Cesarean Section: A Randomised Controlled Trial." *British Journal of Obstetrics and Gynaecology* 111(9): 908–912.
Moynihan R, Doust J, and Henry D. 2012. "Preventing Overdiagnosis: How to Stop Harming the Healthy." *British Medical Journal* 344: e3502.
OECD Indicators. 2019. "Caesarean Sections." In *Health at a Glance 2019: OECD Indicators.* Paris: OECD Publishing. Retrieved 21 January 2022 from https://www.oecd-ilibrary.org/social-issues-migration-health/health-at-a-glance-2019_fa1f7281-en.
Office Fédéral de la Statistique (OFS). 2019a. "Statistique Médicale des Hôpitaux. Accouchements et Santé Maternelle en 2017." *Federal Statistics Bureau of Swit-*

*zerland*, 17 May. Retrieved 28 January 2028 from https://www.bfs.admin.ch/bfs/fr/home/actualites/quoi-de-neuf.assetdetail.8369419.html.

———. 2019b. "Communiqué de Presse. Recul du Recours aux Césariennes et Épisiotomies en 2017." *Federal Statistics Bureau of Switzerland*, 17 May. Retrieved 28 January 2028 from https://www.bfs.admin.ch/bfs/fr/home/actualites/quoi-de-neuf.assetdetail.8369419.html.

Onsea J, Bijnens B, Van Damme S. et al. 2018. "Exploring Parental Expectations and Experiences around 'Gentle' and 'Standard' Caesarean Section." *Gynecologic and Obstetric Investigation* 83: 437–442.

Potter JE, Hopkins K, Faúndes A, Perpétuo I. 2008. "Women's Autonomy and Scheduled Cesarean Sections in Brazil: A Cautionary Tale." *Birth* 35(1): 33–40.

Rochat L. 2017. "Apprendre à s'Attacher: Des Femmes Enceintes et leur Fœtus en Situation de Grossesse à Risque d'Accouchement Avant Terme." *Anthropologie & Santé* 15 (15). Retrieved 30 January 2022 from https://www.researchgate.net/publication/321392343_Apprendre_a_s'attacher_Des_femmes_enceintes_et_leur_foetus_en_situation_de_grossesse_a_risque_d'accouchement_avant_terme.

Rochat L. 2019. *Penser le Lien: Anthropologie de l'Attachement et de la Prématurité dans un Service de* Néonatologie en Suisse. PhD dissertation, University of Lausanne.

Roth-Kleiner M. 2007. "Taux Élevé de Césariennes et Augmentation de l'Incidence du Syndrome de Détresse Respiratoire du Nouveau-né en Suisse." *Paediatrica* 18(5): 47–48.

Rowe-Murray HJ, Fisher J R. 2002. "Baby Friendly Hospital Practices: Cesarean Section is a Persistent Barrier to Early Initiation of Breastfeeding." *Birth* 29(2): 124–131.

Scamell M, Alaszewski A. 2012. "Fateful Moments and the Categorisation of Risk: Midwifery Practice and the Ever-Narrowing Window of Normality during Childbirth." *Health, Risk & Society* 14(2): 207–221.

SGGG (Schweizerische Gesellschaft für Gynäkologie und Geburtshilfe). 2014. *Comment Allez-vous Mettre Votre Enfant au Monde? Une Brochure d'Information sur l'Accouchement.* Berne: La Société Suisse de Gynécologie-Obstétrique. Retrieved 28 January 2022 from https://www.sggg.ch/fileadmin/user_upload/Dokumente/3_Fachinformationen/4_Patienteninformationsblaetter/F_Comment_allez-vous_mettre_votre_enfant_au_monde_2014.pdf.

Smith J, Plaat F, Fisk NM. 2008. "The Natural Cesarean: A Woman-Centred Technique." *British Journal of Obstetrics and Gynaecology* 115: 1037–1042.

Tully KP, Ball HL 2013. "Misrecognition of Need: Women's Experiences of and Explanations for Undergoing Cesarean Delivery." *Social Science & Medicine* 85: 103–111.

World Health Organization (WHO). 2018. *Implementation Guidance. Protecting, Promoting and Supporting Breastfeeding in Facilities Providing Maternity and Newborns Services: The Revised Baby-Friendly Hospital Initiative.* Geneva: World Health Organization.

# CHAPTER 6

# Scoring Women, Calculating Risk
## The MFMU VBAC Calculator

*Nicholas Rubashkin*

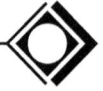

Over the last 30 years, the United States has witnessed a sharp increase in cesareans, which have long accounted for one in three births or 1.2 million pregnant women per year (around 32%). One of the main reasons for this persistently high rate is that vaginal births after cesareans (VBACs) have become less common in the United States, with the current VBAC rate ranging between 10–13% (MacDorman, Declercq, and Menacker 2011; CDC 2019), down from a high of 28% in 1996 (Cunningham et al. 2010). In any given state, some 50% of hospitals don't "offer" VBAC as a supported birth option (Leeman et al. 2013), the reasons for which relate to the issue of using the most invasive technique—cesarean birth—as the solution to the anticipated risks of an attempted VBAC. Due to these significant access issues, around 80,000 US women per year will have a VBAC, compared to 500,000 women who, after having undergone a first cesarean, give birth via what is called an elective repeat cesarean delivery, or ERCD (CDC 2019).

With each subsequent cesarean, the risks of maternal, newborn, and child morbidity and mortality increase (Sandall et al. 2018). Even in California—the state that leads the United States in reducing avoidable maternal morbidity and mortality—40% of all women's avoidable morbidity can be attributed to cesareans, with Black women being the most affected (Leonard, Main, and Carmichael 2019). Due to a combination of structural and interpersonal racism in healthcare settings, Black women experience the most negative effects of unnecessary cesareans (Campbell 2021).

Because of the significant impacts of avoidable cesareans on maternal and child health, in 2010, the National Institutes of Health (NIH) declared increasing the US VBAC rate to be a public health priority. At that time, the NIH also noted that statistical models could accurately predict the probability for a successful VBAC (Cunningham et al. 2010). VBAC prediction models might help increase the VBAC rate if only those women assessed to have the highest probability for a success went on to attempt a VBAC, assuming that a proportion of these women were scheduling repeat cesarean births despite a high probability for success in giving birth vaginally (Metz et al. 2013a).

Starting in 2007, one VBAC prediction model rose to prominence in the United States: the Maternal-Fetal Medicine University (MFMU) Network VBAC Success Calculator. The "VBAC calculator" made its prediction by combining a woman's clinical history with her age, race/ethnicity, and Body Mass Index (BMI) (Grobman et al. 2007). In the calculator's algorithm, Black and Hispanic women had 50% lesser odds of successful VBAC than white women. The VBAC calculator dominated the research literature (Chaillet et al. 2013; Fonseca et al. 2019), appeared in the American College of Obstetricians and Gynecologists (ACOG) national VBAC guidelines (ACOG 2010, 2017), and is or was used in many clinical settings in the United States (Thornton et al. 2020).

In this chapter, I demonstrate how the calculator circumscribed VBAC-interested women's decision-making capacity by putting forth cesarean surgery as the best and only treatment for a predicted low probability of success. VBAC-interested women challenged the calculator with alternative, and often less invasive, approaches to the uncertainty of attempting a VBAC. Because the VBAC calculator explicitly factored in race/ethnicity (as opposed to racism) as an intrinsic risk factor for poor individual health, the calculator put VBAC-interested Black and Hispanic women at risk for cesareans they didn't desire or need (Attanasio, Kozhimannil, and Kjerulff 2019). I also examine how some maternity care providers—more often midwives but also some obstetricians—challenged the calculator's approach and supported VBAC-interested women in a range of birth options. In my Conclusion to this chapter, I will place my findings in dialogue with the movement for the abolition of race-based medicine (Chadha et al. 2020), which recently influenced the MFMU to develop a new VBAC calculator that excludes race/ethnicity as a variable (Grobman et al. 2021).

## A Closed Knowledge System

A central argument of this three-volume book series has been that obstetrics as a field often functions as a closed system of thinking (see

Davis-Floyd, Chapter 1, this volume). Using history as an example, Jo Murphy-Lawless (1998) dated the obstetric tendency toward closed system thinking to the very origins of the profession in 17th-century Ireland (see also Chapter 2 in this volume). Murphy-Lawless (1998:157) went so far as to project the closed nature of obstetrics into the future, writing that "Knowledge formation within obstetrics will always be premised on a closed form of rationality which excludes women yet operates at the expense of women." The fact that obstetric researchers invented a rational object like the VBAC calculator without soliciting input from birthing individuals in the design or the application of the calculator is testimony to the dynamics of closed system thinking. At the same time, the VBAC calculator was designed to engage women as decision makers; thus, the calculator cannot be understood *only* as a closed form of rationality that excludes women.

Statistical instruments, such as randomized controlled trials and prospective cohort studies like the one that informed the VBAC calculator (Grobman et al. 2007) represent a dominant form of rationality in contemporary US obstetrics. Obstetrics uses statistical prediction to justify surgical intervention prior to the onset of labor to avert future maternal and/or fetal risks (Wendland 2007). Far from supporting the judicious use of rigorously tested interventions, the movement for statistical evidence in obstetrics elevated cesareans as the best ways to guard against future danger, and cast vaginal birth as a risky alternative available only to select candidates (Wendland 2007). The application of statistical instruments in obstetrics has expanded the terrain for surgical intervention into normal pregnancies and births (Healy, Humphreys, and Kennedy 2017), in what Melissa Cheyney and Robbie Davis-Floyd (2019:8) have called the "obstetric paradox": "intervene to keep birth safe, thereby causing harm."

For example, the anticipation of risk and the default to apply cesarean to those anticipated risks has significantly impacted the access to VBAC in the United States. In the late 1990s, some obstetricians successfully argued that a scheduled repeat cesarean prior to the onset of labor was the most responsible choice for women to make in order to avert the risk to the fetus of uterine rupture—a rare surgical emergency that can occur during an attempted VBAC (Phelan 1998). These professional shifts away from VBAC and toward repeat cesarean were accelerated by a publication in *The New England Journal of Medicine* by Mona Lydon-Rochelle and colleagues in 2001. This study showed that artificially inducing or augmenting labor during an attempted VBAC increases the risk of uterine rupture. Uterine rupture happens when, during an attempted VBAC, the prior uterine scar separates, and thus, is a surgical emergency. Yet because obstetricians have been more prone to artificially inducing or augmenting labor, the study and the Editorial that accompanied it (Greene 2001) focused on the tripling of the relative risk of uterine rupture, even though in the absolute sense uterine rupture was a rare event, occurring in 0.5% of un-augmented labors and 2% of labors augmented with prostaglandins. Because even the baseline uterine rupture risk represented a three-fold increase compared to repeat cesarean, the scientific and professional consensus shifted strongly to recommend that VBACs should only be attempted in tertiary-level hospitals with obstetricians and anesthesiologists on call 24/7 so that a surgical emergency like uterine rupture could be dealt with at any hour. Thus, VBACs disappeared as an option in community hospitals around the country.

The concerns around the risk of uterine rupture during an attempted VBAC were distinctly focused on the risk to the fetus as compared to the mother. So, while many in the obstetric profession consider the choice between a VBAC and a repeat cesarean to be preference-sensitive, and therefore a decision into which childbearers should have input, the obstetric anticipation of risk in an attempted VBAC can ultimately circumscribe and limit available care options.

## How the VBAC Calculator Worked

An accurate and precise VBAC prediction model could assist providers to counsel and help women make more informed decisions about their mode of birth. In the past, providers quoted VBAC candidates a general population range of success between 60–90%, yet in key interlocuter interviews (see below), members of the MFMU stated that they viewed this approach as imprecise. Their innovative calculator provided a more precise and personalized estimate of the probability for a successful VBAC. In fact, the members of the MFMU believed that they had outlined the contours of a new population science. In their first article (Grobman et al. 2007), they compared the calculator's probability distribution to the population-derived estimates of aneuploidy risk[1] used to counsel women around prenatal genetic diagnosis. By comparing their innovation to prenatal genetic diagnosis, the MFMU elevated their calculator to be on par with genetics, a more established population science, while also arguing for the calculator's universal applicability in prenatal counseling (Rapp 2000).

To calculate the probability for a successful VBAC along with a 95% confidence interval (a statistical measure of uncertainty around an average), a provider entered these six prenatal factors: (1) age; (2) BMI (Body Mass Index); (3) race/ethnicity (coded as mutually exclusive categories as either Black, Hispanic, or "White and others"; see Table 6.1); (4) any previous vaginal delivery; (5) any vaginal delivery since the last cesarean; and (6) a prior cesarean for arrest of dilation or arrest of descent. Greater age and BMI decreased the score. Being categorized as Black or Hispanic, or having a prior cesarean for a labor arrest disorder, resulted in a prediction of 50% lesser odds of VBAC, while any prior vaginal birth (including a VBAC) increased the probability for success. See Figure 6.1 to understand how the original calculator appeared to users on its NIH-hosted website and see Table 6.1 to understand the contribution of each factor, in the form of odds ratios, which were used to calculate the probability for a successful VBAC. In other words, the odds ratios from Table 6.1 were programmed into the web-hosted version of the VBAC calculator, thus facilitating use of the calculator, which combined all the odds ratios into a final score (Figure 6.1.).

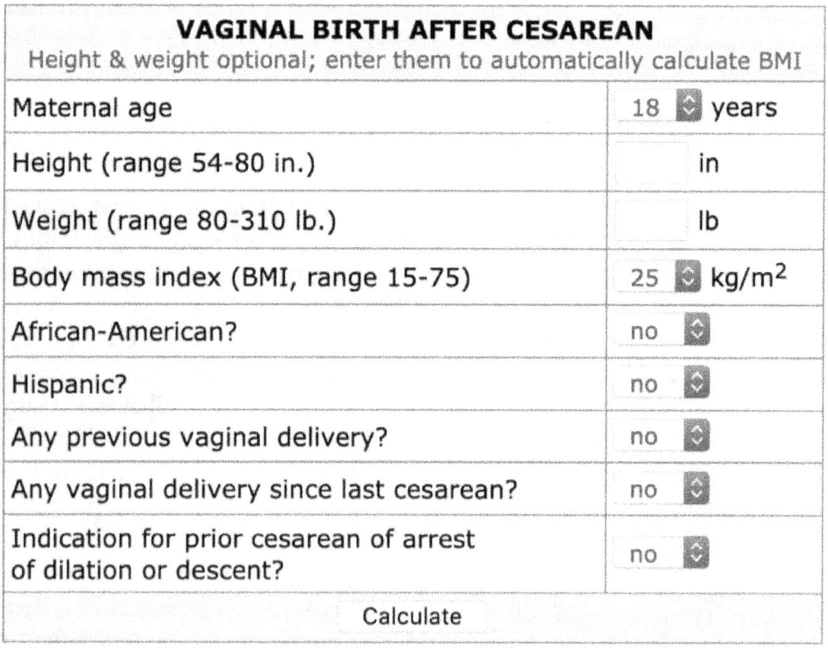

| **VAGINAL BIRTH AFTER CESAREAN** | |
|---|---|
| Height & weight optional; enter them to automatically calculate BMI | |
| Maternal age | 18 ⬍ years |
| Height (range 54-80 in.) | in |
| Weight (range 80-310 lb.) | lb |
| Body mass index (BMI, range 15-75) | 25 ⬍ kg/m² |
| African-American? | no ⬍ |
| Hispanic? | no ⬍ |
| Any previous vaginal delivery? | no ⬍ |
| Any vaginal delivery since last cesarean? | no ⬍ |
| Indication for prior cesarean of arrest of dilation or descent? | no ⬍ |
| Calculate | |

**Figure 6.1.** The MFMU VBAC Calculator as it used to appear on its hosted website. A new calculator that excludes race/ethnicity as a variable has been developed and can be found here: https://mfmunetwork.bsc.gwu.edu/web/mfmunetwork/vaginal-birth-after-cesarean-calculator.

The VBAC calculator worked as much by what it included as by what it excluded. It did not account for the impacts of hospital policies and practices. According to the calculator, comparing women with identical "risk factors," women giving birth at a hospital with a high VBAC rate (defined as the highest quartile) have a 77% greater chance of successful VBAC compared to women who give birth at a hospital with a low VBAC rate (defined as the lowest quartile) (Triebwasser et al. 2019). The calculator also excluded a pregnant person's subjective level of commitment to VBAC, and such commitment predicts attempting a VBAC (Kaimal et al. 2019). Finally, by considering race/ethnicity to be an intrinsic measure of population health, the calculator excluded the possibility that racism explained Black and Hispanic women's lower VBAC rates (Crear-Perry et al. 2020). (See Table 6.1)

In a later analysis, the members of the MFMU wanted to know not only whether their calculator could support more informed decision-making, but also whether the calculator could be used to actually improve maternal and neonatal outcomes. Therefore, the MFMU analyzed whether surgical complications increased with decreasing calculator scores. They found that when calculator scores dropped below 60%, 3.1% of women who attempted a VBAC experienced maternal or neonatal morbidity, compared to 1.5% of women who scheduled a repeat cesarean.[2] The MFMU researchers found this relative risk of 2:1 to be statistically significant, and they proposed that a repeat cesarean may be the safer option for women assessed to have a probability for a successful VBAC of less than 60% (Grobman et al. 2009).

Table 6.1. Factors Associated with Vaginal Birth after Cesarean Delivery, from the original VBAC calculator article © Grobman et al. 2007.

| Variable | Odds Ratio | 95% Confidence Interval |
|---|---|---|
| Maternal age (y) | 0.96 | 0.95–0.97 |
| Body mass index (kg/m2) at first prenatal visit | 0.94 | 0.93–0.95 |
| Maternal race | | |
|     White and Others | Referent | |
|     Latina | 0.51 | 0.44–0.59 |
|     African American | 0.51 | 0.44–0.59 |
| Recurring indication for cesarean delivery | 0.53 | 0.48–0.60 |
| Any prior vaginal delivery | 2.43 | 2.04–2.89 |
| Vaginal delivery after prior cesarean | 2.73 | 2.21–3.36 |

When ACOG (2010) wrote the calculator into national guidelines, the 60% cutoff instructed providers on how they might use the calculator, stating: "Although there is no universally agreed on discriminatory point, evidence suggests that women with at least a 60–70% chance of a VBAC have equal or less maternal morbidity when they undergo TOLAC (trial of labor after cesarean) than women undergoing elective repeat cesarean delivery" (ACOG 2010:454). I agree with Hazel Keedle that the term "trial of labor" conveys a lack of faith in the birth process and connotes that women give birth in front of a judge and jury. The VBAC calculator also used a vocabulary of failure, and thus I've chosen to refer to the "MFMU VBAC Success Calculator" simply as the "VBAC calculator." However, many providers in my study used the term "TOLAC." So, when not directly quoting an interlocutor, I replace TOLAC with "labor after a cesarean" or "planned VBAC" (see Keedle 2020).

Importantly, the guidelines did not similarly suggest that VBAC candidates with scores *above* 70% should attempt a VBAC, thus preserving the option for women with high scores to choose a repeat cesarean. The 60% threshold set a high bar for success for all women, but especially for Black and Hispanic women, and became a new barrier to planning a VBAC (Thornton et al. 2020).

## Materials and Methods

### My Methodological Approach

In conducting this study, I worked from the perspective that science and technology represent situated forms of knowledge (Haraway 1988; Wendland 2007). More specifically, I approached the calculator as a "technology of security"—one that used the concept of risk to manage the future health of populations through prenatal interventions (Weir 2006). My methodological approach for this study was both literature-based and ethnographic. From April 2019 until November 2020, I immersed myself in scientific papers, blog posts, podcasts, visual artifacts, interviews, observations of women engaging with the VBAC calculator, and audio recordings of prenatal visits during which I was not in the room. These recordings really helped me to understand how providers *actually* talked in general about the risk and benefits of different birth options, and specifically how they talked about the VBAC calculator with patients, which was different than with me as a colleague/interviewer. My colleagues didn't feel comfortable having me sit in the room and take notes during VBAC consultations—that felt too embarrassing to them, as if I were going to correct their VBAC counseling or something. But they were open to me leaving a recorder in the room. As an obstetrician, I did not gather data from pregnant or postpartum women who were under my care. The study was approved by the University of California, San Francisco Committee on Human Research.

## Sample

In order to obtain the full range of engagements with the calculator, I interviewed members from three groups: key interlocutors, clinicians, and pregnant/postpartum women. I purposely selected 22 key interlocutors as users and non-users of the calculator based on their research publications or public statements. Many of these key interlocutors held prominent national positions working on issues related to VBAC. In this group, I enrolled researchers, lawyers, hospital risk managers, perinatologists/maternal-fetal medicine [MFM] specialists, general obstetrician/ gynecologists, doulas, certified nurse midwives/CNMs, community midwives (including certified professional midwives/CPMs and licensed midwives/LMs),[3] as well as civil society actors who worked in birth advocacy organizations or who worked on writing national VBAC guidelines. The racial/ethnic breakdown of Group 1, my key interlocutors, was: 15 white; 5 Black; 2 Asian/South-Asian American.

To understand how the calculator worked on the ground, Group 2 of my interlocutors consisted of clinicians who worked in four institutions. I identified clinician-users of the calculator though a short email survey. As the study continued, I reached more clinicians via professional networks and snowball sampling. For Group 2, I interviewed 17 providers, including perinatalologists, general obstetrician/gynecologists, and CNMs. The clinician interlocutors had this racial/ethnic breakdown: 11 white, 3 Hispanic, 2 Black, 1 Asian American.

Group 3 of my research participants consisted of pregnant and postpartum women. I enrolled 31 women who had all undergone a prior cesarean: 27 of these were currently pregnant and four had already given birth. Study recruitment staff approached pregnant women who spoke English or Spanish, who were over the age of 18, and who were willing to participate in at least one interview. I enrolled postpartum women through social media advertisements and through snowball sampling. I purposely sampled pregnant women to obtain a range of birth histories and calculator scores. The sample included four women who already had a VBAC, and the rest had only one birth—a cesarean. Ultimately, as these women progressed through their pregnancies, 13 had VBACs, 10 had unplanned cesareans for a variety of reasons, and 8 had scheduled repeat cesareans. Their racial/ethnic identifications were as follows: 8 white (2 foreign-born); 2 Asian/South Asian (1 foreign-born); 1 Native American; 12 Hispanic (3 foreign-born); 4 African American; and 4 who identified as mixed-African, mixed-Hispanic, or mixed-Asian ancestry. Three women spoke Spanish only and I interviewed them in Spanish. The calculator scores of these interlocutors ranged from a low of 12% to a high of 95%.

## Settings

The clinician interlocutors worked in four different institutions. At two of these institutions—a large academic hospital network in the Northeast and a community hospital in the Southwest—practice policies required that providers use the VBAC calculator to counsel women with scores lower than 60% to have a repeat cesarean. At the two other institutions in Northern California, providers sporadically used the calculator without knowledge of the 60% cutoff. The majority of women interviewed hailed from the two sites in Northern California, with 27 of the 31 giving birth at these sites. Ultimately, two women switched from hospital-based care to planned VBACs with community midwives. ("Community midwives" attend births in homes and in freestanding birth centers.)

## Data Collection

After obtaining informed consent, I conducted 39 semi-structured interviews with key interlocutors and clinicians. I asked participants to detail their involvement with the calculator, to explain how the calculator worked, and to share what they saw as the calculator's benefits or harms. In clinician interviews, I also inquired about their general approach to mode-of-birth counseling and how the calculator did or did not fit into their approach. I also asked clinicians to recount specific cases in which they found the calculator helpful or controversial. Settings for the interviews were in person, on the phone, or via internet video.

After providing informed consent, the 31 pregnant and postpartum women had the option of participating in multiple data collection events, including interviews, observations of them engaging with the calculator, and recordings of prenatal visits. These women participated in a total of 81 data collection events (range 1–5 events per woman).

After a literature search, I designed an initial interview guide. The first interview with each woman was broad, and was focused on understanding the context of mode-of-birth decisions, including the circumstances that led to the first cesarean, their emotional and physical recoveries from the surgery, significant events between pregnancies, and interactions with providers during the current/recent pregnancy. Prior to COVID restrictions, I arranged to observe them in person engaging with the calculator.

If women had not encountered the calculator during prenatal care, I introduced it during follow-up interviews. If the calculator had been introduced, I probed women's thoughts and reactions to the discussions they had with providers. During follow-up interviews, I entered different arrangements of risk factors into the calculator in order to make explicit how age, race/ethnicity, and BMI contributed to the final score. Varying the combinations of factors often elicited discussions about risk, probability, and VBAC. As the study progressed, I altered the interview guides to hone in on emergent findings.

## Data Analysis

The interviews and prenatal visits were transcribed verbatim and analyzed using ATLAS.ti, a qualitative analysis software. Observations were entered into field notes, which were also managed using this software. The analysis followed the method of grounded theory (Charmaz 2014). Analysis began from the very start of data collection and continued throughout. An open coding process was used in order to ascertain preliminary themes, and using the constant comparative method, preliminary themes were tested within and across interviews as more data were gathered. With ongoing data collection, these preliminary themes were assembled into codes; these codes were then merged and clustered through additional re-readings of transcripts. During the analysis, I contrasted the calculator's approach to the ways in which providers from different professional backgrounds and VBAC candidates approached uncertainty, prediction, and VBAC. I analyzed the data thematically on multiple levels to identify points of convergence. I also pursued silences, divergences, and marginal perspectives, as these were all key to defining approaches to the uncertainty of planning a VBAC that differed from the calculator (Clarke 2005). Data saturation was reached as no new information emerged with additional recruitment of participants. In the next section, I present my findings by contrasting different approaches to the uncertainty of planning a VBAC. For the women participants, I present my findings in the form of representative ethnographic cases, using pseudonyms to protect their identities.

## Using an Early Statistical Prediction to Rationalize the Uncertainty of VBAC

The VBAC calculator circumscribed mode-of-birth decisions by favoring an early decision to schedule a repeat cesarean. In designing their calculator, the MFMU proposed that an early statistical prediction using factors known at the first prenatal visit could best alleviate the uncertainty of attempting a VBAC. In interviews, key interlocutors and clinicians reported that they viewed the main benefit of the VBAC calculator as helping women avoid "failure," defined as a cesarean performed after labor started. Providers who used the VBAC calculator followed a "3-box" model of counseling (see Figure 6.2), summarized well by a white general ob: "This is my counseling to my patients: You can have a [scheduled] repeat cesarean section, you can have a successful TOLAC, or you can have a trial and labor, fail and then have a repeat section. The highest number of complications for mom and baby are in the people who fail a trial of labor."

Providers believed that counseling in this 3-box model could lead to better outcomes by preventing women from falling into the third and worst box—a failed TOLAC. The prenatal calculator's prescient predictions induced some providers to imbue the calculator with near mystical powers: "If I had a crystal ball and I knew that you were going to need a c-section for whatever reason, then it's safer to just schedule that c-section. I don't have a crystal ball, so all we have is risk factors" (white general ob). Positioning themselves as both statisticians and soothsayers, clinicians used the calculator's early prediction to peer into the future and save women from the "turmoil" of an unscheduled surgery.

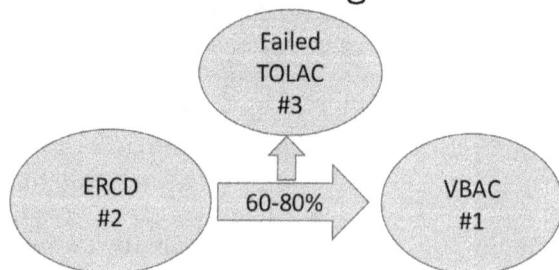

The three-box model of mode-of-birth counseling.

Figure 6.2. The 3-Box Model.

However, for those who considered pregnancy to be an embodied and unfolding process, the calculator's demand for an early decision seemed unfair. One of the interlocutors, a white Licensed Midwife (LM) who sustained a homebirth practice, had never heard of the calculator. After discussing the ideal prenatal use of the calculator in an interview, she hypothesized that the calculator put women in a difficult position: "They are gonna be put in this weird place of having to sort of foresee their own future." This midwife stressed that the individual woman does not yet know how her body will react to labor, and that the spontaneous onset of labor might be an important input for the decision to attempt a VBAC. A Hispanic CNM, who worked primarily with a population of Spanish-speaking Latina immigrants in a hospital setting, concurred. She observed that that the calculator's emphasis on early planning didn't speak to her clients: "In Western ways of thinking about things, there's this very, like, big weight put on anticipating and planning and that kind of thing and that just isn't—I haven't felt that to resonate a lot" (Adams 2009:673).

Paula, one of the pregnant participants, struggled with the decision of whether to attempt a VBAC until the end of her second pregnancy, and the physical experience of reaching full term did enable new ways for her to reason through the uncertainty of attempting a VBAC. Noting Paula's struggle to decide, her perinatologist astutely raised the possibility of waiting and seeing how things unfolded after 39 weeks. "[My perinatologist] said, like, 'Let's just go and see if by week 38 or 39, you want to do a c-section.'" Knowing that she could make her mind up depending on how she felt in the moment helped Paula to relax: "Okay. Let's see how things go. That's what I did. So the baby was born at 40 weeks and 5 days . . . Labor . . . started spontaneously. The baby was head down. Everything looked good. And so I decided, 'Okay. Let's try the VBAC.'" Waiting for normal signs at full term helped Paula to make the final decision, and she ultimately had a VBAC.

The white LM quoted above rephrased the issues of uncertainty and VBAC to be those of confidence and not of statistical prediction. "It isn't 'What is my percent chance of doing this?' The question is 'Can I do this?'" The calculator's early statistical prediction did not address the role of confidence in one's capacity to birth. By forcing an early decision, the calculator neglected the possibility that a woman might need to rebuild her confidence over the course of her pregnancy. The LM continued: "I always feel like these women are so brave to kind of like gather up their kind of confidence and, you know, rebuild their belief in themselves . . . they have to overcome that big hurdle of 'I failed. I failed . . . My body didn't work. My uterus didn't work.'" This LM concluded that the calculator's requirement for an early decision belied a lack of faith in the birth process. "It's sounds efficient and all. You're not gonna have to go through this labor if it's not gonna work . . . as opposed to having, you know, *faith in women* [emphasis mine]."

The VBAC calculator's early prediction intended to mitigate risk through the supposed security of a scheduled cesarean. In contrast, many midwives, some obstetricians, and some VBAC-interested women pursued less invasive approaches, which included waiting and seeing what would happen as the pregnancy progressed, and using cesarean as a back-up option should the need arise. Because the VBAC calculator systematically gave Black and Hispanic women lower probabilities, calculator proponents believed that such women would most benefit from knowing these low scores, helping these women "to express their autonomy" by opting for a repeat cesarean early in pregnancy. By demanding an early decision to schedule a repeat cesarean, the VBAC calculator sliced through other, more qualitative approaches to the uncertainty of planning a VBAC.

## The Problematic Logic of Non-Modifiability

The VBAC calculator narrowed the terrain of decision-making through a problematic logic of non-modifiability. The non-modifiability of the calculator's inputs, the six aforementioned prenatal risk factors, and its output—the estimated probability for a successful VBAC—arose from several related technological priorities and practices. First, the statistical practice of "variable selection" supported the notion that the calculator's variables represented objective truths. One South Asian perinatologist described the practice of variable selection as follows: "With a predictive model really you're wanting the data to guide you. I think that it is really important for predictive modeling not to do variable selection." The MFMU members did not insert their subjective determinations about which variables to include or exclude from their calculator. In essence, they believed that the data that informed the calculator spoke for itself, revealing a hidden and unmodifiable statistical "truth."

Members of the MFMU, as well as many clinician-users of the calculator, considered the inputs of age, race/ethnicity, and BMI to be non-modifiable demographic variables, as opposed to biosocial factors potentially amenable to manipulation (Susser 1998). In particular, the calculator's use of race/ethnicity as a non-modifiable, mutually exclusive, and essential category problematically obscured the ways in which specific histories of racism and ongoing processes of marginalization produce measurable differences among racial/ethnic groups (Crear-Perry et al. 2020).[4] If the calculator needed to be modified at all, it would be because women's risk factors changed over time. A white perinatologist member of the MFMU who worked on validating VBAC prediction models discussed how it would be ideal to "to refine the model every five to ten years or so as the demographics and the . . . pregnant population characteristic changes with time. That will be perfect."

Because only six variables appeared necessary to accurately estimate the probability for a successful VBAC, scientists who validated the VBAC calculator in other domestic and international settings felt that they did not need to alter the calculator's formula to include additional variables. For instance, again, provider and hospital factors contribute to successful or unsuccessful VBACs. Only a Swedish group added a hospital variable (the labor unit cesarean rate) to the VBAC calculator, and adding this variable improved prediction accuracy (Fagerberg et al. 2015). Because the calculator demonstrated the accuracy and precision of its six-variable model in multiple validation studies, it appeared that a non-modifiable statistical logic must be governing women's chances for a VBAC across settings. Finally, if the calculator's inputs were all non-modifiable, then the calculator's output—the probability for successful VBAC—also carried immutable properties. As a result, the members of the MFMU whom I interviewed never asked the scientific question of what could be done to change the probability for a successful VBAC. When I started to interview members of the MFMU in April of 2019, there was no internal agenda within the network to revise the calculator, which at that time was considered "settled science." It wasn't until the social movement to abolish race-based medicine emerged that the MFMU was compelled to revise the calculator's use of race/ethnicity as a non-modifiable and essential variable (Chadha et al. 2020).

The non-modifiability of the calculator's inputs included the "demographic factors" of age, race/ethnicity, and BMI, but also extended to the clinical indication for the prior cesarean. The clinical indication was entered into the calculator as having had a prior cesarean for a labor arrest disorder, or not. As one perinatologist mused about the calculator's inputs, "There's not a lot of modifiable things. Like you can't change what the indication was for a prior delivery." In other words, the calculator's rubric did not account for the contextual circumstances that led to the prior cesarean. When providers didn't interrogate the reasons for the prior cesarean, they unproblematically applied the calculator to all women who had a prior cesarean, treating every prior cesarean as having been clinically necessary, yet many are not. A white LM highlighted the danger of this use of the calculator: "The women right now who are trying to have a VBAC are the product of . . . an obstetrical culture that may not have been doing necessary c-sections." A Black CNM, who had a homebirth practice and who had also worked as labor and delivery nurse, worried that the calculator's model erased the variations in care that result in overmedicalized births for particular populations, especially Black women. "It's like the calculator doesn't take into account that environment in which the primary c-section took place."

The dominance of the prenatal VBAC calculator combined with the logic of non-modifiability to de-emphasize the use of VBAC calculators that incorporate intrapartum variables in addition to the demographic variables used by the VBAC calculator. Intrapartum calculators require variables known only when labor starts, and the MFMU members did develop an intrapartum version of their own calculator (Grobman 2009). Yet providers rarely used the intrapartum calculator, in part because it was more difficult to find, requiring an additional "click" on a small link at the bottom of the prenatal calculator's web page. A white general ob recognized that her use of the intrapartum calculator was unique in her community hospital in the Southwest, which required use of the prenatal calculator: "I do appreciate how the calculator has that option for when they come in and labor. You can reassess if they have a favorable cervix . . . [The intrapartum calculator] was underutilized in our practice, honestly. I think people would sort of make their decision and think 'that's it.'" The demand for an early prediction combined with the problematic logic of non-modifiability meant that a woman's probability for successful VBAC was fixed early in pregnancy and might never be revisited. Finally, providers rarely, if ever, discussed the range of uncertainty around the calculator's statistical estimate. By omitting a discussion about statistical uncertainty, providers reinforced the fixity of the calculator's prediction.

Obstetric discussions around modifying probability contrasted with the conversations that a white CNM shared. In her general approach to discussing mode of birth, this midwife talked about a range of ways to modify one's cesarean risk:

So I talk to them about all the same things that can decrease your risk of cesarean for a nulliparous woman. I talk about being admitted to the hospital at the right time. If you're in labor, not being admitted too early.[5] I talk about labor support, I talk about delivering in a hospital that supports vaginal delivery, I talk about exercise during pregnancy . . . If they want to see a midwife, it is often to have that conversation about "How can I increase my likelihood of having a successful vaginal delivery?"

Ob/gyn residents were trained in the obstetric notion that risk factors were all that were necessary to know about VBAC counseling. Risk became a master narrative that crowded out other counseling elements, as explained by two maternal-fetal medicine (MFM) specialists:

> Yeah, I feel like as a resident, it was part of our checklist of how to think about patients' risk factors for having been unsuccessful in the pursuit of vaginal birth after cesarean section, and so we would calculate the chance of success for every single patient that we would see and particularly in our high-risk obstetric clinics. (Black MFM)

> It was just a part of how we were taught to counsel about TOLAC, so we were required as a part of residency to always put those numbers in. We had to put it as a part of the medical record and then the attending would want to see what their percentage was and then the range, and then we discussed that with the patient. (Middle-Eastern MFM)

Ob/gyn residents strove to practice according to ACOG Guidelines, as they wanted to appear to be evidence-based. The calculator made it possible to make a plan for the mode of birth without first talking to the patient about her prior birth history and her desires for the upcoming birth. Thus, a score could be calculated from the medical record before going into the room, without revealing the score to the woman or how it was calculated.

In many hospitals, the number could follow the woman from her outpatient record and be written up on the management board for labor and delivery. Thus a patient with a low success score faced a barrier after arriving at the labor unit: their providers would have a lower threshold to intervene. A white general ob would often question residents about why someone's score was low, but the residents hadn't given it much critical thought: "Like, literally it is the number, and because I many times say, 'Why is their number so low?' People will be like, 'I think its BMI.' People often don't—there's not even that level [of critical thinking]." Instead of personalized care, a VBAC candidate would get branded with a number and not with her preferences.

And indeed, one of the primary complaints repeatedly voiced by VBAC candidates was that the calculator ignored their level of commitment. In fact, a woman's level of commitment can be statistically modeled and has been shown to predict attempting a VBAC (Kaimal et al. 2019). An Asian American perinatologist suggested that because the calculator excluded (and still excludes in the new version) the meaning that some women associate with a vaginal birth, the calculator might cause long-term harm: "Somebody that really, really wanted a vaginal delivery . . . that's very meaningful to her. That's just not in any of the calculators . . . I think that has potentially long-term mental health and probably physical health implications for the mom, and the baby too." Thus we can see that one of the risks the calculator did not take into account was the psychological risk to the woman who deeply desired a TOLAC but was forbidden to have one. As Davis-Floyd (2022) and others have shown, postpartum depression and even PTSD can result from such denial of deep desire.

At institutions where the VBAC calculator wasn't required per matter of policy, and providers had more leeway in their counseling strategies, some providers were drifting away from using the tool with every patient. They found that the calculator wasn't meaningful to women, especially those who professed a strong preference for VBAC. A Hispanic MFM said, "I think for women with one prior C-section, if they're very motivated from the get-go, if . . . they're very motivated for TOLAC, I find myself not using the calculator very much because it's not [instinctual] . . . I'm not trying to counsel them out of that if they're very motivated." The group of providers who ultimately used the calculator in select cases *started* with women's preferences and would only apply the calculator if the woman had some level of indecision about her options.

Following the calculator's problematic logic of non-modifiability, if a woman with a low probability for successful VBAC actually achieved a VBAC, she simply "got lucky." After all, the calculator's prediction had a range of statistical uncertainty. When providers input every prior cesarean into the calculator as an immutable fact, they sutured that cesarean to a set of non-modifiable demographic factors, thus turning prior cesareans into recurring indications.

In contrast, many VBAC candidates flexibly interpreted the calculator's inputs and did not subscribe to the view that their chances for a VBAC were fixed. VBAC candidates sought to increase their probability for a successful VBAC by transferring care to a new hospital, seeking out "VBAC-friendly" providers, switching to a community birth setting, hiring a doula, or, to the extent that they could, by trying to grow a smaller baby through changes to diet and exercise, postulating that a smaller baby would help labor to move forward more easily. In an era of decreased access to VBACs, some women need to travel long distances to a VBAC-offering hospital. Some providers softened the impact of the calculator's non-modifiable prediction by centering women's preferences, going so far as to withhold the calculator's result from motivated VBAC candidates.

## Selecting "Good" VBAC Candidates

Many providers—most often obstetricians—used the calculator to select "good" VBAC candidates by risk-stratifying them into the three boxes shown in Figure 6.1. Here too, certain uses of the calculator circumscribed women's decisions because their providers counseled—or prohibited—them from attempting a VBAC due to a low score. Women who had low scores, yet still desired to attempt a VBAC, were often made to feel as if they were unreasonable in their desires for a vaginal birth.

Professional guidelines, research, and education all discuss the role of the obstetrician in selecting "good" VBAC candidates through statistical means (ACOG 2010:454, 2019:e112). In their practice bulletin, ACOG (2019:e113) defined good candidates for VBAC as "those women in whom the balance of risks (as low as possible) and chances of success (as high as possible) are acceptable to the patient and obstetrician or other obstetric care provider." The MFMU defined a population of VBAC candidates with the lowest risk and highest probability for success as those women who had calculator scores above 60%. In a tautological explanation, a white perinatologist described perfectly how selecting good candidates was the truest benefit of prediction models: "If we counsel people in a way that more women who actually were going to succeed, tried, and less women who weren't going to succeed, didn't try, then we actually would be impacting outcomes. We would be reducing maternal morbidity and decreasing the c-section rate."

There are several problems, from the statistical to the ethical, with denying VBACs to women below the 60% threshold. For example, many VBAC prediction models—the VBAC calculator included—show decreased predictive ability in the lower score ranges—a decay in precision that the MFMU researchers acknowledged in their first article: "Only when the empirical chance of VBAC is quite unlikely (less than 35%) does the precision of the predictive model deteriorate" (Grobman et al. 2007:811). However, the MFMU researchers dismissed women with low scores as insignificant in view of the greater functioning of the calculator's statistical logic: "Yet, from a clinical standpoint, this imprecision is unlikely to be of great importance because many physicians and their patients would consider any estimate in this range to be a disincentive to attempting a VBAC" (Grobman et al. 2007:811).

Other VBAC prediction researchers have been more measured in their interpretations of low scores, and have explicitly cautioned that a low calculator score should not be used to prohibit a VBAC attempt (Metz et al. 2013b). Moreover, ACOG (2016a) has made strong ethical statements against forced, coerced, and court-ordered cesareans, and in articles that were published contemporaneously with the rise of the VBAC calculator, several bioethicists (Lyerly and Little 2010; Charles and Wolf 2018:466) recommended that the ultimate person to make the decision for or against a mode of birth should be the woman herself. However, in their VBAC guidance, ACOG left open the possibility that the obstetrician would make the final assessment of good candidacy for VBAC. As a result, an obstetric estimate of maternal/fetal safety could take precedence over an individual woman's preference for VBAC.

Because ACOG did not discuss the statistical nuances around the 60% threshold, nor did they explicitly center women's autonomy in mode-of-birth decisions, providers who were familiar with the ACOG Guidelines had only committed to memory that attempting a VBAC with below a score of 60% was "unsafe." When providers lacked knowledge of the above statistical nuances, they were more prone to misapplying the calculator in ways that discriminated against VBAC candidates with low scores, who were more likely to be racialized/ethnicized by the calculator as Black or Hispanic.

In two of the institutions where I gathered data, women with scores below 60% were strongly counseled against or prohibited from attempting a VBAC. As one white general ob discussed the official practice policy in her community hospital in the Southwest, she said: "The policy was you calculate, you get their score and if it's less than 63%, you do a C-section. If it's more than 63%, you can offer them a VBAC." After some VBAC candidates pushed back against this threshold, the hospital altered the policy to include an intrapartum re-assessment of the predicted probability. Depending on whether the woman was in spontaneous labor, for example, her calculator score might increase. However, if the score continued to be below 50%, the ob said that only "really motivated" women could continue in their attempt:

> If they walk in the door, and they're under 63%, you say, "okay, you're going to have a c- section." . . . So if they're between 50 and 63% but they seem really motivated, then we do extra counseling where we say, "We don't feel great about this, but as long as you're giving us . . . good informed consent about risks and benefits and you agreed to all that."

For example, Beatriz planned to give birth at a hospital in the Southwest that had just instituted a cutoff score of 63%. Beatriz identified as mixed-Hispanic/white ethnicity, and when her providers entered all her factors into the calculator, her score reached 61%. Notably, even when her providers categorized Beatriz as white, due her BMI, Beatriz's score did not rise above the practice threshold. Her providers held firm to a 63% cutoff, which they explained as an issue of safety. Beatriz's recollection of the practice's cutoff was 63%; I could never confirm why her providers had chosen this number, as the MFMU's own science proposed 60% as a potential lower limit. I did interview a provider in the obstetric practice where Beatriz was a patient who said that Beatriz's case caused such a controversy that the group decided that a well-counseled woman could make an informed decision to attempt a VBAC when her score ranged between 60–70%. Below 60%, the practice held a firm line.

After repeated counseling sessions, during which Beatriz's providers contrasted her birth options as between the security of a scheduled cesarean or an untimely death should she attempt a VBAC, Beatriz incredulously summarized the dearth of presented options: "I just want a chance to labor, this isn't like vaginal birth or death!" Beatriz spelled out how her clinicians used the calculator to magnify risk and present repeat cesarean as the best solution to that risk. Her providers made Beatriz feel that she was unreasonably risking her life in a planned VBAC. Beatriz entertained the notion of driving 200 miles to find a VBAC-friendly provider, yet she eventually found a supportive provider closer to home and had a successful VBAC.

A white general ob interlocutor worked at an institution in the Northeast that also had a policy of steering women with low scores toward repeat cesarean. This ob had a continuity relationship with a Black woman, Destiny, who desired a VBAC despite having a low score of 12%. Her ob spent a significant number of visits discussing mode-of-birth options with Destiny, and after all this counseling, Destiny was very clear that she still wanted a VBAC. I interviewed Destiny, who had suffered from a difficult recovery from her first cesarean yet desired a larger family. When she arrived at the labor unit for an induction of labor, the on-call ob phoned to consult with Destiny's primary ob: "The colleague contacted me that she was going to go along with the plan, however, she did not think that the patient had been appropriately counseled." If a provider supported a woman like Destiny in a planned VBAC, who at 12% had an extremely low score, the provider's clinical judgment could be called into question. Destiny did progress through her induction of labor and pushed her way to a successful VBAC.

The pressure and coercion to have a repeat cesarean that women with low scores experienced was often intense. Few ob providers commented on the contradiction present in the ACOG Guidelines and in the policies that counseled (or forbade) women with low scores from attempting a VBAC. Namely, no similar policies came into effect to counsel (or force) women with high scores to attempt a VBAC. An Asian American perinatologist pointed out this contradiction: "Because the standard of care at this point, at least in the US, is if somebody wants a repeat section, they can have one. . . . Even if they predict success scores over 90, they can still have a repeat section if they want, which is funny." The contradiction is "funny" because a woman's autonomous decision to have a VBAC is circumscribed around those who are good candidates for vaginal birth, but even good candidates for vaginal birth can elect to have a cesarean birth. While I am of course not advocating that women with high scores should be forced into vaginal births they don't desire, I am saying that the contradictory approaches to "good" and "bad" VBAC candidates demonstrate that the protected form of autonomy in obstetrics is when a patient "elects" for a cesarean birth, and not the other way around.

The calculator set up a "rational" choice between an obstetrically defined version of safety and the "irrational" choice of putting oneself at greater risk through an attempted VBAC. In hospitals where use of the calculator was more sporadic and where a range of mode-of-birth decisions were supported, a provider might have the space to support a preference-sensitive approach. As a white ob put it: "I think that the calculator—the way that I always saw it was, you have to have a conversation with the patient about what their goal is and how committed they are to try and have a vaginal delivery or how scared they are to have a vaginal delivery. That really needs to be kind of the forefront of the counseling." A *preference-sensitive* approach to counseling would say that a good VBAC candidate is anyone who wants to have a VBAC.

## Discussion: The Authoritative Status of Obstetrics

The VBAC calculator marginalized certain women by enrolling them into a well-circumscribed risk analysis that proposed surgical birth as the only solution to the probability of failure. Due to the multiple ways in which the calculator circumscribed decisions, the VBAC calculator can be understood as an example of "information packaging" (Altman et al. 2019). Through selective sharing of information, the calculator drew from and perpetuated the authoritative status of obstetrics as the modern science supposedly best equipped to deal with risks in childbirth through invasive procedures.

As a result, certain uses of the calculator expanded, rather than shrank, the terrain for surgical intervention, perpetuating obstetric dominance through racialized surgery mandates. The VBAC calculator was structured by a distinct and narrow vision of mode-of-birth counseling, namely, by an obstetric desire to deal with risk in advance through surgery. In turn, the VBAC calculator transformed the structure of mode-of-birth counseling, introducing the notion that many, if not most, women should share the obstetric desire to control risk in advance. The VBAC calculator was designed to support only one kind of decision, neglecting the diversity of the ways in which VBAC-interested women and their supportive providers approached the uncertainty of planning a VBAC (Berg 1997:676).

To address the discriminatory impacts of the race-adjusted VBAC calculator on Black and Hispanic women, the MFMU researchers recently published a model that does not use race/ethnicity as a variable (Grobman, Sandoval et al. 2021), the pictoral form of which is too diffuse to be replicated in print, but can be found at the Maternal-Fetal Medicine Units Network.[6] The eight variables in this new calculator include maternal age, height, weight, pre-pregnancy weight, BMI, obstetric history, arrest disorder indication for prior cesarean, and treated chronic hypertension (yes/no). Most unfortunately, these variables again do not include women's preferences nor their level of commitment to VBAC.

If the analysis in this chapter is correct, *any* VBAC prediction tool that exclusively relies on individual risk factors, including the new VBAC calculator, will potentially be used to circumscribe mode-of-birth decisions, especially if one prediction model dominates clinical care. The dominance of one *prenatal* VBAC prediction model narrowed the terrain of counseling, and the new calculator continues to rely only on prenatal factors.

A woman-centered approach to discussing the probability for a successful VBAC recognizes that prediction is not a relevant frame for many VBAC candidates, and therefore should not play an outsized role in counseling these women. For those VBAC candidates who desire a numeric estimate of their probability for a successful VBAC, providers should delve into a robust conversation about the multiple hospital, provider, and individual factors that influence successful VBACs. Providers should also discuss what can be done to potentially increase the probability for success, thus challenging the problematic logic of non-modifiability. Women who have low probabilities for success should be afforded a range of birth options, not just a cesarean. Finally, *no VBAC-interested person should be denied a VBAC based on what providers perceive to be a low score.* The denial of VBAC as an option for women with perceived low scores has much to do with how providers perceive risk and use cesarean surgery as the only viable intervention to deal with that risk. Those providers who use the VBAC calculator to coerce women into a surgery that has life-long reproductive and personal consequences demonstrate the need for further provider education on the statistical methods that inform VBAC prediction, on the limitations of VBAC prediction models, and on how best to translate these models into clinical practice.

In a systematic review of the 94 studies that investigated which individual factors predict VBAC, Wu and colleagues (2019:361) boasted that "the probability of successful vaginal birth is one of the most crucial factors in the decision-making process during the prenatal counseling" of women with a prior cesarean. Contrary to this assertion, I have shown in this chapter how the probability for a successful VBAC is an *obstetric* project that works for those providers and for some women who value surgical control over the uncertainty of planning a VBAC. In the realm of VBAC prediction, cesarean surgery plays a starring role, swooping in before birth gets "too risky." On the other hand, some providers and VBAC-interested women in this study advocated that cesarean surgery should play a supporting role—a back-up option only if and when the need should arise.

**Nicholas Rubashkin** is a Clinical Professor in the Department of Obstetrics, Gynecology, and Reproductive Sciences at the University California San Francisco (UCSF). He completed a PhD in Global Health Sciences, also at UCSF, where his dissertation research focused on algorithmic racism and cesarean births in the United States. Nicholas is of Hungarian descent, and in 2014 he was a Visiting Scholar at the Institute of Behavioral Sciences at Semmelweis University in Budapest, where he conducted survey research concerning Hungarian women's experiences with evidence-based and respectful care. Since 2015, Nicholas has sat on the board of directors for the international non-profit Human Rights in Childbirth.

## Notes

1. "Aneuploidy" refers to a range of conditions characterized by an abnormal numeric complement of chromosomes that are commonly evaluated during prenatal care using either screening or diagnostic testing, including: evaluation of maternal serum (e.g., cell-free fetal DNA, maternal analytes), ultrasonographic markers (e.g., nuchal translucency), amniocentesis, or chorionic villus sampling. The nuchal translucency scan (also called the NT scan) uses ultrasound to assess fetal risk of having Down syndrome and some other chromosomal abnormalities, as well as major congenital heart problems. The NT scan measures the clear (translucent) space in the tissue at the back of the fetal neck. The maternal

serum screen is a prenatal screening test that analyzes proteins excreted from the pregnancy in the maternal blood. The maternal serum screen can tell a pregnant person if their baby has an increased chance of Down syndrome; trisomy 18 (Edwards Syndrome); neural tube defects; and abdominal wall defects. An innovative technology in the past 20 years is cell-free fetal DNA, which evaluates the presence of DNA excreted from the pregnancy in maternal serum; similar to the maternal serum screen, it can evaluate for common aneuploidies, as well as sex chromosomal abnormalities (e.g., XO, or Turner's syndrome). Finally, invasive prenatal diagnosis—either through CVS or amniocentesis—can directly assess any evidence of chromosomal abnormality, inclusive of deletions and duplications in fetal genetic material; furthermore, it can also test for single-gene disorders (e.g., cystic fibrosis), which other screening modalities can incompletely evaluate, at best (see ACOG 2016b).

2. In order to compare total morbidity rates across groups, the MFMU researchers combined minor maternal (puerperal fever, blood transfusion, wound infection), major maternal (hysterectomy, operative injury), and neonatal morbidity (Apgar <4 at 5 minutes, umbilical cord arterial pH <7.00, NICU admission, hypoxic-ischemic encephalopathy, death; see Grobman et al. 2009). Their use of this composite outcome informed providers using the calculator to forbid a VBAC for reasons of safety when scores fell below 60% (see Thornton et al. 2020). Composite outcomes are much used in obstetrics and have significant limitations. To effectively use composite outcomes, the assembled outcomes should be both clinically important and of similar importance (e.g., in terms of numeric frequency). For an extended discussion on composite outcomes in obstetrics, see Herman et al. 2021.

3. Community-based Licensed Midwives (LMs) obtain their CPM certification first, then may drop it after they become state-licensed to avoid the expense of keeping it, as CPM certification must be renewed every three years. There are around 3,000 CPMs or former CPMs currently in practice in the United States (Robbie Davis-Floyd personal communication with Ida Darragh, Chair of the Board of the North American Registry of Midwives—the organization that certifies CPMs, September 22, 2022). Certified nurse-midwives (CNMs) are also LMs; according to the American College of Nurse-Midwives (personal correspondence with Robbie Davis-Floyd, September 22, 2022), there are around 14,000 CNMs currently in practice. The vast majority of them attend only hospital births; only around 200 CNMs attend community births—births at home and in freestanding birth centers. Thus there are around 17,000 LMs in the United States as compared to around 35,000 ob/gyns. (See Davis-Floyd 2022.)

4. The consequences of treating race/ethnicity as "non-modifiable" variables are so significant that I will take up the calculator's racial politics in another publication.

5. Active labor is defined as starting at 6 cm of cervical dilation. The latent phase of labor, before 6 cm, can safely take hours or days. Going to the hospital while still in latent labor greatly increases the chances of Pitocin augmentation and cesarean birth (see, for example, Palatnik and Grobman 2015).

6. Maternal-Fetal Medicine Units Network. "Vaginal Birth After Cesarean." Retrieved 8 November 2022 from https://mfmunetwork.bsc.gwu.edu/web/mfmunetwork/vaginal-birth-after-cesarean-calculator.

# References

ACOG. 2010. "ACOG Practice Bulletin No. 115: Vaginal birth after Previous Cesarean Delivery." *Obstetrics & Gynecololgy* 116(2 Pt 1): 450–463.

———. 2016a. "Refusal of Medically Recommended Treatment during Pregnancy: Committee Opinion No. 664." *Obstetrics & Gynecology* 127: e175–182.

———. 2016b. "Practice Bulletin No. 163: Screening for Fetal Aneuploidy." *Obstetrics & Gynecology* 127(5): e123–e137.

———. 2017. "Practice Bulletin No. 184: Vaginal Birth After Cesarean Delivery." *Obstetrics & Gynecology* 130: 217–233.

———. 2019. "Practice Bulletin No. 205: Vaginal Birth after Cesarean Delivery." *Obstetrics & Gynecology* 133(2): e110–127.

Adams V, Murphy M, Clarke AE. 2009. "Anticipation: Technoscience, Life, Affect, Temporality." *Subjectivity* 28(1): 246–265.

Altman MR, Oseguera T, McLemore M, et al. 2019. "Information and Power: Women of Color's Experiences Interacting with Health Care Providers in Pregnancy and Birth." *Social Science and Medicine* 12(238): 112491.

Attanasio LB, Kozhimannil KB, Kjerulff KH. 2019. "Women's Preference for Vaginal Birth after a First Delivery by Cesarean." *Birth* 46(1): 51–60.

Berg, M. 1997. *Rationalizing Medical Work: Decision-Support Techniques and Medical Practices*. Cambridge MA: MIT Press.

Campbell C. 2021. "Medical Violence, Obstetric Racism, and the Limits of Informed Consent for Black Women." *Michigan Journal of Race & Law* 26. Retrieved 8 November 2022 from https://repository.law.umich.edu/mjrl/vol26/iss0/4/.

CDC. 2019. *National Vital Statistics Reports: Births, Final Data for 2018*. Hyattsville MD: U.S. Department of Health and Human Services.

Chadha N, Kane M, Lim B, Rowland B. 2020. *Toward the Abolition of Biological Race in Medicine*. Berkeley: Othering & Belonging Institute.

Chaillet N, Bujold E, Dubé E, Grobman W. 2013. "Validation of a Prediction Model for Vaginal Birth after Caesarean." *Journal of Obstetrics and Gynaecology Canada* 35(2): 119–124.

Charles S, Wolf AB. 2018. "Whose Values? Whose Risk? Exploring Decision Making about Trial of Labor after Cesarean." *Journal of Medical Humanities* 39: 151–164.

Charmaz K. 2014. *Constructing Grounded Theory*. Thousand Oaks CA: Sage.

Cheyney M, Davis-Floyd R. 2019. "Birth as Culturally Marked and Shaped." In *Birth in Eight Cultures*, eds. Davis-Floyd R, Cheyney M, 1–16. Long Grove IL: Waveland Press.

Clarke AE. 2005. *Situational Analysis: Grounded Theory after the Postmodern Turn*. Thousand Oaks CA: Sage Publications.

Crear-Perry J, Correa-de-Araujo R, Lewis Johnson T, et al. 2020. "Social and Structural Determinants of Health Inequities in Maternal Health." *Journal of Womens' Health* 30(2): 230–235.

Cunningham FG, Bangdiwala SI, Brown SS, et al. 2010. "NIH Consensus Development Conference Draft Statement on Vaginal Birth after Cesarean: New Insights. NIH Consensus Statement." *Science Statements* 27(3): 1–42.

Davis-Floyd R. 2022. *Birth as an American Rite of Passage*, 3rd ed. Abingdon, Oxon: Routledge.

Fagerberg MC, Marsal K, Kallen K. 2015. "Predicting the Chance of Vaginal Delivery after One Cesarean Section: Validation and Elaboration of a Published Prediction Model." *European Journal of Obstetrics, Gynecology, and Reproductive Biology* 188: 88–94.

Fonseca JE, Rodriguez JL, Salazar DM. 2019. "Validation of a Predictive Model for Successful Vaginal Birth after Cesarean Section." *Colombia Medical* (Cali, Colombia) 50(1): 13–21.

Greene M. 2001. "Editorial: Vaginal Delivery after Cesarean Section: Is the Risk Acceptable?" *New England Journal of Medicine* 345: 54–55.

Grobman WA, Lai Y, Landon MB, Spong CY, et al. 2007. "Development of a Nomogram for Prediction of Vaginal Birth after Cesarean Delivery." *Obstetrics & Gynecology* 109(4): 806–812.

———. 2009. "Can a Prediction Model for Vaginal Birth after Cesarean Also Predict the Probability of Morbidity Related to a Trial of Labor?" *American Journal of Obstetrics & Gynecology* 200(1): 56 e1–6.

Grobman WA, Lai Y, Landon MB, et al. 2009. "Does Information Available at Admission for Delivery Improve Prediction of Vaginal Birth after Cesarean?" *American Journal of Perinatology* 26(10): 693–701.

Grobman WA, Sandoval G, Murguia Rice M, et al. 2021. "Prediction of Vaginal Birth after Cesarean Delivery in Term Gestations: A Calculator without Race and Ethnicity." *American Journal of Obstetrics and Gynecology* 225(6): 664.e1–664.e7.

Haraway D. 1988. "Situated Knowledges: The Science Question in Feminism and the Privilege of Partial Perspective." *Feminist Studies* 14(3): 575–599.

Healy S, Humphreys E, Kennedy C. 2017. "A Qualitative Exploration of How Midwives' and Obstetricians' Perception of Risk Affects Care Practices for Low-Risk Women and Normal Birth." *Women and Birth* 30(5): 367–375.

Herman D, Lor KY, Qadree A, et al. 2021. "Composite Adverse Outcomes in Obstetric Studies: A Systematic Review." *BMC Pregnancy and Childbirth* 21(1): 107.

Kaimal AJ, Grobman WA, Bryant A, et al. 2019. "The Association of Patient Preferences and Attitudes with Trial of Labor after Cesarean." *Journal of Perinatology* 39: 1340–1348.

Keedle H. 2020. *The Experiences of Women Planning a Vaginal Birth after Cesarean (VBAC) in Australia.* PhD dissertation, Western Sydney University: School of Nursing and Midwifery.

Leeman LM, Beagle M, Espey E, et al. 2013. "Diminishing Availability of Trial of Labor after Cesarean Delivery in New Mexico Hospitals." *Obstetrics & Gynecology* 122: 242–247.

Leonard SA, Main EK, Carmichael SL. 2019. "The Contribution of Maternal Characteristics and Cesarean Delivery to an Increasing Trend of Severe Maternal Morbidity." *BMC Pregnancy and Childbirth* 19(1): 16.

Lyerly AD, Little MO. 2010. "Toward an Ethically Responsible Approach to Vaginal Birth after Cesarean." *Seminars in Perinatology* 34: 337–344.

Lydon-Rochelle M, Holt VL, Easterling TR, Martin DP. 2001. "Risk of Uterine Rupture during Labor among Women with a Prior Cesarean Delivery." *New England Journal of Medicine* 345: 3–8.

MacDorman M, Declercq E, Menacker F. 2011. "Recent Trends and Patterns in Cesarean and Vaginal Birth after Cesarean (VBAC) Deliveries in the United States." *Clinical Perinatology* 38(2): 179–192.

Metz TD, Stoddard GJ, Henry E, Jackson M, et al. 2013a. "How Do Good Candidates for Trial of Labor after Cesarean (TOLAC) Who Undergo Elective Repeat Cesarean Differ from Those Who Choose TOLAC?" *American Journal of Obstetrics and Gynecology* 208(6): 458 e1–6.

———. 2013b. "Simple, Validated Vaginal Birth after Cesarean Delivery Prediction Model for Use at the Time of Admission." *Obstetrics & Gynecology* 122(3): 571–578.

Murphy-Lawless J. 1998. *Reading Birth and Death: A History of Obstetric Thinking.* Bloomington: Indiana University Press.

Palatnik A, Grobman WA. 2015. "Induction of Labor versus Expectant Management for Women with a Prior Cesarean Delivery." *American Journal of Obstetrics and Gynecology* 212(3): 358.e1–6.

Phelan JP. 1998. "Point/Counterpoint: II. The VBAC 'Con' Game." *Obstetrical & Gynecological Survey* 53(11): 662.

Rapp R. 2000. *Testing Women, Testing the Fetus: The Social Impacts of Amniocentesis in America.* New York: Routledge.

Sandall J, Trib RM, Avery L, et al. 2018. "Short-Term and Long-Term Effects of Caesarean Section on the Health of Women and Children." *Lancet* 392(10155): 1349–1357.

Scott KA. 2021. "The Rise of Black Feminist Intellectual Thought and Political Activism in Perinatal Quality Improvement: A Righteous Rage about Racism, Resistance, Resilience, and Rigor." *Feminist Anthropology* 2(1): 155–160.

Susser M. 1998. "Does Risk Factor Epidemiology Put Epidemiology at Risk? Peering into the Future." *Journal of Epidemiology and Community Health* 52(10): 608–611.

Thornton P, Liese K, Adlam K, et al. 2020. "Calculators Estimating the Likelihood of Vaginal Birth after Cesarean: Uses and Perceptions." *Journal of Midwifery and Womens Health* 65(5): 621–626.

Triebwasser JE, Kamdar NS, Langen ES, et al. 2019. "Hospital Contribution to Variation in Rates of Vaginal Birth after Cesarean." *Journal of Perinatology* 39(7): 904–910.

Weir L. 2006. *Pregnancy, Risk, and Biopolitics: On the Threshold of the Living Subject.* New York: Routledge.

Wendland CL. 2007. "The Vanishing Mother: Cesarean Section and 'Evidence-Based Obstetrics.'" *Medical Anthropology Quarterly* 21(2): 218–233.

Wu Y, Kataria Y, Wang Z, et al. 2019. "Factors Associated with Successful Vaginal Birth after a Cesarean Section: A Systematic Review and Meta-Analysis." *BMC Pregnancy and Childbirth* 19(1): 360–372.

CHAPTER 7

# On Risk and Responsibility
## Contextualizing Practice
## among Mexican Obstetricians

*Vania Smith-Oka and Lydia Z. Dixon*

## Introduction

Anthropologists have been increasingly interested in understanding the ontology of behaviors, beliefs, and practices within professional categories. There has also been a growing body of literature on women's experiences with obstetric care. However, less attention has been paid to the intersection of these fields: for example, the ways in which obstetricians as professionals come to behave, believe, or practice as they do. In this chapter, we draw on our combined years of experience studying reproduction in Mexico to consider how Mexican obstetricians perceive and react to national efforts to improve maternal health care, and to illustrate the importance of taking obstetricians' perspectives into account when trying to make sustainable changes.

Mexico has long been concerned with improving maternal health, implementing several efforts over the past two decades to achieve this goal, especially aiming to reduce high rates of cesareans (Althabe et al. 2004), maternal morbidity/mortality (Freyermuth, Muñoz, and Ochoa 2017; Williams 2020), and, most recently, violence toward women in obstetric encounters—known primarily as *obstetric violence* (Sadler et al. 2016; Montoya et al. 2020; see also Volume III of this series, *Obstetric Violence and Systemic Disparities* [Davis-Floyd and Premkumar 2023b]). Much of this work has been spurred in part by activist and scholarly efforts. Here, we examine Mexican obstetricians' explanations for the persistence of high cesarean rates and the use of obstetrically violent practices. Our data show that obstetricians in Mexico view activists' efforts to reduce cesareans and eliminate obstetric violence with a degree of trepidation. While some agree in principle that these efforts are noble, they may view them as interconnected with entrenched social, cultural, structural, and economic factors beyond their control, and may also push back against what they see as narratives pinning responsibility on individual obstetricians themselves.

Our argument here is twofold. First, we argue that Mexican obstetricians justify cesareans and obstetrically violent practices with discourses of *risk* and *responsibility*, which are at odds with activists' rights-centered discourse. As we describe below, obstetricians frequently see cesareans as necessary to combat what they understand to be risky bodies and pregnancies in a context of resource scarcity. Similarly, obstetricians see routine practices increasingly deemed "obstetric violence" as justified because they are believed to mitigate potential risk. In addition to discourses of risk, obstetricians discuss cesareans and obstetric violence in relation to ideas of responsibility—their responsibility for their patients and their perception of patients' lack of responsibility are both used to justify obstetricians' actions. Second, we argue that if significant, sustainable changes are to be made to cesarean rates and obstetric violence, we must take obstetricians' perspectives and the realities of their medical practices into account.

In the next sections, we briefly describe how global movements to reduce cesareans and eliminate obstetric violence have played out in the Mexican context, tying these to anthropologists' responses to growing narratives of responsibilization and risk management in obstetrics. We then draw from our ethnographic research to describe how obstetricians in hospitals in two Mexican cities interpret and respond to these movements in practice. Finally, we discuss the importance of integrating the perspectives of all stakeholders—including obstetricians—into structural and policy changes moving forward.

## Cesareans, Risk, and Obstetric Violence in Mexico: An Overview

Cesareans are lifesaving when medically necessary, yet medically risky when done unnecessarily or under subpar conditions. Mexico stands out as one of the countries with high cesarean birth (CB) rates; for comparison, Mexico's CB rate is above 45% (Uribe-Leitz et al. 2019), which is more than 10% higher than the US rate of almost 32% (Osterman et al. 2022) . In 2015, WHO published a study supporting their long-standing position that CB rates above 10–15% do not contribute to a reduction in maternal mortality and emphasizing the increased additional risks of unnecessary cesareans. One study in Mexico concluded that only 16.6% of CBs had an adequately supported indication, and that 55% of CBs were not medically necessary (Aranda-Neri et al. 2017). Many factors contribute to the increasing CB rates, including rising maternal age, socioeconomic factors (Soto-Vega et al. 2015), financial incentives, fears of malpractice lawsuits, physician convenience, and women's choice (Ronsmans, Holtz, and Stanton 2006). Addressing the causes behind rising rates is vital because of the additional risks that unnecessary CBs carry to the mother (especially in subsequent pregnancies) and to the child (Keag, Norman and Stock 2018). Risks to the mother and baby include uterine rupture, wound infection, stillbirth (in the setting of uterine rupture), preterm birth, and risks of obesity and asthma for the baby, among many others (Sandall et al. 2018). Recovery can be lengthy, exhausting, and painful (Declerq et al. 2008). There are physical, social, and economic impacts to cesareans, especially for women who lack social support or who have no time to heal before having to return to work (Lobel and DeLuca 2007; Shah et al. 2015).

Because CB rates are largely the result of obstetricians' decision-making, a focus on obstetricians' perspectives allows us to better understand some of these factors and, ultimately, to design interventions that address them in targeted, sustainable ways. Some studies have examined the power differences between patients and practitioners, in which doctors' medical expertise and authority are important factors in shaping women's decisions (Jenkinson, Kruske, and Kildea 2017). Maternal requests for CBs are equally shaped by their restricted control over childbirth and their agency (or lack thereof) within the biomedical system (Kuan 2014). Anthropologists Kristin Tully and Helen Louise Ball (2013) concluded that indications for CBs can be misrecognized: both doctors and patients may not be aware of the benefits of labor to a fetus's transition to the extra-uterine environment; patients often expect to be in control of their births; and providers are often not trained in more complicated vaginal delivery scenarios, such as breech and twin deliveries.

As concerns over rising CB rates have grown in Mexico, so too have broader concerns about how women are treated during birth. "Obstetric violence," which has become an umbrella term referencing various harmful practices, conditions, and attitudes women face in obstetric care (see Savage and Castro 2017 for a review of scholarship on the mistreatment of women in childbirth), has been well documented in Mexico (Smith-Oka 2015; Zacher Dixon 2015; Castro and Frías 2020). Examinations of obstetric violence bring together studies of the med-

icalization of birth with studies of gender inequality and gender violence. Obstetric wards incorporate much technology, ritual, and routine
(Davis-Floyd 2003, 2018a, 2022) that engender contestations over the
appropriate degree of biomedicalization (Brauer 2016). Stakes are frequently high for practitioners (with life and death often coexisting and
competing, where teamwork must be effective), and yet their jobs feel
simultaneously underappreciated, as obstetrics in Mexico is not a particularly prestigious career; it can be low paid and often necessitates
long hours. Maternity wards can be highly fraught with emotions and
contradictions. Activists and midwives across Mexico have rallied for
legislative changes to render obstetric violence illegal and hold practitioners accountable (GIRE 2015). A life free from obstetric violence fits
into the national narrative about women's rights and the right to a life
free from violence more generally.

In Mexico, there has been an increased emphasis in obstetrics on
risk and risk management. "Responsible" patient choices in reproduction
are those that are seen to best mitigate risk. A growing topic of interest
to anthropologists of reproduction is how reproductive risk is framed
as something that is scientifically measurable and that can be mitigated
through technology and behavioral modifications—a perspective that
reinforces risk as a consequence of patient choices (Fordyce and Maraesa 2012). Scholars have begun to point out how obstetricians also fall
into regimes of risk management and responsibilization. That is, it is
not just patients' choices, but rather, "all decision-making in maternity
care is deeply embedded in social and cultural narratives of risk" (Hallgrimsdottir et al. 2017:617). In this chapter, we examine how Mexican
obstetricians frame their patients as risky and in need of risk mitigation,
while also making choices that they see as mitigating potential risks to
their own careers.

## Methods

We have both worked as ethnographers in Mexico for a number of years,
interacting with various healthcare practitioners (midwives, nurses, general practitioners, obstetricians) and have seen the (sometimes differing)
ways in which they conceptualize the pregnant and laboring body, as
well as how their practices and views have changed over time. Most
recently, we have begun ethnographic data collection for a collaborative project examining, in part, obstetricians' decision-making processes
in Mexican hospitals. Both of us had our research cleared through our
own institutional review boards (IRBs) and through the local Mexican

hospital ethics review committees. We use pseudonyms to protect the identities of all involved, except, of course, for ourselves.

I (Vania) have carried out ethnographic research projects in hospital settings since 2007, the bulk of these in Puebla, a large city in central Mexico. Over this time, I have seen how healthcare workers have treated their patients, sometimes with kindness and sometimes without. In 2013, I began to specifically investigate the latter topic, first working with 86 young medical students in their university classes, and in later years (2014 and 2016) with 40 more senior students who were undergoing a year-long hospital internship. My most recent hospital ethnography (in 2018) was with 12 obstetric residents, where I aimed to understand how they made decisions about CBs. For this research, I worked in a high-density public hospital that attends to approximately 500 births a month, about 52% of which are CBs. The obstetric residents I worked with attended to many patients over the course of their shifts. The data I describe in this chapter come from this latter population.

I (Lydia) have conducted ethnographic research in Mexico since 2009, focusing on maternal health and midwifery. For years I studied Mexican midwifery education and practice and was always interested in how midwives perceived the obstetricians they knew, worked with, and learned from. It became increasingly common for midwives to describe the routine medical practices they observed in the hospitals as "obstetric violence," though they believed that hospital-based providers did not see them as such. In 2019, I began to conduct research in a public hospital in central Mexico, where I was interested in understanding what happened on the obstetrics ward from the perspectives of the obstetricians. The data I describe herein are drawn from my observations on that ward and from in-depth interviews with seven obstetricians.

## Reducing Cesareans versus the Realities of Obstetrics Wards

In my (Vania) interviews, the obstetrics residents brought out several themes that highlighted their concerns with decision-making. They identified a tension between the need to reduce cesareans and the realities of the obstetrics ward that created circumstances that increased the number of CBs they performed. All reported that they preferred vaginal birth over cesarean birth, stating that it was a gentler, more normal form of birth. They emphasized risk as a key factor impacting their patients' health and, consequently, their medical decision to intervene surgically. Risk appeared in a twofold manner: the perception of the extreme risk of childbirth (where a normal situation could turn dangerous in an instant) as well as the riskiness of patients themselves. Participants described patient persistence in requesting CBs and how, as doctors, they often felt compelled to acquiesce, even if there was no medical indication for these surgeries, because of their fear of being sued—a potential risk as well, which they preferred to avoid.

Doctor Javier,[1] a third-year resident with short black hair and a well-groomed beard, said during our interview that cesarean indications were well established when a CB would "improve the prognosis for the mother and baby." All the residents interviewed distinguished between "absolute" and "relative" cesarean indications. Doctor Rubén, a fourth-year resident, defined the difference between these, stating that in absolute indications, "there is no doubt" that a CB must be performed, while for relative ones, a vaginal birth could take place "unless [a cesarean] is necessary for a patient." He elaborated: "So, like I tell you, for absolute indications there is no turning back, right? . . . The resolution of the pregnancy must be via cesarean." Absolute indications listed by the interlocutors included acute fetal suffering, eclampsia, and placental abruption (detachment), among others.[2] One fourth-year resident, Doctor Manuel, spoke at length about risk indicators, listing several absolute indications, including placenta previa ("when the placenta comes before the baby") and placenta accreta, which is a serious condition when the:

> placenta invades tissue it shouldn't. Normally the placenta detaches when the baby is born. But when it's accreta, it invades the deeper parts of the uterus—the myometrium—and can even reach the serosal [layer]. In those cases, the placenta will not detach, and if you try to tear it out, the patient will experience massive bleeding. So, you must do a cesarean. And once you do the cesarean you have to remove her uterus, [you have to] do a hysterectomy.

It's important to note that the main cause of accreta spectrum disorder is multiple cesarean births (Cahill et al. 2018). Doctora Pamela, a third-year obstetric resident with an intense stare and a worried expression, said that "If a patient arrives with placental abruption, I'm not going to tell her, 'I'm going to give you a vaginal birth.' I know that's an indication for a cesarean. So in that case I tell her, 'So, I can't offer you a vaginal birth. The indication is for cesarean, and it's urgent.'"

Within relative indications, participants listed conditions such as pre-eclampsia, HIV+ status, gestational diabetes, chronic hypertension, some pathologies (renal, pulmonary), as well as certain fetal presentations (occiput-posterior, breech, etc.) in which the obstetrician's expertise would greatly influence the mode of birth. It is worth noting that these indications for cesarean may not hold in other contexts (Spong et al. 2012). As Doctor Rubén said, "If one doesn't have sufficient experience to get the [baby] out pelvically, they can instead perform a cesarean . . . but it's not an absolute indication." Doctor Manuel said, "So, we know that some patients have risk factors: they have oligohydramnios [too little amniotic fluid], whose membranes have broken, and they are not starting labor. Sometimes the only way to interrupt that is . . . the cesarean, primarily to prevent future risks." Doctor Javier added nuance to these definitions, while also emphasizing the benefits of cesareans: "So, the choice is up to each of us, but there are clear indications of what one must do. So, it's not like, 'Ah, well, let's operate on this one because I want to.' No. We will operate on [a patient] because she has this risk factor where it's demonstrated that the cesarean improves the risk, or . . . it provides more benefits to the mother and fetus." As Amali Lokugamage (2011) showed in her research on UK obstetricians' fears of risk, these doctors also emphasized that risk was ever-present and, though CBs carried their own forms of risk, they could also reduce overall risk.

What was interesting to us was that, despite residents distinguishing between absolute and relative indications, in their narratives there was sometimes a less-discrete boundary between them. Most participants would describe situations with relative indications, and then within a few sentences would elaborate on how rapidly situations could worsen and there would be an absolute need for a CB. Doctor Rubén's narrative illustrates this situation; he described how gestational diabetes or gestational hypertension were

[i]n general, not indicative, at all, for cesarean. That is, they are not absolute indications for cesarean. But any poor metabolic control or a serious [lack of] control in a hypertensive patient can take us to an immediate resolution. So, as such, [these diseases] are not data for an elective cesarean; but their complication . . . according to maternal wellbeing, one may evaluate their resolution via cesarean.

Though Doctor Rubén overtly described the differences between relative and absolute as discrete, through his words he inadvertently showed the gray areas between these categories, whereby CBs were sometimes the default mode of birth. Interestingly, both pathologies mentioned above do not "immediately resolve" but can take up to six weeks after delivery to resolve (ACOG 2018; 2020).

It is important to note that this hospital had a specific policy, aligned with national efforts, aimed at reducing its CB rate. Doctora Leticia, a reserved third-year resident with light brown hair tied back, who wore the required white scrubs complemented by small silver earrings and a pendant, said that though patients often arrived expecting a CB, doctors had to justify all cesareans to the government. Doctor Javier added that: "Elective cesarean exists, and can be performed if [the patient] requests it. However, in this hospital, there is a policy of prioritizing vaginal birth, so, not because a patient wants a cesarean will she be given it." Several of the residents stated that patients arrived wedded to the idea of having a cesarean, with one resident calculating that about 20% requested an elective CB. Participants gave many explanations for this request, including that private hospitals (where patients might receive prenatal care) "sold them on the idea of surgery" or that the referring primary care doctors incorrectly diagnosed the need. When interlocutors determined that there was no indication for CB, they said that "there would be complaints" from the patients about their care. They added that patients in labor would experience much pain and would "scream for a cesarean." Under those circumstances, the doctors would explain that pain was a normal part of labor as well as the risks of cesareans "so they understand that they don't have any indication to be operated on." Doctora María Elena, who wore her dark brown hair in a braid and seemed genuinely interested in humanized birth, said that when their pleading did not result in the desired CB, patients would accuse doctors of wanting "to see them suffer" by not intervening, "when in reality, in fact, if all goes well, you don't have to do much more than monitor the correct evolution" of the labor. Most public hospitals in Mexico have a scarce amount of epidural analgesia, which is reserved for CBs, so most patients labor without epidurals, but with the regular use of Pitocin (artificial oxytocin), which increases the magnitude and frequency of contractions, making labor much more painful than it would otherwise be. Doctora María Elena stated that when patients accuse her of causing their suffering, they are not entirely wrong, meaning that the structures of care (the routine procedures and the lack of epidurals), rather than the doctors' intention, cause suffering.

However, despite government or hospital policies, obstetricians spoke about feeling compelled to acquiesce to patient requests when possible. Ironically, given the issues with obstetric violence, Doctor Rubén said that hospital policy dictated that doctors should avoid obstetric violence, and so if a patient requested a CB, "in theory . . . her decision has to be respected." In an odd reversal to the "obstetric paradox": intervene to keep birth safe, thereby causing harm (Cheyney and Davis-Floyd 2019:8), the doctors could cause harm by respecting patient requests; they could find themselves performing unnecessary procedures (which are considered to be obstetrically violent; see Liese et al. 2021) while acquiescing to patient requests (and aiming to reduce obstetric violence). In addition to fearing being accused of obstetric violence, obstetricians also felt compelled to acquiesce to patient requests because they considered patients and their family members to be aggressive and litigious. Doctor Pablo, a fourth-year resident, said that patients would try to influence medical decisions by going to other doctors and hospitals "so that their [chart reflects] an indication [that she should have] an elective cesarean," so they could request a CB on arrival and not undergo labor for a vaginal birth. His words illustrate how obstetricians often placed the blame on the patients for excess CBs. Doctora Constanza, a fourth-year resident with glasses who wore her curly light brown hair in a ponytail, said that they would try to explain to these patients the reasons why CBs were performed or not, "but the relatives think that we will do a cesarean, [but] here we evaluate [the patient] and [might] do a vaginal birth." Doctor Manuel added that even when they explained to a patient's relatives about the potential risk of complications from CB, these relatives would sometimes "also get aggressive when things don't go well." Doctor Pablo said that relatives would often appear with lawyers if things went wrong, with an attitude of "let's sue them; because of poor care, she died." While death is the most tragic outcome possible, doctors also voiced concerns over being sued for other reasons, including mistreatment or incorrect diagnoses. As Doctora Pamela concluded, linking obstetric practice to potential legal consequences, when patients requested CBs without indication, the obstetricians would explain the risks:

> "To undergo a surgical procedure, it's the same as if I tell you I will operate on your heart. There's anesthesia. . . there's medications, everything." The patient doesn't understand and tells you, "No, I want a cesarean," and so you as a doctor are forced to sign off on something that might not be indicated, the patient has a complication, and you end up in jail.

These data show how the participants framed their narratives as ones in which they were the *victims* of the story, even though it has been shown by other scholars that cesareans are often performed without clear patient consent (for examples, see El Kotni 2018).

## Eliminating Obstetric Violence versus Managing Risk: The Manual Uterine *Revisión*

As the topic of obstetric violence gains traction in Mexico, obstetricians' decisions and behaviors are increasingly being scrutinized by activists, scholars, and midwives. Women have reported a wide range of types of obstetric violence in Mexican hospitals, including verbal abuse, physical abuse, and non-consensual care (Castro and Frías 2020). The doctors whom I (Lydia) interviewed were aware of the term and of allegations of violence being made by women and activist groups, but they had mixed feelings about the implications for them personally and for their profession. They agreed that some practices, such as non-consensual insertions of IUDs or verbal abuse of patients, were unacceptable. Some obstetricians also recognized that many practices deemed obstetric violence persisted because they continued to be part of doctors' official and unofficial curricula.

When I asked Doctor Flores, a senior doctor known locally as a midwifery supporter, whether he agreed that practices deemed obstetric violence needed to change, he agreed enthusiastically; he was especially concerned with routine practices done without basis in evidence. He recognized that his colleagues' reluctance to adopt updated norms for practice—such as letting laboring women drink water or walk around—was indeed problematic, but he was unsure how to change entrenched practices among his peers. Other obstetricians felt that many practices conducted in the name of risk reduction were being incorrectly marked as "dangerous" or "criminal"—in these cases, the obstetricians were defensive and sometimes angry that their expertise was being questioned. They felt justified in continuing with practices that they had learned as risk reduction strategies especially necessary for populations deemed high risk.

Doctor Valdez, another senior attending on the ward, scoffed when I mentioned the term "obstetric violence," arguing that:

> The definition is too broad, which is dangerous for patients and doctors. Everything is obstetric violence now: if the patient cannot eat, is left in bed, gets an episiotomy, has a uterine cavity *revisión* without anesthesia, if we leave them there too long, if we give them Pitocin, if we ask them about birth control too much . . . It's all considered obstetric violence. It's like they want us to leave them to lie there and not do anything! But if we don't do anything, they are like, "Why didn't you help me?" So it's like we cannot win.

Doctor Valdez went on to posit that criminalizing doctors' choices was a slippery slope: the evocation of obstetric violence undermined his professional training and practice, rendering him unable to act (or not act) without critique (and potential legal repercussions). He felt that this put his patients at risk because he might be constrained in treating them; it also put him at risk because he felt that he was under increased scrutiny.

A quintessential example of a practice deemed by some to be "obstetric violence" and by others to be "necessary" is the *revisión de cavidad uterina manual* (manual uterine cavity revision), which I refer to herein as a *revisión*. This routine practice, done postpartum in the name of reducing hemorrhage risk, involves inserting a gloved hand into the uterus to scrape out any placental remains while massaging the abdomen with the other hand. In addition to this practice being excruciatingly painful for the woman, studies have shown that it is unnecessary unless the placenta is not complete when delivered, and that it may introduce the risk of bacterial infection (Epperly, Fogarty, and Hodges 1989; Alvirde-Álvaro and Rodríguez-Anguíñiga 2009).

Like the routine use of episiotomy, the routine use of the *revisión* is common across Latin America (Camacaro Cuevas et al. 2019). In Mexico, it has long been documented in public hospitals; Matthias Sachse-Aguilera and Omar Calvo-Aguilar (2013) showed how a methodologically-problematic 1991 study supporting its benefits may have been used to reinforce the practice, despite later studies refuting that finding and revealing potential dangers. A recent review of the literature revealed that no substantial research has been done on women's qualitative responses to anesthesia or analgesia during *revisiones*, and its authors emphasized the need for better evidence to establish best practices (Kongwattanakul et al. 2020).

Obstetrician interlocutors varied in their perspectives on the routine use of the *revisión*. Doctor Flores explained that: "I don't do them unless I need to, so that is how I teach the interns as well. But I tell the interns, 'With me, you do not have to do them unless it is medically indicated. But with other doctors . . . do whatever they tell you.'" His colleagues, he said, did not all follow the same guidelines when it came to *revisiones* or episiotomies. He sighed and said that "even when the evidence exists, the studies exist, it is hard to change minds. The doctors still say: 'That's how I learned, that's how they taught me.'"

Doctora Laura, an intern, echoed Doctor Flores. "The doctors are all different," she told me. "Doctor Flores rarely does *revisiones*, but some always do them, like Doctor Valdez or Doctora Garza. You learn quickly what to do with each of them." Curious, when Doctor Valdez was next on shift I asked about his use of *revisiones*. Contrary to Doctora Laura's experience, he assured me that he didn't always do them, though he explained that he felt pressure both from the activist side *not to* do them and from the legal side *to do* them.

Doctor Valdez said, "The *parto humanizado* movement says not to do *revisiones*, or to only do them if the placenta looks incomplete, and to always use anesthesia." For Doctor Valdez, the fact that *revisiones* were the norm meant that he had to carefully document why he *did not* do one. He said that he always checked the placenta and, if it was complete, marked in the chart that he did not do a *revisión* because of the complete placenta. This step was important because "if the woman comes back with an infection a few days later, I can point at the chart and say, 'I didn't do a *revisión* because the regulations say not to for complete placentas.'"

Doctor Valdez said he only did *revisiones* when he saw any potential for concern (again contrary to what Doctora Laura thought about him). Yet he found it nearly impossible to comply with activists' mandate to only do them under anesthesia: "That sounds good, but what am I going to do, wait there half an hour for the one anesthesiologist at the hospital to show up and prep her and do an epidural? No. I just tell the woman that I am going to do it and that it is going to hurt, and I do it quickly."

Doctor Valdez's account shows that he agrees with the evidence for when a *revisión* is indicated, but still expressed fear that not doing one could be risky, potentially landing him in trouble if an infection developed—despite the fact that, again, *revisiones* can themselves cause infections. Further, he agreed with the goal of using anesthesia, but found it impossible to comply because they generally had only one anesthesiologist per shift. Doctor Valdez viewed the choice to do the *revisión* quickly and get it over with as a pragmatic one that reduced risk to the patient and to himself, carried out in a setting of less-than-ideal resources.

Doctora Garza had a reputation for being one of the obstetricians who always performed the *revisiones and* taught her interns to do the same. Moreover, she instructed them to employ active management in the third stage of labor, including cord traction to extract the placenta quickly, rather than waiting for the body to expel it—a method that may sometimes decrease blood loss postpartum but can also be dangerous, especially if done by inexperienced practitioners (Güngördük et al. 2018).

I was observing one day when a patient, Juana, delivered vaginally. From my place near her head, I watched as Doctora Garza told Doctora Ana, an intern, to put traction on the umbilical cord while massaging the woman's uterus from above. At first, Doctora Ana seemed timid, worried to push or pull too hard, but Doctora Garza moved close to her and asserted that she needed to do it right. Turning this into a teaching moment, she asked, "Where on the uterus do the contractions start?" Ana ventured, "Um, the top?" to which Doctora Garza nodded. Doctora Ana massaged the top of Juana's abdomen, hard, while Juana writhed in pain, moaning. Doctora Garza said, "We have to do this, it will be over soon." Doctora Ana pulled on the cord and massaged, and suddenly sat back, yelping "Doctora! The cord broke!" This is one of the major risks of this procedure, as a broken cord can cause a postpartum hemorrhage, and while the uterus generally delivers the placenta on its own within 30 minutes, the WHO suggests waiting up to 60 minutes before attempting to remove it manually (Urner, Zimmerman, and Krafft 2014).

Doctora Garza hurried over, found the end of the cord, and continued putting traction on it, massaging the patients' abdomen even harder, and finally the placenta slithered out. She showed it to Ana, explaining how to check that it was complete and affirming that it was. Despite this conclusion, Doctora Garza abruptly reached her whole forearm into Juana's vagina to do a *revisión*, telling her to pant. Juana cried out even louder as she tried to push herself away from the pain. Once Doctora Garza was satisfied that the uterus was empty, she stood up and let Ana take over again, telling her that Juana had agreed to a Mirena IUD (a hormone-containing IUD; see Evans, this volume) and that she should insert it now.

Later that month, a nurse showed me the register of births; something that jumped out at me was the column noting whether a *revisión* had been conducted. During my time there, 134 (91%) of the 148 women who had vaginal births had received a *revisión*. If Doctor Flores' goal of increasing evidence-based practices was going to encompass updating practices related to *revisiones*, he clearly had an uphill battle ahead of him. When I asked him what it would take to change his colleague's routine use of *revisiones*, he sighed and said that ideally, science would change their minds, but that "not everyone reads the evidence, or has the disposition to change the way they practice even if they do read it." While the WHO notes that uterine revision is customary in some countries after every birth (as is the case across much of Latin America), they argue that "There is not the slightest evidence that such policy is useful; on the contrary, it can cause infection or trauma or even shock" (WHO 1996:34). Doctor Flores' concerns reveal a disconnect between widespread practice and available evidence-based recommendations.

## How Risk, Responsibility, and Resource Scarcity Shape Decision-Making

Why do many obstetricians continue to routinely employ outdated and potentially dangerous practices like *revisiones* or elect to perform medically contraindicated CBs? To some Mexican activists, the answer is that obstetricians and Mexican hospitals are not interested in women's experiences or autonomy. For example, an outspoken critic of hospital-based obstetrics in Mexico, who had co-founded a well-known midwifery school, told me (Lydia) that "practices like these continue because women's bodies and choices are simply not respected." She admitted that some small gains had been made in hospital-based obstetrics, but argued forcefully that the overuse of *revisiones*, episiotomies, cesareans, and other practices revealed that obstetric violence was still rampant and was based on an underlying disregard for women. This perspective was shared among many birth activists and midwives, who saw the efforts of some obstetricians—like Doctor Flores, who regularly worked with local midwives—as admirable, but ineffective at addressing the underlying issues that allowed obstetric violence to persist. These activists insist that systemic change needs to occur to halt unnecessary, dangerous, and violent practices across the obstetric realm.

Discussions about humanizing practice, making it evidence-based, and reducing unnecessary CBs are increasingly common in Mexico, and have led to various new laws, hospital policies, and procedures. Yet it is not enough to simply add layers of bureaucracy that signal superficial change. I (Lydia) observed this on the ward in the form of a new state nursing form that gave space for providers to indicate the humane, "friendly birth" actions that were taken (giving the woman fluids to drink, letting her walk, giving her a massage, etc.). Although this form took up a large section of the paperwork for laboring women, it was largely ignored. Nurses and doctors explained that they did not have the resources to do all of that for women, and pointed out that many of the "friendly" practices, such as walking, eating, and drinking, were, in their opinions, risky. In Puebla, Doctora Leticia told me (Vania) that it was very hard to care for patients if they were mobile because "if the baby is born and it falls, that, well, then it's the doctors' responsibility." Her words reveal some of the trainees' potential lack of skills in obstetric care, as well as their perceptions about patients' lack of embodied knowledge about the imminence of their births. Similarly, the hospitals where we worked had been explicitly tasked with examining their CB statistics and trying to keep rates low to align with national priorities, though the obstetricians we interviewed argued that they were *already* only doing CBs when necessary. The interlocutors in Puebla felt that though they preferred vaginal births and the hospital was requiring them to reduce CBs, the realities were not conducive for them to achieve these bureaucratic expectations.

Concerns over issues of risks and resources motivated many of the decisions obstetricians made on the wards where we conducted our research. Risk takes many forms for the obstetricians with whom we worked; these include:

1. Their concern with risky patients who, doctors believed, engaged in risky practices, such as improper antenatal care or family planning, or whose social conditions, such as living in remote areas, placed them at greater risk;
2. Their belief that all pregnancies and births are underscored by risk, evidenced by the quotes and vignettes we included above that emphasize doctors' concerns with how quickly a normal situation could turn dangerous;
3. The concern with risk reduction and preventing future risks through timely obstetric interventions, such as CBs, cord tractions, or uterine *revisiones*;
4. Risk from patients themselves, specifically the risk of being sued by them.

We can see that these obstetricians' actions were motivated by ideas of risk and responsibility that frequently did not align with the medical literature and guidelines for maternal care, but rather, as we have shown elsewhere (Dixon, Smith-Oka, and El Kotni 2019; see also Davis-Floyd 1987, 2018b), were uncritically passed on from teacher to student.

In relation to the procedures discussed herein, resource scarcity shaped both the justifications for their routine use and the ways in which they were done. That is, doctors justified the need for *revisiones*, even when the placenta was complete, because they argued that their patients often lived risky lives in rural, far-flung communities, and any retained piece of placenta could lead to a deadly hemorrhage. They justified the lack of anesthesia during the procedure by explaining that there simply weren't enough anesthesiologists on duty to numb all their patients for what they saw as a brief (if painful) process. Waiting for an anesthesiologist would, they posited, put the patient at risk because of the delay, but would also put the rest of the ward at risk, because the ob would not be able to attend to other patients while waiting. They justified the use of CBs via their perceptions of inherent risk in pregnancy and birth, because the boundaries between absolute and relative indications are not always clear, and also because of the constraints due to scarcity—of beds, of pain medication, of supplies. Given the specter of risk and the lack of resources (real and perceived), many obstetricians argued that their responsibility to prevent harm superseded a responsibility to comply with activists' anti-obstetric violence demands.

What we both saw across our sites was that the fear of potential future risks—medical or legal—motivated many obstetricians to opt for higher risk procedures like CBs and *revisiones*. In their decision-making, they not only weighed the potential outcomes of future risks against those of immediate risks (e.g., their fears of long-term risk of uterine rupture versus the immediate need to save a life), and sometimes determined that the immediate risks were worth it, but they also weighed different risks to decide which ones were more acceptable than others (e.g., the fleeting pain of a *revisión* versus a potential future hemorrhage). Their decision-making was shaped by their training as well as by their medical expertise. Many of them also had mixed feelings about obstetric violence, considering it an important concern but also feeling paralyzed by the potential risk to their careers of being accused of violence by intervening too much or too little. The question of timing and choice of interventions is taken up in Melissa Cheyney and Robbie Davis-Floyd's (2020) advocacy for what they call RARTRW care—the right amount at the right time in the right way—as opposed to care that is TMTS (too much too soon) and TLTL (too little too late) (Miller et al. 2016).

Even though some of the practices at these hospitals are considered outdated or even dangerous by international standards, many of them remain due to a combination of socialization and inertia (for example, obstetricians say things like, "This is how I was trained and how things are done") and fears of unexpected risk, such as when they ask, "What would happen if I don't do this?" In her chapter in this volume, Davis-Floyd refers to the effects of these attitudes as "Stage 1 naïve realism"—a position from which obstetricians come to view their way as the only possible way. This naïve realism helps to explain why practitioners such as Doctor Flores and Doctora María Elena, who were deeply concerned with changing the practices within their hospitals, would often find themselves having to justify why they were *not* engaging in these routine practices. Davis-Floyd (Chapter 1, this volume) would label such doctors "Stage 4 humanistic practitioners," as they are among those proposing that "there must be better ways that honor everyone's human rights."

## Conclusions: Listening to Obstetricians to Achieve Systemic Change

In this chapter, we have paid close attention to what our Mexican obstetrician interlocutors do and what they say about their obstetric care. Though it can be tempting to categorize their practices as unnecessary, harmful, and as obstetric violence, our aim here has been to be more nuanced in our approach. These doctors find themselves pressured from both sides: national policies aimed at reducing unnecessary CBs and obstetric violence restrict their "normal" practices and make them doubt themselves, while patients may sue them if they do not acquiesce to their requests for CBs. However, we want to make clear that we do disagree with many of these practices; denying patients water, food, and movement, and/or subjecting them to painful uterine *revisiones* are undoubtedly problematic. Many obstetricians across Mexico agree with the need for broad, humanistic reforms to hospital-based maternity care and, as some interlocutors expressed above, recognize that many of their colleagues are not willing to change how they practice obstetrics. Blaming individual doctors or trying to change behavior at the individual level will not work, especially when problematic practices are intrinsic to the educational system and are reinforced through embodied apprenticeship training on the maternity wards.[3] Additionally, the public hospital system in Mexico and how the country allocates resources strains the ability of many biomedical institutions and their practitioners to carry out their work while following international obstetric standards of care. To reduce high rates of CBs and incidences of obstetric violence, change must happen on a systemic level.

For systemic changes to occur, we must understand doctors' decision-making rationales and take their fear-based perspectives about risk and responsibility into account, while also paying attention to the concerns raised by scholars and activists. Currently, many obstetricians fear that changing how they practice will open them (and their patients) to increased risks, yet the activist, scholarly, and governmental push to reduce CBs and eliminate obstetric violence has illuminated the urgent need for change. Because of the strained system, obstetricians cannot always practice in evidence-based ways; indeed, paradoxically, they believe that following the (risk reducing) international guidelines (minimizing CBs and *revisiones*) would actually *increase* risk—a belief contrary to the scientific evidence and to the opinions of reproductive scholars.

Bridges must be built between the evidence and obstetricians' and scholar/activists' perspectives and goals. Activists and scholars have increasingly called on obstetricians to reduce CBs, to take concerns about obstetric violence seriously, and to change their practices to create more humane treatment. Given obstetrician participants' awareness of the movement for humanized birth and against obstetric violence, as expressed above, it is clear that these calls to action have been heard—and yet the ob interlocutors felt themselves stuck between "a rock and a hard place"—between their perceptions of risk and women's and the government's desires for them to engage in what they perceive as risky behaviors, such as lowering CB rates and stopping the performance of *revisiones*. Linking these broader concerns is a call for obstetrics to get with the times: to recognize the evidence linking humanistic obstetric care to better quantitative and qualitative outcomes.

However, there is also a need to allow doctors to comply with evidence-based best practices without fear of legal repercussions, and to find ways to increase the quality of care even within resource-poor settings. By listening to obstetricians' concerns, we can better arrive at creative solutions that allow them to do their jobs while also improving care. For example, despite cramped quarters on the ward, privacy curtains could be drawn to allow patients to bring in partners or family members who can support them. Adding that support would reduce patient stress, and potentially also reduce the constant monitoring and interventions performed. Reporting protocols could be changed so that doctors who conduct *revisiones* have to justify *why* they did so, rather than having to justify why they do *not* do them. Hospitals could incorporate CB monitoring systems (such as the Robson Classification, supported by the WHO, which is a system designed to help practitioners understand childbirth patterns based on several factors, such as a woman's obstetric history, gestational age at delivery, fetal presentation, parity, etc.) into their practices to track not only the number of CBs, but also which patients receive them and why (Vogel et al. 2015). These are just a few minor changes that could have major impacts on patients and on biomedical interns and residents learning in the maternity wards. Continued research into the perspectives of the obstetricians and nurses working on the front lines is needed to develop further changes, as are re-socialization courses that train them in how to facilitate normal physiologic births. By including their buy-in and input, they can be central to attempts to ensure much-needed systemic changes.

**Vania Smith-Oka** is an Associate Professor of Anthropology at the University of Notre Dame. Her work addresses questions of obstetric violence, medical decision-making, cesareans and incisions, medical spaces, and medical training in Mexico and Kenya. Her first book, *Shaping the Motherhood of Indigenous Mexico* (2013) explores how state programs used conditional cash programs to develop "good motherhood" and "good citizenship"; her second book, *Becoming Gods: Medical Training in Mexican Hospitals* (2021) examines the ways in which medical students developed the skills, attitudes, and practices of biomedicine within a shaky biomedical system.

**Lydia Z. Dixon** is an Assistant Professor of Health Science at California State University, Channel Islands. Trained as a medical anthropologist at the University of California, Irvine, she has worked in the field of reproductive health in Mexico for two decades and publishes on topics related to midwifery, childbirth, obstetric violence, and global development. Her book *Delivering Health: Midwifery and Development in Mexico* (2020) examines how midwifery education in Mexico addresses various global development, health outcomes, and human rights concerns related to reproduction and gender inequality.

## Notes

1. We use the gendered "Doctor" (masculine) and "Doctora" (feminine) as used in Mexico. Further, we use first names for residents and last names for attending physicians, as was the convention in these hospitals.
2. Obstetricians in Mexico use the terms "fetal suffering" and "asphyxia" to indicate the same thing.
3. Some of the chapters in Volume I of this series (Davis-Floyd and Premkumar 2023a) show what happens to individual obstetricians when they go against the technocratic grain by shifting to humanistic or holistic practice (see Cooper 2023; Fontes 2023; Geréb and Fábián 2023; Jones 2023); such obstetricians inevitably experience ostracism, and often persecution, by their technocratic colleagues, and are generally unable to create any kind of systemic change.

## References

Althabe F, Belizán JM, Villar J, Alexander S, et al. 2004. "Mandatory Second Opinion to Reduce Rates of Unnecessary Caesarean Sections in Latin America: A Cluster Randomised Controlled Trial." *Lancet* 363(9425): 1934–1940.

Alvirde-Álvaro O, Rodríguez-Anguíñiga G. 2009. "Revisión Rutinaria de Cavidad Uterina en el Postparto Inmediato." *Archivos de Investigación Materno-Infantil* 1(2): 58–63.

American College of Obstetricians and Gynecologists (ACOG). 2018. "Practice Bulletin No. 190: Gestational Diabetes Mellitus." *Obstetrics & Gynecology* 131(2): e49–e64.

———. 2020. "Practice Bulletin No. 222: Gestational Hypertension and Preeclampsia." *Obstetrics & Gynecology* 135(6): e237–e260.

Aranda-Neri JC, Suárez-López L, DeMaria LM, Walker D. 2017. "Indications for Cesarean Delivery in Mexico: Evaluation of Appropriate Use and Justification." *Birth* 44(1):78–85.

Brauer S. 2016. "Moral Implications of Obstetric Technologies for Pregnancy and Motherhood." *Medicine, Health Care and Philosophy* 19(1): 45–54.

Cahill AG, Beigi R, Heine RP, Silver RM, Wax JR. 2018. "Placenta Accreta Spectrum." *American Journal of Obstetrics and Gynecology* 219(6): B2–B16.

Camacaro Cuevas M, Arismendi Serrano M, Orellana Cabrera E, Pinto Ramos M, Naranjo M. 2019. "Voces de Mujeres que Denuncian la Violencia Obstétrica: Revisión Manual Uterina Como Rutina." *Revista Inclusiones: Revista de Humanidades y Ciencias Sociales* 6: 14–35.

Castro R, Frías SM. 2020. "Obstetric Violence in Mexico: Results from a 2016 National Household Survey." *Violence Against Women* 26(6–7): 555–572.

Cheyney M, Davis-Floyd R. 2019. "Birth as Culturally Marked and Shaped." In *Birth in Eight Cultures*, eds. Davis-Floyd R, Cheyney M, 1–16. Long Grove IL: Waveland Press.

Cheyney M, Davis-Floyd R. 2020. "Birth and the Big Bad Wolf: A Biocultural, Co-Evolutionary Perspective, Part 2." *International Journal of Childbirth* 10(2): 66–78.

Cooper J. 2023. "An Awakening." In *Obstetricians Speak: On Training, Practice, Fear, and Transformation*, eds. Davis-Floyd R, Premkumar A, Chapter 5. New York: Berghahn Books.

Davis-Floyd R. 1987. "Obstetric Training as a Rite of Passage." *Medical Anthropology Quarterly* 1(3): 288–318.

———2003. *Birth as an American Rite of Passage*, 2nd edn. Berkeley: University of California Press.

———. 2018a. "The Rituals of Hospital Birth." In *Ways of Knowing about Birth: Mothers, Midwives, Medicine, and Birth Activism*, Davis-Floyd R and Colleagues, 45–60. Long Grove IL: Waveland Press.

———2018b. "Medical Training as Technocratic Initiation." In *Ways of Knowing about Birth: Mothers, Midwives, Medicine, and Birth Activism*, Davis-Floyd R and Colleagues, 107-140. Long Grove IL: Waveland Press.

———. 2022. *Birth as an American Rite of Passage*, 3rd edn. Abingdon, Oxon: Routledge.

Davis-Floyd R, Premkumar A, eds. 2023a. *Obstetricians Speak: On Training, Practice, Fear, and Transformation*. New York: Berghahn Books.

Davis-Floyd R, Premkumar A, eds. 2023b. *Obstetric Violence and Systemic Disparities: Can Obstetrics Be Humanized and Decolonized?* New York: Berghahn Books.

Declercq E, Cunningham DK, Johnson C, Sakala C. 2008. "Mothers' Reports of Postpartum Pain Associated with Vaginal and Cesarean Deliveries: Results of a National Survey." *Birth* 35(1): 16–24.

Dixon LZ, Smith-Oka V, El Kotni M. 2019. "Teaching about Childbirth in Mexico: Working across Birth Models." In *Birth in Eight Cultures*, eds. Davis-Floyd R, Cheyney M, 17–47. Long Grove, IL: Waveland Press.

El Kotni M. 2018. "Between Cut and Consent: Indigenous Women's Experiences of Obstetric Violence in Mexico." *American Indian Culture and Research Journal* 42(4): 21–41.

Epperly TD, Fogarty JP, Hodges SG. 1989. "Efficacy of Routine Postpartum Uterine Exploration and Manual Sponge Curettage." *Journal of Family Practice* 28(2): 172–176.

Fontes R. 2023. "Repercussions of a Paradigm Shift in the Professional and Personal Life of a Brazilian Obstetrician." In *Obstetricians Speak: On Training, Practice, Fear, and Transformation*, eds. Davis-Floyd R, Premkumar A, Chapter 6. New York: Berghahn Books.

Fordyce L, Maraesa A. 2012. "Introduction: The Development of Discourses Surrounding Reproductive Risks." In *Risk, Responsibility, and Narratives of Experience*, eds. Fordyce L, Maraesa A, 1–13. Nashville TN: Vanderbilt University Press.

Freyermuth MG, Muños JA, Ochoa, MP. 2017. "From Therapeutic to Elective Cesarean Deliveries: Factors Associated with the Increase in Cesarean Deliveries in Chiapas." *International Journal for Equity in Health* 16(1): 1–15.

Geréb A, Fábián K. 2023. "Hungarian Birth Models Seen through the Prism of Prison: The Journey of Ágnes Geréb." In *Obstetricians Speak: On Training, Practice, Fear, and Transformation*, eds. Davis-Floyd R, Premkumar A, Chapter 8. New York: Berghahn Books.

GIRE (Grupo de Información en Reproducción Elegida). 2015. *Obstetric Violence: A Human Rights Approach*. Mexico City: Grupo de Información en Reproducción Elegida, A.C. Retrieved 8 November 2022 from https://gire.org.mx/wp-content/uploads/2020/02/ObstetricViolenceReport.pdf.

Güngördük K, Olgaç Y, Gülseren V, Kocaer M. 2018. "Active Management of the Third Stage of Labor: A Brief Overview of Key Issues." *Turkish Journal of Obstetrics and Gynecology* 15(3): 188–192.

Hallgrimsdottir H, Shumka L, Althaus C, Benoit C. 2017. "Fear, Risk, and the Responsible Choice: Risk Narratives and Lowering the Rate of Caesarean Sections in High-income Countries." *AIMS Public Health* 4(6): 615–632.

Jenkinson B, Kruske S, Kildea S. 2017. "The Experiences of Women, Midwives and Obstetricians When Women Decline Recommended Maternity Care: A Feminist Thematic Analysis." *Midwifery* 52: 1–10.

Jones R. 2023. "The Bullying and Persecution of a Humanistic/Holistic Obstetrician in Brazil: The Benefits and Costs of My Paradigm Shift." In *Obstetricians Speak: On Training, Practice, Fear, and Transformation*, eds. Davis-Floyd R, Premkumar A, Chapter 7. New York: Berghahn Books.

Keag OE, Norman JE, Stock SJ. 2018. "Long-Term Risks and Benefits Associated with Cesarean Delivery for Mother, Baby, and Subsequent Pregnancies: Systematic Review and Meta-Analysis." *PLOS Medicine* 15(1): e1002494.

Kongwattanakul K, Rojanapithayakorn N, Laopaiboon M, Lumbiganon P. 2020. "Anaesthesia/Analgesia for Manual Removal of Retained Placenta." *Cochrane Database of Systematic Reviews* 4: CD013013.

Kuan CI. 2014. "'Suffering Twice': The Gender Politics of Cesarean Sections in Taiwan." *Medical Anthropology Quarterly* 28(3): 399–418.

Liese K, Davis-Floyd R, Stewart K, Cheyney M. 2021. "Obstetric Iatrogenesis in the United States: The Spectrum of Unintentional Harm, Disrespect, Violence, and Abuse." *Anthropology & Medicine* 28(2): 1–16.

Lobel M, DeLuca RS. 2007. "Psychosocial Sequelae of Cesarean Delivery: Review and Analysis of Their Causes and Implications." *Social Science & Medicine* 64(11): 2272–2284.

Lokugamage A. 2011. "Fear of Home Birth in Doctors and Obstetric Iatrogenesis." *International Journal of Childbirth* 1(4): 263–272.

Miller S, Abalos E, Chamillard M, et al. 2016. "Beyond Too Little, Too Late and Too Much, Too Soon: A Pathway Towards Evidence-Based, Respectful Maternity Care Worldwide." *Lancet* 388(10056): 2176–2192.

Montoya A, Fritz J, Labora A, Rodriguez M, Walker D, Treviño-Siller S, González-Hernández D, Lamadrid-Figueroa H. 2020. "Respectful and Evidence-Based Birth Care in Mexico (Or Lack Thereof): An Observational Study." *Women and Birth* 33(6): 574–582.

Osterman MJK, Hamilton BE, Martin JA, Driscoll AK, Valenzuela CP. 2022. "Births: Final Data for 2020." National Vital Statistics Reports, 70(17). Retrieved 25 November 2022 from https://www.cdc.gov/nchs/products/index.html.

Ronsmans C, Holtz S, Stanton C. 2006. "Socioeconomic Differentials in Caesarean Rates in Developing Countries: A Retrospective Analysis." *Lancet* 368(9546): 1516–1523.

Sachse-Aguilera M, Calvo-Aguilar O. 2013. "Indicaciones de la Revisión Manual de la Cavidad Uterina durante la Tercera Etapa de Trabajo de Parto: Revisión de la Evidencia." *Revista CONAMED* I(1): 31–36.

Sadler M, Santos MJDS, Ruiz-Berdún D, et al. 2016. "Moving Beyond Disrespect and Abuse: Addressing the Structural Dimensions of Obstetric Violence." *Reproductive Health Matters* 24(47): 47–55.

Sandall J, Tribe RM, Avery L, Mola G, et al. 2018. "Short-Term and Long-Term Effects of Caesarean Section on the Health of Women and Children." *Lancet* 392(10155): 1349–1357.

Savage V, Castro, A. 2017. "Measuring Mistreatment of Women During Childbirth: A Review of Terminology and Methodological Approaches." *Reproductive Health* 14(138): 1–27.

Shah NT, Golen TH, Kim JG, Mistry B, et al. 2015. "A Cost Analysis of Hospitalization for Vaginal and Cesarean Deliveries." *Obstetrics & Gynecology* 125(91S).

Soto-Vega E, Urrutia-Osorio M, Arellano-Valdez F, López-Begines IY, Hernández-Romero CH. 2015. "The Epidemic of the Cesarean Section in Private Hospital in Puebla, México." *Obstetrics & Gynecology International Journal* 2(6): P.00058.

Smith-Oka V. 2015. "Microaggressions and the Reproduction of Social Inequalities in Medical Encounters in Mexico." *Social Science & Medicine* 143: 9–16.

Spong CY, Berghella V, Wenstrom KD, Mercer BM, Saade GR. 2012. "Preventing the First Cesarean Delivery: Summary of a Joint Eunice Kennedy Shriver National Institute of Child Health and Human Development, Society for Maternal-Fetal Medicine, and American College of Obstetricians and Gynecologists Workshop." *Obstetrics & Gynecology* 120(5): 1181–1193.

Tully KP, Ball HL. 2013. "Misrecognition of Need: Women's Experiences of and Explanations for Undergoing Cesarean Delivery." *Social Science & Medicine* 85: 103–111.

Uribe-Leitz T, Barrero-Castillero A, Cervantes-Trejo A, Santos JM, De La Rosa-Rabago A, Lipsitz SR, Basavilvazo-Rodriguez MA, Shahf N, Molinaf RL. 2019. "Trends of Caesarean Delivery from 2008 to 2017, Mexico." Bulletin of the World Health Organization 97 (7): 502.

Urner F, Zimmermann R, Krafft A. 2014. "Manual Removal of the Placenta after Vaginal Delivery: An Unsolved Problem in Obstetrics." *Journal of Pregnancy* 2014: 274651.

Vogel JP, Betrán AP, Vindevoghel N, Souza JP, et al. 2015. "Use of the Robson Classification to Assess Caesarean Section Trends in 21 Countries: A Secondary Analysis of Two WHO Multicountry Surveys." *Lancet Global Health* 3(5): e260–e270.

WHO. 1996. *Care in Normal Birth: A Practical Guide*. Report of a Technical Working Group. Retrieved 8 November 2011 from https://www.mhtf.org/document/care-in-normal-birth-a-practical-guide/.

———. 2015. *WHO Statement on Caesarean Section Rates*. Geneva: World Health Organization. Retrieved 25 November 2022 from https://www.who.int/publications/i/item/WHO-RHR-15.02.

Williams SA. 2020. "Narratives of Responsibility: Maternal Mortality, Reproductive Governance, and Midwifery in Mexico." *Social Science & Medicine* 254(112227): 1–9.

Zacher Dixon L. 2015. "Obstetrics in a Time of Violence: Mexican Midwives Critique Routine Hospital Practices." *Medical Anthropology Quarterly* 29(4): 437–454.

# CHAPTER 8

# Crossing Bodily, Social, and Intimate Boundaries

## How Class, Ethnic, and Gender Differences Are Reproduced in Medical Training in Mexico

*Vania Smith-Oka and Megan K. Marshalla*

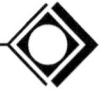

How are social, intimate, and physical boundaries crossed during certain interactions? What factors structure the ways in which these boundaries can be crossed and by whom? What determines whose boundaries are crossed and whose are not? And how do bodies interact to create and reconfigure knowledge about boundaries and their crossings? In this chapter we address these questions, using data from our research on biomedical training in Mexico.[1] Drawing on frameworks of embodied learning (Cohen 2010; Downey 2010; Prentice 2013; Harris 2016) and of sensory skills in training (Rose 1999; Van Dongen and Elema 2001; Van Drie 2013), we unpack how, among Mexican biomedical obstetric practitioners and students, knowing and being known, seeing and being seen, touching and being touched, and feeling and being felt are stratified in particular ways by the broader political economy. The obstetricians and obstetric trainees we interviewed repeatedly emphasized that their biomedical practice and expertise did not mean simply diagnosing, providing a prognosis, and establishing treatment, but also encompassed a "grounded cognition" (Cohen 2010:S194) in the development, maintenance, and refinement of the ability to use their bodies to touch, examine, probe, or cut the bodies of their patients. As Sheila Kitzinger (1997) reminded us, touch in childbirth can be classified according to its social function, whether that is instrumental or affective. As we show below, the forms of touch used by the obstetrician (ob) trainees we met were almost entirely instrumental—as a means to perform a task.

Medical trainees (who included interns and residents, whom we define below) seemed to grapple with the acquisition of such skills, appreciating the ability to engage in practice but also acknowledging how complex it was to learn these skills. Though hands were key parts of their practices, they also used many other parts of their bodies—including fingers, arms, ears, noses, and backs (see below)—in their clinical interactions with patients. All of these body parts served as social objects connecting bodies (those of patients and practitioners) that crossed multiple boundaries—the physical boundaries of the skin, the social boundaries of class, race, or gender, and the sensory boundaries of the emic patient body and the etic physician body. Abstract medical knowledge is internalized through what we have termed *somatic translation*, meaning the embodied processes of learning, repeating, and making the body (of both patient and physician) legible. This "embodiment approach" emphasizes the bidirectionality of the material, neural, and physical realms with the conceptual, behavioral, and perceptual realms (Cohen 2010; Downey 2010). As bodies are trained to know and perceive, they change and are shaped by this knowledge and these perceptions (Harris 2016), in what Greg Downey (2010) has called "an alteration of the organic architecture of the body." That is, embodiment entails a complete interior change—from neural and perceptual to anatomical—so that biomedical trainees can "accomplish tasks, that, prior to enskillment, were impossible" (Downey 2010:S35).

In this chapter, we analyze how somatic translation and the oft-repeated term among our interlocutors of *manitas* (meaning being hands-on—but this term also carries a deeper meaning, as we elaborate later on) intersect with the broader political economy (particularly with gender, skin color, and class differences). We address the effects of this intersection on the bodily practices of obstetricians when they interact with their patients, asking: What social effects do these practices produce? In this manner, we elaborate on how class and ethnic differences are learned and perpetuated through medical bodies. We analyze how these deeper structures that shape the social lives of medical hands also somatically translate biomedical expertise and care toward particular types of social difference. Building on Rachel Prentice's (2005) work on "mutual articulation," Janelle Taylor's (2005) concept of "surfacing the body's interior," Byron Good's (1994) analysis of how medicine constructs its objects, and Anna Harris's (2016) study of how bodies are configured through multisensory practice, we deepen the scholarly analysis of embodied practice by adding a broader political economic framework to examine how skillful practice is cultivated, is deeply embedded in the clinical and diagnostic process, and is part of obstetric

196 ◆ Vania Smith-Oka and Megan K. Marshalla

encounters. In places such as Mexico, with deep fissures between vulnerable and agentive populations, the bulk of the patients upon whom medical trainees learn are economically or socially vulnerable, or both; their bodies are seen to have fewer boundaries—or more permeable or breachable boundaries—and are more likely to receive treatment by unskilled and unpracticed biomedical trainees.

Hands and body parts are perceptual instruments, meaning that they can sense while they act (Anderson and Dietrich 2012); a central part of biomedical training is learning to cultivate and discipline the body's senses (Hirschauer 1991), including touch, sight, sound, and smell (leaving only taste outside of the current biomedical approach). While the "clinical hand" is often the first point of contact between a patient and biomedical care, and is very much in use in biomedical practice, obs use many parts of their bodies in complex ways to examine their patients—through observation, palpation, percussion, and auscultation. ("Percussion" is a method of tapping body parts with fingers, hands, or small instruments for certain types of diagnosis; percussion of a body part produces a sound that can be heard by ear or, more usually, via a stethoscope. "Auscultation" in obstetrics means listening to the fetus's heartbeat.)

Obs' medical bodies can connect or create distance, cross boundaries as allowed through social scripts, and wield technology and implements to cut, suture, examine, puncture, touch, or heal a patient's body. Medical trainees can learn to break the social rules they are accustomed to and to touch people in ways they would not in non-clinical encounters, or in ways with which they are not yet familiar.

Our study focuses not only on the role of the *medical body*, but also on the boundaries that body is allowed to cross. "Medical bodies" are what Etienne Wenger (2010:128) refers to as *boundary objects*: they find their value in being able to connect across boundaries. As we discovered during our interviews, body parts, such as hands, fingers, or ears, become instruments that allow biomedical practitioners to move across boundaries—a surgeon's hands can move an assistant's hands while cutting a patient's body; a first-year obstetrics resident's fingers can do a pelvic exam on a woman in labor; an intern's hands can palpate a patient's pregnant belly to determine fetal position while their ears can hear the fetal heartbeat. But not just any bodies can cross these boundaries; only medical bodies can do so, because of social conventions and because clinicians are experts who have the requisite skills and are socially expected to touch their patients. As we discovered, not all clinicians can cross the same social, physical, or sensory boundaries. As a tool of the trade, the "medical body" (the body of the biomedical practitioner) acts as a mediator, closing the social distance between obstetrician and patient. Obstetricians come to *know* their bodies during their training, understanding them as extensions not only of themselves but of their community as well.

## Ethnographic Encounters

We conducted the research on which this chapter is based between 2013 and 2016 in the city of Puebla, Mexico, which has slightly more than 1.5 million people living within the city limits (INEGI 2017) and perhaps another 300,000 to 400,000 people in the larger metropolitan area, of whom almost half have no medical insurance (INEGI 2014). We conducted this research in two locations in Puebla: a public hospital ("Hospital Salud") and a private hospital ("Hospital Piedad"). (All names of institutions and people have been changed for privacy and confidentiality.) Hospital Salud's lower-middle-class and working-class patients were enrolled in this hospital's care because they or one of their family members worked for the government. Hospital Piedad was a small private teaching hospital that served middle- and upper-middle-class patients, as well as some less-affluent patients whose companies provided them with health insurance.

Our participants included 50 medical interns from Hospital Salud and 26 from Hospital Piedad; three obstetric residents from Hospital Salud; and three obstetricians from Hospital Piedad and one from Hospital Salud. Though in the United States and other countries, "intern" refers to a first-year resident, in Mexico these are two distinct categories of trainees. Interns are students in their fifth year of medical school who engage in a year-long internship rotation at a hospital, which is followed by their sixth and last year: a mandatory year of social service. (In Mexico, all professionals must spend one year after graduation performing a social service of some kind; medical doctors are often assigned to serve in rural clinics that have no permanent doctors.) Residents have been accepted into a residency program in their chosen specialty after passing the national residency exam. Our ethnographic research consisted of observations of their practices and of formal classes, clinical rounds, and case history presentations. We spent time with them during procedures in the surgery and ob/gyn wards, as well as in the emergency room, and carried out unstructured and semi-structured interviews with them, during which we discussed their perceptions of life as biomedical practitioners, their expectations and experiences with mentorship, and how they had learned certain skills.

## Traversing Bodily and Social Boundaries

As we examined the responses we collected, it became increasingly clear to us that obstetricians learned to use their bodies as medical implements by converting theory (book knowledge) into practice (practical, skill-based knowledge). In this "situated learning" (Lave and Wenger 1991), medical trainees shifted from acquiring transmitted knowledge to constructing knowledge through practice in embodied ways. In the process, they also learned (without realizing it) how to cross boundaries. We first became interested in exploring the roles of bodies in obstetric training after our participants began elaborating on the processes of *meter mano* and *hacer manitas*, which on the surface mean putting one's hands into or onto someone's body, yet also implies getting them "dirty" through practice. Interns stated that "*hacer manitas* [is] where you are allowed to *touch* the patient." Yet these phrases go beyond simply hands and touch, instead emphasizing the crossing of bodily boundaries and of entering the bodies of others by using a multisensorial approach. Both expressions can also carry a more sexual innuendo, especially the sense of "groping around," which also conveys a sense of dirtiness, though of a different kind. In accordance with Mary Douglas's (1966) definition of dirt as "matter out of place," some of this dirtiness also involves the discomfort of crossing bodily and intimate boundaries. "It smells bad," was what one male intern said regarding patients in ob/gyn (though he was unconcerned about the odors in urology, his dream specialty). The meaning of *manitas* suggests the use of hands and other body parts to cross boundaries to become sensorially familiar with another's body. *Manitas* allow obs to "get dirty" by touching a patient; they can directly detect "unseen problems" by linking to another's body with their own (Hinojosa 2002:23), by "surfacing the body" (see below) (Taylor 2005), which allows them to understand sensory experiences such as the "feel of a scalpel on human flesh" (Wendland 2010:91). Similar to the doctors in Harris's (2016) work, who were learning percussion techniques (see below), the trainees in our research learned, through *manitas*, embodied techniques for identifying bodily sensory differences and similarities; they also developed a greater awareness and sensibility of their own bodies and those of their patients—what Harris (2016:51) called "the strangers within." Through *manitas*, the bodies of obstetric practitioners traverse conventional skin and social boundaries, as well as structural boundaries of gender, race, and class. They also cross boundaries through what we term *somatic translation* in order to see, feel, and sense others' bodies with their own.

During training and biomedical encounters, the interns we observed were taught to traverse conventional boundaries. By "conventional," we mean boundaries that most people are not usually allowed to cross but that clinicians can because of their training and their positions in society. These are boundaries of the skin (through cutting skin or entering orifices), of intimacy (viewing, touching, or cutting genitals or other private parts), of social interaction (such as objective "detached touch"), or of whose bodies can or cannot be touched (as stratified through class, gender, ethnicity, and race). These boundaries are both individual and overlapping; that is, some forms of touch might only breach the boundaries of the skin, while others might simultaneously breach multiple boundaries.

The boundaries of the skin can be breached by radiological images, by cutting, or by percussion and palpation, which search for information below the skin's surface, materializing it (see Rice 2008; Howes-Mischel 2016). These processes of "seeing" the body are invasive (Good 1994), making the internal body knowable. Seeing the body is part of the process of what Taylor (2005) called "surfacing"—bringing to the surface the things that lie beneath it by troubling and disrupting the body's outer boundaries, bringing hidden things into public view. Taylor added that the term "surfacing" suggests a dynamic tension between movements and performances that simultaneously create and breach surfaces. We can "surface" the social body as well as the individual body; by troubling the boundaries present in society, we can identify the tensions that exist in the sociopolitical structure.

Several interns said that their mentors physically guided their hands during procedures so they could learn the motions and begin to internalize—to embody—the knowledge. Yoselin, an intern at Hospital Piedad, said that "in case there is a complication with something, [the doctors] help us, they move our hand, they guide us." In their different rotations in the hospital, interns increasingly learned how to touch patients' bodies. Trainees learned the "duality of touch" (Van Dongen and Elema 2001), which includes the utilitarian and practical (e.g., the correct placement and movement of their hands, ears, or eyes), as well as the intimate or emotional, acquiring biomedical values transmitted by the mentors alongside these technical skills.

Touching patients as a means of diagnosis requires that interns practice in order to learn. The interns we interviewed learned to breach skin, bodily, and social boundaries by conquering their hesitations about whether to touch or not, and by developing "skilled bodies" (Harris 2016) that were not awkward when touching others. César, an intern at Hospital Piedad, said that he was usually fearful when he had to do a procedure for the first time, and that the only way he lost that fear was by "doing the things" he had to do. Gabriela told us, "When I say 'practice' I mean just that: to touch the patients . . . so you . . . move your hands properly, right? Sometimes you are afraid, you don't know if you touch or don't touch." These interns had to learn how to appropriately *listen to the body*, because touch risks being misinterpreted (Van Dongen and Elema 2001). When people first learn a new skill, they are bound by rules, carefully and actively thinking through them, in what Gabriela and César referred to as "fear" or "hesitation." Downey (2010) suggested that bodily training shifts in and out of consciousness when the learner focuses on technique before the practice becomes embodied and, thereby, habitually automatic. In the case of interns, these new practices might consist of asking how to touch, where to touch, when to touch, and where or when not to touch. The interns whom we observed learned what Katherine Young (1997:3) referred to as an "etiquette of touch" through which they took over the bodies of their patients, while those patients simultaneously ceded their bodily autonomy over to strangers. A social contract of sorts develops at this juncture, where intimate, yet objective, touch is allowed in biomedical encounters.

This ceding of patient autonomy was evident in many of the labors and births we witnessed, where the clinician never asked the patient, "Can I touch you?" before doing pelvic exams. Instead, they would inform the patient, "You'll feel a touch, ma'am." This type of touch crosses physical, social, and personal boundaries, as it penetrates the body of a patient without asking for her consent. These "territories of the self" (Goffman 1997:45) formed by the skin are blurred in these interactions; the body and its sheath of skin belong to the patient, but its territory is laid claim to by the clinician in medical interactions. In the process, the social boundary separating patient from physician is blurred. The skin becomes a permeable zone of exclusion, serving as a boundary not only for a person's interior, but also for where decisions come into being about who can touch it and in what ways.

Each culture has tactile norms (Van Dongen and Elema 2001). For instance, obstetricians can touch patients by following sociocultural scripts (Henslin and Biggs 1971) in ways and in places that would not be allowed in other contexts or by other people. Social scripts make medical actions seem "normal" that in other situations would be socially unacceptable. For example, as patients we can be unclothed in the presence of a medical team and touched in ways that are acceptable in that context. These social scripts occur in a liminal context. These same interactions would rarely (if ever) be acceptable outside of the medical space, even with the very same members of the medical team and within minutes of the prior encounter. The touch of medical hands within a medical space transforms intimate touch into objective, detached touch. The medical body is different from the non-medical body or, even to some degree, from the bodies of medical trainees. The medical body is constituted by an assemblage of factors: the medical implements picked up and handled, the patient body physically examined and interviewed, the social roles and scripts within the institution of medicine, or the expertise of the medical practitioner. All of these factors allow the medical body to cross boundaries that other bodies cannot, or are not supposed to.

## Crossing Structural Boundaries of Race, Gender, and Class

The most significant boundaries crossed in the medical contexts we observed were not just of skin or social etiquette, but were also structured by class, gender, and race/skin color. As Prentice (2007) has pointed out, medical training simultaneously embodies technical and social lessons. In these settings, the social lessons consist of learning the roles of rank and hierarchy, how to touch, whom one can touch, and in what ways. In the process, these lessons also (unintentionally) impart information on which bodies matter and which ones do not.

The care at public and private Mexican hospitals clearly illustrates this breach of boundaries, as, during the time of our research and ongoing, medical interactions are very different in each type of hospital. Social and economic differences are often mapped onto hospital types and spaces, which frequently reflect the intertwinings of class and color. Public hospitals are government funded and generally serve the lower socioeconomic sectors of the population. These institutions tend to be quite large, usually have a high patient load and concomitant low doctor-to-patient ratio, and often (though not always) operate in run-down facilities and with older technologies. In contrast, the private medical system is reserved for those who can afford to pay the premiums or whose employers pay a private insurance company for their employees' care. The political economy of health care in Mexico structures factors such as patient volume, infrastructure, access to health care, and patient agency. In high-volume public hospitals, interns have ample exposure to more cases and more experiential learning because there are not enough full-time (and skilled) clinicians to care for all the patients. But these advantages can be counterbalanced by the facts that in these public hospitals, trainees have less time to rest and less direct guidance from superiors, potentially leading to an increase in mistakes and to obstetric iatrogenesis. In private hospitals, the workload is lower, as these hospitals place much greater emphasis on high patient-to-clinician ratios and on protecting the rights of paying patients. In these spaces, obstetric trainees are not allowed to touch patients as freely as in public hospitals. Interns in private hospitals may get less sink-or-swim practice but do receive greater guidance on developing their techniques and skills, and more time to study to pass their residency exams.

Many interns told us that public institutions provide excellent ways to practice without the worry of patients refusing treatment, whereas patients in public institutions have little to no choice about some of the medical procedures they undergo, or about the number (and experience level) of the practitioners who can touch them (Smith-Oka 2021). These differences in patient agency greatly affect how doctors cross boundaries. The interns we interviewed emphasized that their ability to do *manitas* was much greater in public hospitals. In fact, many of them chose public hospitals precisely *because* they could practice as much as they wanted to, with little attention to patient choice. Carmen, from Hospital Salud, said that she specifically chose not to do her internship in a private hospital because "there are not many patients and [the doctors] don't let you *meter mano* (put in a hand), because in a private one the patients don't want that." An intern at Hospital Piedad also saw this difference as a potential advantage:

> In public hospitals, sometimes cases go there that you will never see in your life, and in the private ones you probably have less opportunity to do that. But, well, they both have their pros and cons. In the private ones you can read, you can continue studying and preparing for . . . the national exam [akin to the US Boards written examinations]. And in the public ones you can *hacer manitas*.

Samantha's case illustrates the troubling breaching of boundaries in learning medicine. Samantha was an intern at Hospital Piedad who participated in a month-long external rotation at a public hospital to gain more experience in ob/gyn. A few days after she returned to Piedad, we sat down in the hospital's cafeteria for coffee and to chat about her experiences during that month. She told us how one day the labor ward was very full, with many of the patients slated for cesarean births (CBs). In order to triage the care of patients, on that day, the residents went into the operating rooms to perform those CBs, leaving the bulk of the management of labor and vaginal deliveries to the interns. During our conversation, Samantha said that she had previously participated as an assistant in a few vaginal births but had no actual experience attending one, especially by herself. Despite this lack of experience, she said that a female resident told her, "You know what? You can attend [a vaginal birth] alone."

Samantha told us that she prepared for the delivery while the resident was in the other room attending to a CB and calling out instructions to her. One of the first instructions was to do an episiotomy (a perineal cut used to enlarge the vaginal opening, routine in most hospitals in Mexico). Samantha told us that she had never done an episiotomy before, "And I'm, like, 'Ay! . . . Oh well, I'll do it.'" She added that she then thought to herself, "The problem isn't doing it, but rather afterwards when I have to repair [suture] it. How will I do that?" She said that the obstetric residents had explained to her how to do the procedure earlier, but that it "was the first time I did it without someone observing what I was doing." With little guidance from more experienced obstetricians, she proceeded to figure out how to suture the patient's incision. Preferring to err on the side of caution, she asked one of the other interns in the hospital to help her. However, the other intern was also unsure of how to suture an episiotomy, and so together they figured it out as best they could. She shrugged and said, "I mean, I'm not sure if it was a good job, but . . ."

What is perhaps most salient about Samantha's narrative is the fact that she seemed to have little concern about the effects of her untrained hand suturing a very intimate area of a woman's anatomy where, if the sutures were badly placed and the incision did not heal properly, the procedure could cause the patient significant and/or long-term pain or discomfort, as well as other morbidities (such as infection, fecal incontinence, or pain during sex) (Karaçam and Eroğlu 2003). We asked her whether any of the residents or obstetricians inspected the sutures afterward. Samantha replied, seeming unsure, "I think they might have examined her in recovery. . . . But, yeah, it was only us interns who attended to this patient." We probed more deeply into some of the implications of her involvement in the patient's delivery, especially whether she felt that she did a good job. Samantha replied by focusing on the immediate symptoms of infection rather than on whether she had the skills to do a good job for the patient's long-term wellbeing, "Yes, yes, it was good, because the worry is whether she develops a fever while in recovery, or she is bleeding, like if I didn't do something right."

The broader concerns in situations such as Samantha's go beyond the fact that procedures performed by untrained practitioners can have significant consequences for patients; this situation also brings up important aspects of whose bodies are used as training and practice grounds for physicians. As Julieta, an intern at Piedad, stated, "The thought is that you can do what you want in a public [hospital]. And the patients don't insist on their right to complain." When we asked Samantha about whether she ever thought about the ethical questions regarding her and other interns doing procedures with little training, she replied, "I think that because there are so many patients there, the [residents] don't notice. And, well, at least the ones who already trusted us would ask us to attend to the [patients]." Her focus was less about the ethics of learning on certain bodies or even about the unassailable fact that the high volume of patients necessitated someone to care for them (even if they were unskilled), and more about gaining the respect and trust of residents who would subsequently allow her to carry out procedures. In this example, a tension exists between two modes of touch. On the one hand, touch closes the physical distance between clinicians and patients, while on the other, touch symbolically re-instantiates this distance through the process of performing and suturing episiotomies without concern for the patient's long-term wellbeing.

In private hospitals, the interns' practices are much more supervised and guided. Mauricio stated that all the moments of guidance at Piedad had helped him to learn how to practice, adding, "Not only in a cesarean, but also in a surgery they let you do one or two sutures. . . . So you begin acquiring a certain *maña* (knack), well, technique, but also *maña*." Doctor Luna, an ob whom we met at the private hospital (but whose second job was at a high-volume public hospital in the city), bemoaned the training undertaken by the interns in private hospitals. He believed that all interns needed many more skills before they left for their mandatory year of social service. He said that interns should know how to:

> attend a birth, do an episiotomy, repair it. They need to know how to begin treatments of all pathologies . . . They also need to know how we attend [a birth], and we let them do it little by little. Here it is difficult for them to *meter mano*. In teaching hospitals they are told, "You figure it out." The problem is that this is both a teaching *and* a private hospital. The workload is very scant compared to [public hospitals].

In vaginal births with private hospital patients, the trainee interlocutors told us that they shifted from the center of the action to the periphery, in contrast to the experiences of interns like Samantha in public hospitals, where trainees could carry out many of the procedures themselves. In the private hospital, the majority of the procedures were done by the attending obstetricians, and only occasionally would an intern carry out a pelvic exam or other procedure. Mauricio stated, "It depends upon the attending physician. There are some who tell you, 'You know what? Not today.' And others who do let you." But the private patient's permission was always requested prior to an untrained hand working on them. In contrast, and as previously noted, permission from patients in public hospitals was not sought. Rarely did these facilities disclose or discuss with patients the fact that interns did many of the procedures. Indeed, because clinicians all wear similar clothes (scrubs or long white coats), only a patient familiar with medical hierarchy and status would know who was an intern, who was an obstetric resident, and who was an obstetrician.

Our data make it clear that training in these public spaces did not emphasize learning skills in the "right" way, but rather was about the repetition of techniques without quite knowing the what, how, or why behind them. Almost all the interns reported that public hospitals were for learning through practice and private hospitals were for learning through observation. As Mauricio said of public hospitals, "They teach you two, three times, and *órale* (go)!" Indeed, when we discussed patient care and rights with him, especially comparing the care between both types of hospitals, he stated, "It's kind of like in a private hospital one has to be a bit . . . more careful of the patients, right? They are paying. And in the public sector, [the practitioners] are a little bit more careless that way." César added, "I believe that in a private [hospital], they look after the patient better (*cuidan un poco más al paciente*)." (Here, the term *cuidar*—"to take care of"—can refer to the quality of care but also to careful care.) He paused and said, "The attention is more personalized, the nurses are more attentive. And many times with private patients, they don't allow students to practice as much, right?" He added that in public hospitals, an intern could do rounds with the obstetrician and be allowed to do examinations on pregnant women, "and you can also do the gynecological examination and such—but not so much in a private one."

In these interns' words, we find an interesting dynamic between two forms of care: careful and careless. The "careful" practice in private hospitals suggests a physical distance in which the patient body is not touched by just anyone, evidencing a form of tactile respect. There is a simultaneous social closeness that is marked by politeness and respect for a certain amount of bodily autonomy. The "careless" practice in public hospitals, on the other hand, is almost the reverse: a physical closeness between patients and clinicians resulting from being touched by more people, where patients' boundaries are breached more easily and where the lack of patient bodily autonomy reflects a social distance between the patients and the clinicians. In fact, we argue that the bodies of patients in public hospitals are seen to have more porous or fluid social boundaries, given that these boundaries can be breached with greater ease. In contrast, the bodies of private hospital patients are more socially rigid and less able to be breached.

We also argue that medical interactions between patients and physicians in public hospitals cross stratified socio-structural boundaries. The bodies being penetrated and touched belong to patients with less agency—created through an intersection of structural aspects like gender, skin color, and class. These patients are used as "training wheels" for interns and residents who need more practice in certain techniques. The external rotation at the public hospital for interns from Piedad (the private hospital) is very illustrative of this dynamic, because these interns would be unable to learn the requisite skills with paying patients (who would rarely allow untrained hands to touch them). Instead, in the public hospital (Hospital Salud) with non-paying patients, interns were able to practice these skills. In these public hospital settings, there can sometimes be an unintended lack of regard for the welfare of the patient, since there is no time and there are few staff members to do this kind of in-depth, careful work. This situation is evidenced by the lack of direct observation of Samantha's suturing technique, which can be contrasted with the ways in which Mauricio, César, and other interns at Piedad were closely observed and supervised as they learned.

In addition to the fact that the bodies being practiced upon in the public hospital are mostly poor and darker-skinned, and have little, if any, agency, is the troubling reality that those practicing on such women are usually middle class, lighter-skinned, and educated. The purpose of this system is to export practices from private hospitals to public ones, leveraging the high patient volume in the public hospital to doctors'/ trainees' own advantage and bypassing legal, ethical, or moral concerns. Underprivileged patients are vital to the production of biomedical competence. A similar structure can be found in the global health and biomedical programs in resource-rich countries that send their students for practicums to resource-poor countries, which Claire Wendland (2012:110) refers to as "clinical tourism." In her analysis, Wendland argues that "the wretchedness of clinical practice" depends on "a contrast with medicine as practiced elsewhere, remembered or imagined" (2012:113). Such social hierarchies have historically played a role in defining who gets to be the practitioner and who gets to be practiced upon. In these contexts, in speaking of international medical "voluntourism" (the mixture of tourism with short-term volunteering), Noelle Sullivan (2018) states that doctors are able to justify the practices and interventions (like those in the public hospital) that would be wholly unacceptable at home (like those in the private hospital). And as Susan Erikson and Claire Wendland (2014) state, these systems replicate patterns of (dis)advantage, where impoverished and/or darker-skinned populations enter medical engagements as test subjects on which others may learn—a deeply racialized phenomenon that has characterized the development of obstetrics since its beginning, including the experiments that the now-notorious obstetrician J. Marion Sims performed on Black slaves to learn how to repair vaginal/anal fistulas; his techniques are still practiced today (Owens 2017). Erickson and Wendland (2014) argue that ultimately, these maternity care systems look increasingly like colonial, rather than decolonized, medicine. (On decolonizing medical education, see Chapter 6 [Lokugamage, Ahillan, and Pathberiya 2023] in Volume III of this series [Davis-Floyd and Premkumar 2023].)

## Crossing Boundaries through Somatic Translation

Doctor Marco, one of the ob residents at Hospital Salud, was our first participant to frame the idea of using the body as a tool alongside other biomedical technologies, such as sutures or stethoscopes. One of the primary duties of junior obstetric residents was to manage the early stages of labor and to measure how dilated a patient was by conducting a cervical exam, which in Mexico is called a *tacto* (translated as a "touch"). Describing this technique, Doctor Marco said, "Our tools are our hands; hence, one always has to know, and it's what I have always told the interns, they have to know what their hand measures." For him, knowing one's measurements directly translated to efficacy and practice when crossing patients' bodily boundaries. The body functions as an instrument that provides doctors with the opportunity to perform a technique, developing their bodily practice while also obtaining tactile data from their patients (Rose 1999).

Doctora Valentina, a third-year obstetric resident at Hospital Salud, said that she learned to measure dilation by doing *tactos* in medical school using mannequins, which help obstetric trainees begin to learn to manually understand the boundaries of the body by using their sense of touch in situations where they cannot see what they are touching. These students translated touch and sensation into knowledge and understanding of the body. In hospitals with an actual patient, the only way for interns and residents to do a *tacto* was by inserting their fingers into a patient's vagina to measure her cervix. These *tactos* are very intimate—traversing social and physical boundaries that are not allowed for just anyone. And yet, they are also remarkably commonplace. In every birth we observed, each patient in labor was subjected to *tactos*—in many cases repeatedly and by different clinicians—even though they can be very painful for the laboring woman. Julieta stated, "different people are *tactando* the patient every half-hour, and that is super contraindicated; it should not happen." Samantha said that in the obstetrics ward in the public hospital, all the patients receive multiple *tactos*, adding that "the resident would tell me, 'Come and feel this, and these are the normal characteristics, and these are the characteristics of when she is in labor,' and so forth. So he would tell me that and then tell me, 'Do the *tacto*.'" Doctor Marco emphasized to the interns under his care that to make accurate measurements, they had to know "how long their hand is, how wide their hand is, and they have to know this when they open up [their hand]. Because after all, what for me might be 7 centimeters, for someone [else] could be 8, right? But the [interns] have to learn what their hand measures." As Victoria noted, holding up her fingers to show their dimensions, "Like this it is 2 centimeters, because my fingers are little. But there are fatter fingers where this is already 3 centimeters. But mine are like this; I would calculate this as 2 [centimeters]. Like that."

Again, we refer to this process of learning, repeating, and measuring as *somatic translation*. Somatic translation is a way for physicians to read the patient's body with their own, in the process crafting their own bodies. This process equates the bodies of patients and physicians as they both become objects of measurement. The more interns practice, the more they learn the "feel" of what they are doing and learn to do it correctly (Prentice 2007). They might be aware of the measurement of their hands or fingers prior to inserting them into the vagina of a patient, but they really grow to know them as tools once they use them inside a patient's body. Somatic translation provides them with information that is very different from the information provided by technology. A *tacto* is about the dilation and the texture of the cervix, its thickness, or its "feel"—qualities that cannot be conveyed by an instrument and whose minutiae must be bodily learned in order to understand what exactly is being felt and how to turn it into words (Rose 1999). In this process of doing a *tacto*, clinicians' bodies become "boundary objects" (Wenger 2010) that cross boundaries of skin and intimacy, and their authoritative knowledge about their own bodies supplants the information gleaned from technology, while also closing the physical distance between themselves and their patients.

These clinicians argued that a basic understanding of one's own bodily dimensions makes the medical body a better measurement tool. In this process, obstetricians and obstetric trainees converted their non-standard units of measurement—their bodies—into standard units of measurement (in this case, centimeters) used in biomedical contexts across the world. Knowing their bodies and their measurements also allowed these practitioners to translate a highly intimate form of touch (genital touching) into a detached form of touch (cervical exam). A juxtaposition exists between the invasiveness of a *tacto* and the ways that obs learned to delimit and de-erogenize certain forms of intimacy, especially when the patients are all female and the practitioners are often male. This process is created by other forms of translation, such as anonymization—in which physicians translate a person into a patient—or fragmentation, in which a whole person (the "patient") is translated into particular body parts. The interns we interviewed did not feel that they were touching a patient in an intimate way, but instead were examining the cervix and vaginal walls of a body in a detached, clinical, and impersonal manner.

Near the end of her internship at Hospital Piedad, Gabriela reflected on the process by which she had trained her body to cross boundaries. Using the metaphor of sightedness, she said that it was only by practice that she learned to "see." Combining both the senses of sight and touch in reference to inserting an intravenous needle, she claimed, "At first it's like having blind hands. You can't find the veins. And so *hacer manitas* for me [means] that you try to insert once, you try twice, you try three times, and you start getting skilled with your hands, you more easily identify the structures that you have to know to carry out these procedures." Describing the first time she touched the belly of a pregnant patient, she recounted that "my *compañero* (workmate) told me, 'This is a contraction.' I couldn't feel anything. But [afterward] I would touch [patients], and touch one and [then] another and another. And each time it was easier [to see]." For Gabriela, the process of crossing bodily boundaries was inseparable from touching and seeing. The more she touched, the more tissue she stretched and handled, the more she was able to see and cross the boundaries of the body, and the more she "saw," the more information she was able to glean from her touch. The translational process of seeing is initiated the moment the boundary between the physician's body and the patient's body is crossed.

Through the process of conducting these cervical examinations, the clinician's own medical bodies have "synthesized the look, feel, and motions" (Prentice 2013:175) of the patients' bodies, allowing them a clearer view and understanding of those bodies below their surfaces. Our analysis shows that the interns we observed eventually shifted from seeing the whole body they were touching, cutting, or suturing, to focusing intently on the part of the body they were examining, going less by sight and more by feel and understanding of the ways in which the body tissues are set up—like Gabriela's increased understanding of how a contraction felt from the outside. This process of crossing these boundaries translates into an ability to "see" with one's body. One might argue that this is one of the most profound forms of boundary crossing, producing a type of *embodied cohabitation*, commingling the bodies of physician and patient.

## Conclusion: Why Crossing Bodily Boundaries Matters

In this chapter, we have shown that because medical bodies can traverse social, physical, structural, and intimacy boundaries that are normally more delineated, they become good instruments for understanding the reproduction of health inequalities through somatic translation and practice. These medical bodies cross various boundaries in ways that map onto and reproduce social differences. This process, in turn, tells us about how certain populations are viewed and treated by society in the form of treatment by society's representatives—medical doctors (see Davis-Floyd 2022). The processes of *manitas* and *tacto* that we have described mirror a disconnection between what we term the *violence of knowing* (how knowledge about the body can come at the expense of someone's dignity) on the one hand, and the importance of touch as a legitimate mode of care on the other. This tension matters, because this form of tactile and sensorial learning entails not only a form of boundary crossing that is medically useful, but also a form of boundary crossing that "surfaces" various social inequalities in Mexico by taking advantage of them. We can think of this process as *surfacing the social body's interior*, which unveils and makes visible the various frameworks and structures of society. The ways in which the boundaries are crossed become indicators for the structure of a population that are reproduced within a hospital space. The interactions between practitioners and patients in these clinical spaces both materialize and penetrate these boundaries. To recap from above, in this process, we can identify how and why different patient "types" receive different treatment and care from physicians and medical trainees. The boundaries of their bodies are seen to be different, with different social rules attached to them. Namely, bodies that belong to female, raced, or impoverished populations are seen to be more permeable—their boundaries are more easily breached and have fewer social rules attached to them—while bodies belonging to male, white, or wealthier populations are seen to possess stronger, more impermeable boundaries that can only be breached in certain contexts and by certain people.

And yet, the knowledge of these boundaries might be unconscious. The deeper meaning of *manitas*—as reproductions of social difference and of boundary crossing—is also developed unconsciously by doctors, part of a hidden curriculum (see Hafferty and Franks 1994) that is never explicitly taught or learned in practice. This process is produced through the combination of publicly available symbols—of biomedicine, of class or skin color, of gender, of doctors as gods, etc.—and the invisible schema of cognition and action, consisting of factors regarding what is being learned as well as how, why, and under what circumstances—what Loïc Wacquant (2005) refers to as "out there" and "in here," respectively.

In sum, in Mexico, as elsewhere, biomedical practitioners traverse social and class boundaries regarding which bodies can be touched (and practiced upon) and which ones cannot. Indeed, medical bodies in these contexts *reinforce* class boundaries, due to which impoverished or darker-skinned patients cannot refuse to be touched as they risk being scolded—or worse, losing their access to health care. Conversely, middle- and upper-class (or lighter-skinned) patients do have the agency to refuse to be touched by a trainee and, in private hospitals, routinely do so. Medical trainees in these contexts do not simply learn about biomedical techniques; they also learn about the principles and values of these medical institutions in their daily practices. They learn about the perceived value and worth of different populations. They learn that some patients are fair game for practice, while others can be touched only by skilled clinicians and under certain contexts. The medical body becomes a vehicle for personifying skills and articulating practice, ultimately embodying the broader structural forces and political economy of any given place.

The process of crossing boundaries can tell us about hierarchy and position in professional communities of practice. The rank a practitioner carries and the type of training they have can determine the boundaries that they can cross. In our research, though interns could cross some boundaries as allowed by their training and by their mentors, more advanced trainees (such as residents) had more leeway for boundary crossing, as they were more practiced. Obstetricians could cross many more boundaries, as allowed by their status and authority. Obstetric trainees learned not only what their own bodies were meant to do in any given context, but also to use their bodies in these multiple roles while simultaneously being aware of and evaluating the bodies of others.

**Vania Smith-Oka** is an Associate Professor of Anthropology at the University of Notre Dame. Her work addresses questions of obstetric violence, medical decision-making, cesareans and incisions, medical spaces, and medical training in Mexico and Kenya. Her first book, *Shaping the Motherhood of Indigenous Mexico* (2013) explores how state programs used conditional cash programs to develop "good motherhood" and "good citizenship"; her second book, *Becoming Gods: Medical Training in Mexican Hospitals* (2021) examines the ways in which medical students developed the skills, attitudes, and practices of biomedicine within a shaky biomedical system.

**Megan K. Marshalla** is an obstetrics and gynecology resident at Rush University Medical Center. She has a BA from the University of Notre Dame (2015) and an MD from the University of Illinois at Chicago (2019).

## Notes

1. This chapter is reprinted here in revised and updated form. Reproduced by permission of the American Anthropological Association from *American Anthropologist* 121(1) (2009): 113–125. https://doi.org/10.1111/aman.13174. Not for sale or further reproduction.

## References

Anderson N, Dietrich M. 2012. *The Educated Eye: Visual Culture and Pedagogy in the Life Sciences*. Lebanon NH: Dartmouth College Press.

Cohen E. 2010. "Anthropology of Knowledge." *Journal of the Royal Anthropological Institute* 16: S193–202.

Davis-Floyd R. 2022. *Birth as an American Rite of Passage*, 3rd ed. Abingdon, Oxon: Routledge.

Douglas M. 1966. *Purity and Danger: An Analysis of Concepts of Pollution and Taboo*. New York: Routledge and Kegan Paul.

Downey G. 2010. "'Practice without Theory': A Neuroanthropological Perspective on Embodied Learning." *Journal of the Royal Anthropological Institute* 16: S22–40.

Erikson SL, Wendland C. 2014. "Exclusionary Practice: Medical Schools and Global Health Clinical Electives." *Student British Medical Journal* 22: 1–5.

Goffman E. 1997. *The Goffman Reader*, eds. Lemert C, Branaman A. Maiden MA: Blackwell.

Good BJ. 1994. *Medicine, Rationality, and Experience*. Cambridge: Cambridge University Press.

Hafferty FW, Franks R. 1994. "The Hidden Curriculum, Ethics Teaching, and the Structure of Medical Education." *Academic Medicine* 69(11): 861–871.

Harris A. 2016. "Listening-Touch, Affect and the Crafting of Medical Bodies through Percussion." *Body & Society* 22(1): 31–61.

Henslin JM, Biggs MA. 1971. "Dramaturgical Desexualization: The Sociology of the Vaginal Exam." In *Studies in the Sociology of Sex*, ed. Henslin JM, 243–272. New York: Appleton-Century-Crofts.

Hinojosa SZ. 2002. "'The Hands Know': Bodily Engagement and Medical Impasse in Highland Maya Bonesetting." *Medical Anthropology Quarterly* 16(1): 22–40.

Hirschauer S. 1991. "The Manufacture of Bodies in Surgery." *Social Studies of Science* 21(2): 279–319.

Howes-Mischel R. 2016. "'With This You Can Meet Your Baby': Fetal Personhood and Audible Heartbeats in Oaxacan Public Health." *Medical Anthropology Quarterly* 30(2): 186–202.

INEGI. 2014. "Anuario Estadístico y Geográfico de Puebla 2014." *Instituto Nacional de Estadística y Geografía*. Retrieved 16 March 2017 from http://www.datatur.sectur.gob.mx/ITxEF_Docs/PUE_ANUARIO_PDF.pdf.

———. 2017. "México en Cifras." *Instituto Nacional de Estadística y Geografía*. Retrieved 20 March 2017 from http: //www.beta.inegi.org.mx/app/areasgeo graficas/?ag=21.

Karaçam Z, Eroğlu K. 2003. "Effects of Episiotomy on Bonding and Mothers' Health." *Journal of Advanced Nursing* 43(4): 384–394.

Kitzinger S. 1997. "Authoritative Touch in Childbirth: A Cross-Cultural Approach." In *Childbirth and Authoritative Knowledge: Cross-Cultural Perspectives*, eds. Davis-Floyd R, Sargent CF, 209–232. Berkeley: University of California Press.

Lave J, Wenger E. 1991. *Situated Learning: Legitimate Peripheral Participation*. Cambridge: Cambridge University Press.

Lokugamage A, Ahillan T, Pathberiya SDC. 2023. "Decolonizing Medical Education in the UK." In *Obstetric Violence and Systemic Disparities: Can Obstetrics Be Humanized and Decolonized?* eds. Davis-Floyd R, Premkumar A, Chapter 6. New York: Berghahn Books.

Owens, DC. 2017. *Medical Bondage: Race, Gender, and the Origins of American Gynecology*. Athens: University of Georgia Press.

Prentice R. 2005. "The Anatomy of a Surgical Simulation: The Mutual Articulation of Bodies in and through the Machine." *Social Studies of Science* 35(6): 837–866.

———. 2007. "Drilling Surgeons: The Social Lessons of Embodied Surgical Learning." *Science, Technology, and Human Values* 32(5): 534–553.

———. 2013. *Bodies in Formation: An Ethnography of Anatomy and Surgery Education*. Durham NC: Duke University Press.

Rice T. 2008. "'Beautiful Murmurs': Stethoscopic Listening and Acoustic Objectification." *The Senses and Society* 3(3): 293–306.

Rose M. 1999. "'Our Hands Will Know': The Development of Tactile Diagnostic Skill—Teaching, Learning, and Situated Cognition in a Physical Therapy Program." *Anthropology & Education Quarterly* 30(2): 133–160.

Smith-Oka V. 2021. *Becoming Gods: Medical Training in Mexican Hospitals*. New Brunswick: Rutgers University Press.

Sullivan N. 2018. "International Clinical Volunteering in Tanzania: A Postcolonial Analysis of a Global Health Business." *Global Public Health* 13(3): 310–324.

Taylor JS. 2005. "Surfacing the Body Interior." *Annual Review of Anthropology* 34: 741–756.

Van Dongen E, Elema R. 2001. "The Art of Touching: The Culture of Body Work in Nursing." *Anthropology & Medicine* 8(2–3): 149–162.

Van Drie M. 2013. "Training the Auscultative Ear: Medical Textbooks and Teaching Tapes (1950–2010)." *The Senses and Society* 8(2): 165–191.

Wacquant L. 2005. "Carnal Connections: On Embodiment, Apprenticeship, and Membership." *Qualitative Sociology* 28(4): 445–474.

Wendland CL. 2010. *A Heart for the Work: Journeys Through an African Medical School.* Chicago: University of Chicago Press.

———. 2012. "Moral Maps and Medical Imaginaries: Clinical Tourism at Malawi's College of Medicine." *American Anthropologist* 114(1): 108–122.

Wenger E. 2010. "Conceptual Tools for CoPs as Social Learning Systems: Boundaries, Identity, Trajectories and Participation." In *Social Learning Systems and Communities of Practice*, ed. Blackmore C, 125–143. London: Springer.

Young KG. 1997. *Presence in the Flesh: The Body in Medicine.* Cambridge MA: Harvard University Press.

CHAPTER 9

# The Limitations of Understanding Structural Inequality
Obstetricians' Accounts of Caring for Substance-Using Patients in the United States

*Katharine McCabe*

## Introduction and Background

Problematic substance use is often categorized in one of two ways. Addiction[1] is typically viewed either through a disease lens as a chronic, recurring medical condition, or through a personal responsibility lens wherein problem substance use reflects poor decision-making, moral weakness, and/or a proclivity toward criminality. Social scientists have argued that practitioners' opinions about substance use disorder tend to fall between these two approaches—neither completely medicalized as a disease nor entirely viewed as a moral failing (Campbell 2012; Tiger 2013). What researchers often do not examine are the ways in which addiction is understood and viewed as a "structurally determined" social problem. Both the disease model and the personal responsibility view highlight the tendency to focus on individual-level causal explanations for addiction, when in practice, professionals and people who have struggled with problem substance use often have a situational understanding of addiction that is contextualized in and through a wide range of social experiences.

Drawing from interviews conducted with obstetricians (obs), the findings presented in this chapter demonstrate that addiction is often framed as a socio-structural problem that exists among a web of other complex situations and adversities. Counter to the ways in which social scientists think about "structural competency"—an approach that seeks to instill awareness of "upstream" structural causes of health in clinicians—my study results reveal that structural understanding does not always result in more compassionate or patient-centered care. In fact, what I refer to as *structural-causal thinking* may result in providers adopting attitudes or strategies that *negatively* affect the health and well-being of pregnant and postpartum people with complex needs. In this chapter, I examine how obs' structural understandings of inequity affect their care and their attitudes toward stigmatized groups. My research asks: When providers express concerns about the structural underpinnings of illness, do they also provide more thoughtful and empathetic care resulting in better patient outcomes?

## From Culture to Structure

Over the past 30 years, there has been an evolution of responses within biomedicine to address "biocultural" or "fundamental" causes of health and disease. In the 1990s, biomedical schools and training programs began to integrate curricula that better prepared clinicians to interact across socio-demographic differences. Referred to as "cultural competence," the approach encouraged providers to interact with patients from dissimilar racial-ethnic and cultural backgrounds with open-mindedness and empathy, and to consider how cultural factors—e.g., diet, worldview, language, religious beliefs, and culturally produced stigmas—impact compliance with biomedical care (Kleinman and Benson 2006).

Although sometimes useful for preparing providers for the realities of patient interactions, cultural frameworks have been critiqued for reproducing racial/ethnic stereotypes in care interactions (Kleinman and Benson 2006; Shepherd 2019). Critics argue that cultural sensitivity, in and of itself, does not appear to improve the provision of care, reduce implicit biases, or enable providers to grasp institutional and structural factors affecting health (Harris Interactive 2002). Furthermore, studies suggest that clinicians are especially uninformed about the ways in which the US healthcare system itself perpetuates inequities and illnesses (Kendrick et al. 2015; Britton et al. 2016).

Public awareness of inequity, racism, and stratified opportunities has deepened over the past decade in response to social movements in the United States that have emphasized economic inequity and racial injustice. Clinicians, training programs, and biomedical institutions have had to upgrade how they approach interacting across differences.

In 2015, the Association of American Medical Colleges made changes to the MCAT (Medical College Admissions Test) requiring test takers "to demonstrate aptitude in the influences of culture and community on health behaviors and outcomes, basics of the U.S. healthcare system, social determinants of health, and changes in health policy" (Metzl, Petty, and Olowojoba 2018:191). In response, colleges and universities across the United States have created curricula and programs for pre-clinical students that cut across the social and behavioral sciences to emphasize the macroeconomic, environmental, and social factors influencing biomedicine, health, and the healthcare system.

Concomitant with this sea change in biomedical education and training, a new generation of social scientists has advocated for the adoption of "structural competency"—an approach that "emphasizes diagnostic recognition of the economic and political conditions that produce health inequalities in the first place" (Metzl and Hansen 2014:127). Structural competency calls on providers and students to recognize "upstream" causes of health and illness, such as how "institutions, markets, or healthcare delivery systems shape symptom presentations," and encourages providers "to mobilize for correction of health and wealth inequalities in society" (Metzl, Petty, and Olowojoba 2018:190). Structural competency, along with numerous similar emergent concepts such as "structural vulnerability," "social determinants of health," "fundamental cause theory," and "social diagnosis" are all a part of a changing lexicon in biomedicine that seeks to capture the ways in which risk is "extra-corporal." This new approach stresses that health is determined as much by one's zip code, educational background, and skin color as by one's individual behaviors or genetic makeup.

## Structural Analyses of Substance Use During Pregnancy

Biomedical maternity care still has much work to do to integrate better structural understandings of addiction and substance use during pregnancy and the postpartum period (Knight 2020). Contemporary responses to substance use during pregnancy have been largely shaped by policies and laws that were created during the height of the war on drugs.[2] Khiara Bridges (2020) argues that the punitive bent of these policies is inextricable from the racial animus that infused drug policy during the 1980s and 1990s. Moreover, while lay and biomedical attitudes toward addiction have shifted somewhat, responses within perinatal health care remain punitive, and privilege surveillance over healing and therapeutic treatments. This pattern persists despite clear guidance from professional organizations such as the American College of Obstetricians and Gynecologists, which has come out in opposition to punitive and coercive approaches to substance use during pregnancy by biomedical providers (see ACOG 2020).

Various scholars and health advocates have argued that the policy landscape constitutes a structural barrier to maternal care (ACOG 2011; Roberts and Pies 2011; Knight 2020). Punitive federal and state-level policies, such as mandated reporting for substance use during pregnancy, deter many pregnant women from seeking prenatal care (Roberts and Pies 2011; Stone 2015) and encourage them to make exceedingly risky decisions—including attempting to self-detox (i.e., cease use of substances without the guidance of a trained specialist) during pregnancy (ACOG 2011). Researchers have also found that punitive state policies aimed at substance-using women negatively impact newborn health outcomes (Faherty et al. 2019; Subbaraman and Roberts 2019).

Pregnant substance users face additional stigmas that may translate into structural harm within biomedical systems. For instance, because maternal substance use is often regarded as a lack of fitness to parent (Terplan et al. 2015), substance-using women face a higher risk of becoming system-involved through their interactions with clinicians who drug test and report women based on criminal-legal suspicion (McCabe 2021). One reason why these structural barriers have not been adequately addressed is that they are largely endemic to maternal and perinatal biomedicine, which suggests that providers may have blind spots for harmful processes that they produce and are active in enacting in clinical practice.

In this chapter, I consider the tensions that arise between health education models that promote structural competency and real-world applications of structural thinking in clinical settings. The following findings explore the ways in which clinicians discuss and engage in what, again, I refer to as "structural-causal thinking." Presenting data collected from in-depth interviews with obs practicing in Chicago, Illinois, I argue that obs frequently couch perinatal substance use as a structurally produced and embedded phenomenon. However, such framing is not necessarily conducive to patient-centered care, as it is often leveraged as evidence that little could be done to clinically care for patients with substance use issues. These findings demonstrate that structural-causal thinking leads to justifying intensive and coercive forms of intervention, including non-consensual drug testing, retracting normative care, referring patients to child welfare agencies, and coerced drug treatment.

## Data and Methods

The data presented herein derive from a qualitative study examining multisystem collaboration in response to perinatal substance use in the city of Chicago, Illinois. I draw upon in-depth interview data from 13 obstetricians, all of whom were attendings (attending physicians have completed residency and practice their specialty in hospitals or clinics); the following analysis is also informed by ethnographic and qualitative interviews conducted with more than 70 professionals across the fields of medicine, law, child welfare administration, and substance treatment. In addition, I draw upon insights gained from interviewing 28 mothers who had personally experienced a child welfare intervention due to their substance use during pregnancy. All provider interviews were semi-structured and were centered around understanding the provision of care for substance-using patients, including questions regarding how substance use was determined, drug screening and testing practices, hospital procedures and protocols for treating this population, professionals' attitudes toward substance-using patients, biomedical interventions for maternal substance use, and child welfare involvement. All interviews were transcribed verbatim. Data were coded and analyzed using Atlas. Ti qualitative analysis software. Participants were given pseudonyms to protect their identities. I analyzed this data inductively, following a grounded approach (Charmaz 2014). My interviews first underwent a series of open codings to determine preliminary themes within and between subpopulations of professions and interlocutors. I then generated codes from these initial thematic clusters and re-analyzed the interviews, this time applying these focused codes to determine salient patterns (Charmaz 2014). Ethical approval to conduct this research was obtained through the appropriate institutional review board. All names used in this chapter are pseudonyms.

## The Alliance between Obstetrics and Child Welfare

Attitudes toward addiction and substance use disorders have shifted dramatically over the past 20 years. Both the opioid crisis and the growing movement to legalize marijuana have resulted in a shift in public opinion toward the criminalization of drug use and in more widespread acceptance of the biomedical model for treating substance use disorders (Pew Research Center 2014). However, in maternal biomedicine, punitive responses to substance-using pregnant and postpartum patients have become more commonplace than they were during the height of the crack cocaine panic of the 1980s–1990s. In various states, giving birth to a substance-exposed infant can result in criminal prosecution and incarceration (Paltrow and Flavin 2013). In addition, the number of states that categorize substance use during pregnancy as a form of child abuse or neglect (23 states + DC) and require that medical providers report suspected prenatal drug use (25 states + DC) has steadily increased since the 1980s (Guttmacher Institute 2021). To further complicate matters, federal laws and spending provisions, such as the Child Abuse and Prevention and Treatment Act and the Comprehensive Addiction and Recovery Act, encourage biomedical and child welfare systems to work together to assess newborns in ways that normalize and routinize child welfare involvement at birth based on substance exposure alone.

Obstetricians and other biomedical staff play key roles in detecting and channeling substance-using women to outside authorities, such as law enforcement and child welfare services (Paltrow and Flavin 2013; McCabe 2021). In this chapter, I explore how biomedical providers' decisions to drug test patients are rarely based on clinical criteria, and note that many standard norms in biomedicine must be circumvented to carry out forensic/criminal-legal investigatory tasks. For example, when suspicion of illicit substance use is present in the clinic, medical care is retracted, informed consent and shared decision-making disappear, and diagnostic norms are scaled back (Paltrow and Flavin 2013; McCabe 2021).

Child welfare interventions for perinatal substance use are not a form of "light-handed" state intervention. Since drug exposure in utero poses an ambiguous risk and is not analogous to other forms of child maltreatment, child welfare interventions for fetal substance exposure are usually unpredictable, and the severity of the response often varies on a case-by-case basis (Roberts 2002; Reich 2005). Child welfare workers are not typically trained in the fundamentals of substance dependency and treatment norms. Some ob interlocutors expressed frustration that child welfare staff struggled with basic concepts and terminology, such as not knowing the difference between methamphetamines and methadone—a pain-relieving opioid drug that is often used by doctors to help treat people with opioid use disorder—or not being familiar with clinical diagnostic terminology. Moreover, the consequences of being reported for substance use during pregnancy vary drastically. In states like South Carolina, a positive toxicology test and hotline call from a doctor, midwife, or other medical staff can land patients on a local child abuse registry (ABA 2021) alongside individuals who have physically abused and sexually assaulted children, creating a significant barrier to attaining employment and housing. While out-of-home placement and the permanent removal of children from their parents is generally considered the most unfavorable outcome of Child Protective Services (CPS) involvement, other CPS interventions can also hugely impact women's lives. For example, the "service provision" function of CPS is notably intensive and often requires parent(s) to actively engage in numerous programs and forms of surveillance to maintain custody of their children (e.g., frequent and random drug testing; psychological evaluations; participation in parenting classes, anger management classes, and 12-Step programs; involuntary substance use treatment and residential recovery programming; and other intensive programs [see D'Andrade 2015]). These sorts of compliance regimes create extraordinary stressors for new parents struggling with substance use issues (Sangoi 2020). Moreover, parents caught up in intensive compliance regimes risk losing custody of their children, not for physically abusing or neglecting them, but for being bureaucratically non-compliant—for example, for missing appointments or group meetings, no matter how good the reason. Given the range of possible negative system-related outcomes, biomedical professionals should consider that child welfare interventions can profoundly affect patients' lives.

The question of *why* providers drug test and report patients to the state could be answered in a number of ways. For one, despite efforts to de-stigmatize substance use disorders (SUDs) and to promote the biomedical approach of considering addiction as a disease, most maternal healthcare settings are ill-equipped or unable to provide treatment to patients with SUDs during pregnancy (SAMHSA 2016). As a result, biomedical staff may rely on outside actors, such as child welfare workers, to connect patients to local substance treatment options. Doctors and nurses may equate fetal substance exposure with child abuse, or they may presume that substance use during pregnancy predicts future child maltreatment (McCabe 2021). Moreover, providers may genuinely view child welfare as a helpful partner that can be called upon to take over the management of patients deemed "difficult" or socially "risky" (Fong 2020).

It is this latter concern with containing "social risk" factors that my analysis seeks to unpack. Could the ways in which risk is embodied by patients and interpreted by biomedical staff predict whether or not patients will be drug tested and reported to the state? And do providers' structural understandings of social risk play a protective role, or do they exacerbate the likelihood of criminalization within healthcare settings? My findings focus on how "structure" is discussed by providers. This analysis is not intended to discourage or critique providers for thinking about and considering how structures might affect their patients, nor is it intended to "throw the baby out with the bathwater" in regard to structural competency as a learning and training modality; rather, I intend this analysis to provide insight into important blind spots in care and the limitations of structural thinking.

## Chaos Requires Order

As previously noted, the binary most often presented in discussions about addiction poses substance dependence as either a moral flaw or as a disease. In reality, addiction is often regarded by professionals and practitioners as a socially embedded problem, a problem of environment, structures of opportunity, family influences, and social networks. The ob interlocutors were conscious, and often conscientious, of the structural underpinnings of addiction. The ob quoted below, Dr. Kuar, worked at a safety net hospital; I recall being impressed by how "in tune" she seemed to be with patients' lived experiences as she listed off the types of barriers that keep them from care. Her ability to engage in structural-causal thinking, however, enabled her to draw conclusions that justified a more coercive approach to care. In the extract below, she shares her impressions of her substance-using patients and the ability of "structured recovery programs" to address their needs:

> I like the structure that recovery programs give. And not just the pharmacologic substitution, but the whole, like, "let's get your GED" and "let's practice interviewing" . . . So many patients come from chronically chaotic lives. To present something different, in a setting that is "You don't have to figure out how to make this happen—we have this in place for you"—I think it's really important about the structured long-term recovery, because something was missed . . . or something was never there to get people to the point where they did. Now that is very different . . . than . . . the opioid epidemic of a doctor starting you out with an inappropriate script for oxy. Okay? I'm talkin' about people that are just in chronically chaotic, poverty, substance use, unemployment, miseducation . . . all of that. There's that, and then there's the suburbanized user. And I think the structured programs are probably much more valuable for people that haven't had a lot of structure in their lives or come from an intermittently, maybe poorly resourced structure, where you have programs that come into communities and then go away.

Informed by her observations on working with low-income pregnant populations, this obstetrician understands that patients who come from "chronically chaotic" lives have intensive needs; they are often burdened with multiple adversities such as "poverty, substance use, unemployment, miseducation." It is all too easy to define such patients by their lacks—born into "poorly resourced structures," "something was missing," or perhaps "was never there" to provide stability for such patients. Unfortunately, this line of thinking followed by Dr. Kuar can result in justifying coercive interventions that strip patients of their autonomy and rights. One of the limitations of structural-causal thinking is that, in the process of trying to understand the innumerable material and symbolic social constraints that shape their patients' lives, those in helping professions may easily confuse "order" with "support."

There are significant barriers to accessing appropriate substance treatments for pregnant and parenting women. However, the "structured recovery programs" that Dr. Kuar recommends reflect the two-tier treatment and rehabilitation landscape—wherein private boutique rehabilitation centers cater to class-privileged clients, and structured, often court-mandated, treatment centers manage low-income, marginalized clients. Highly structured treatment and recovery programs, referred to by sociologists Theresa Gowan and Sarah Whetstone (2012) as "strong-arm rehabs," are sites of intensive surveillance, coercion, and control. Several ethnographies conducted by feminists have demonstrated that the logics of strong-arm rehab are more aligned to the carceral system than to biomedicine and that such programs often blend punitive and psychologically abusive techniques with pseudo-therapeutic approaches (McKim 2008; McCorkel 2013).

It is likely that Dr. Kuar was not fully aware of the numerous ways in which structured recovery programs curtail clients' liberties and lives. However, the perception that such sites are providing resources for housing, education, and employment opportunities is an attractive lure for obstetricians and other maternity care practitioners who see "chaos" as the foundational problem in patients' lives. By this logic, if lack of structure is the root problem, then more structure is the solution; if the home, familial, or community environment is the root problem, then removing patients from their environments is the solution. In practice, however, "order" has little to do with "support." The most common complaint from the women I interviewed who were in structured recovery programs was that their basic needs and instrumental forms of support were often ignored. From lack of childcare, to restrictive rules and curfews that kept women from attending school or finding employment, to staff intentionally withholding access to supplies like diapers and baby wipes as a way to instill "self-sufficiency" in clients (i.e., mothers were expected to demonstrate that they could materially support themselves and would not become dependent on the program for meeting their material needs), over and over again women related stories in which order trumped support and care.

Although the ob interlocutors often remarked upon a lack of support, and regarded this lack as problematic for patients, appropriate institutional supports were often difficult to locate. For example, several obstetricians and other care providers mentioned pregnancy as a "window of opportunity." A refrain familiar to obs, this "window" refers to the period of time during prenatal care when patients receive routine care and are provided with medical counseling regarding their own and their future infants' health and wellbeing—in other words, when they are under the surveillance and control of the biomedical system. In the context of substance-using patients, the "window of opportunity" was often described in a way that aligned closely with extra-clinical surveillance, rather than with the provision of care or resource allocation. An ob interlocutor, Dr. Hill, explained:

> There are obviously a lot of stigmas and I think there probably have been instances where mothers who maybe fall into this category [of opioid dependence] are judged more harshly. I think that that is probably difficult. Not all, but many women who have substance abuse issues have other socioeconomic burdens that make it difficult for them to be able to seek care—like poor transportation access and poor family support. And sometimes they're having to work too much, you know, to be a mom working two jobs or something like that. I really do think that that's probably a large reason why a lot of these women sometimes don't get any care, and then they just show up in labor or they show up having an emergency and then if we're not doing a good job to screen or catch them while they're there, they just, they come in, they come out, and you know, they're back out, feeling like they don't have any support again.

Similar to the "chaos requires order" line of structural-causal thinking, this ob identifies a lack of support as the underlying problem facing women with SUDs. Placing herself in the shoes of the patient, Dr. Hill considers that several practical limitations exist for patients to be able to regularly access prenatal care. However, when she specifies the role of biomedicine in supporting patients, she focuses on the limitations of detecting, "screening" or "catching" substance-using patients while they are in the biomedical system. This view of the ways in which providers can support patients narrowly imagines biomedicine's role through the lens of institutional "capture," while specific forms of support and care are left unarticulated.

In general, the ob interlocutors viewed referral to child welfare as the most expeditious route to connecting patients to services and to ensure that risky patients are monitored (Fong 2020). For several of the ob interlocutors, child welfare was seen as a decent enough proxy for institutional support. For example, in the exchange below, an ob, Dr. Parker, explains that the child welfare system plays an essential role in surveilling families, particularly when biomedicine lacks sufficient supports for mothers with SUDs:

> *Parker:* Even if it does come to that point where we have to notify [child welfare], it's not punitive, it's making sure that every resource that is needed in every situation is available.

> *McCabe:* Do you feel like [child welfare] is a service provider, that they're connecting women to services that you all as medical providers are not able to connect them to? Or how does [child welfare] come in in a non-punitive way?

> *Parker:* I think because oftentimes there'll be, once we get past that six-week postpartum visit, they're kind of done with us. And so to make sure that you have that continuity to make sure that there's someone out there following this patient—because we know that in the year following delivery, that's where you have the highest rates of maternal deaths, overdose. And is there someone checking in with them? . . . So just trying to have as many safety nets as possible to pick these patients up who may need extra help, and then providing it for them and understanding what those resources that are available for these patients are, so we can just plug them in as fluidly as possible.

This obstetrician expresses the belief that structural deficits in health care, such as the postpartum lack of continuity of care, can be resolved by the child welfare system, which can "follow" patients and "check in on them." Dr. Parker imagines that CPS may be a resource for preventing overdose deaths through their surveillance function. Indeed, the postpartum period is an especially vulnerable time, and research shows that the risk of fatal overdose does increase in the year after giving birth (Schiff et al. 2018). However, there is no evidence to suggest that CPS interventions reduce overdose deaths, and some recent studies show that CPS involvement may create unique stressors that *precipitate* re-lapse and overdose (see, e.g., Cleveland et al. 2020).

Obs and other healthcare providers who are familiar with the lim-itations and rigidity of for-profit medicine may optimistically view the child welfare system as a dynamic service provider that can flexibly adapt to the needs of families in ways that biomedical systems cannot. The opacity of the child welfare system, and reforms in the last 30 years that emphasize keeping families intact through service provision, enable these sorts of assessments. However, the belief that CPS is better able to address the structural problems that substance-using mothers face pro-motes an underperformance in biomedical maternity care. When obs de-fer to child welfare, they miss opportunities to provide essential care to people with SUDs—for example, by counseling patients and providing referrals to treatment early in pregnancy, or by employing harm reduc-tion strategies such as appropriate information and resources to manage overdose risk during prenatal and postnatal care (for an extensive re-view of perinatal harm reduction strategies, see Kurzer-Yashin and Sue 2020), or by obtaining waivers to provide medication treatment them-selves.[3] In fact, by routinely engaging with CPS through the practices of testing and reporting, providers are likely deterring substance-using patients from seeking medical care when they need it most. Not only have studies shown that fear of CPS has a chilling effect on prenatal care utilization (Roberts and Pies 2011; Stone 2015), but research also suggests that the fear of punitive system involvement results in system avoidance (Brayne 2014) and can have long-term and profound effects on women's health, as they may avoid contact with healthcare settings for extended durations of time (Knight 2015).

In my interviews, the desire to "oversee" families was a common refrain. One provider explained: "When the child goes home, there's not really anybody overseeing that family system. And my experience is most of the time [when] a baby is born substance-exposed, there's a lot of social risks." Another ob emphasized the safety of the newborn as she endorsed postpartum CPS surveillance: "We have to protect the babies. We don't know the circumstances outside of the hospitals that that baby might be exposed to. So even though we, you know, prefer not to get child welfare involved, we have to for the protection of the baby." There was a sense among the interlocutors that the home environment posed an unknown—but likely dangerous—threat to the newborn. This variation on the "chaos requires order" theme reflected that for some obs, drug use *was* a symptom of a larger set of social maladies rooted in patients' homes, relationships, and communities, and it was those non-biomedical risk factors that needed to be contained, managed, and disciplined by a differently qualified set of experts.

## Too Distal to Treat

In 1995, Jo Phelan and Bruce Link introduced "fundamental cause theory" as a new way to understand morbidity as causally linked to socioeconomic status. This theory proposed that epidemiological models had become too subsumed with "proximal" causes of illness, or causes within an individuals' control, and that underlying "distal" (systematic, endemic, structural) causes that shape the social, economic, and political context are too often neglected, resulting in an inability to adequately address enduring morbidities. In the findings that follow, I explore the ways in which obs discussed distal causes of health. My findings reveal that, although providers seem to understand that distal factors such as socioeconomic status (SES), education, and other opportunity structures directly impact the health and wellbeing of mothers with SUDs, it is precisely the distal nature of substance use disorders that places low-income patients beyond the scope of medical intervention. When patients fall into the drug use *plus* social risk category, their substance use is deemed to be too socially determined to interrupt through individual, behavioral, and corporal approaches within biomedical maternity care models. In the quote below, obstetrician Sharon Jenkins defines the boundaries of her role as a physician, and explains that her work ends where patients' "social issues" begin:

> My job as a physician kinda ends after the safe delivery of the baby and the clinical postpartum care of the mom. When I start adding all of the other social issues—because there's usually so many of them—I would spend the majority of my time . . . because there will be patients with so many problems. And the visitors have problems. And they're very demanding and they don't have car seats, and they have family and they've got domestic violence . . . So substance abuse is just one of the many things that we're dealing with.
>    I feel like I have to make sure clinically that my patients are okay from the time they walk in here until the time that they leave. And if I get too involved with the social issues . . . then I risk missing other things. So it's important for me to stay focused. And as much as I would like—when I've made my rounds postpartum—if I have patients who are using methadone or who have . . . admitted to . . .

eight bags of heroin a day, I let my nursing staff kinda deal with that . . . I just cannot sacrifice my mental time and energy there. So we have to be conscious of what we're dealin' with so that we can connect patients with the services that they need, rather than trying to manage those issues on our own.

As Jenkins indicates, the structural issues affecting patients are heterogenous. The "problems" range from a lack of important resources like car seats to domestic violence and substance use. The complex issues, demands, and social relationships with which patients enter the clinic are challenging for providers. Some obs may attempt to cordon off the social from the clinical aspects of their work. Although the binary between "social" and "medical" is certainly a false one, such compartmentalization may be a kind of self-preservation tactic for obs who practice in settings that serve high-need patient populations. Dr. Jenkins, the ob quoted just above, describes the volume of social "problems" as "distractions" that prevent her from providing effective clinical care—or would if she allowed them to. A patient receiving medication treatment is on the same plane of consideration as a patient with an eight-bag-a-day heroin addiction, both construed as a drain on the ob's "mental time and energy," which she would have to "sacrifice" to deal with such "distractions." By homogenizing the complexities of patients' "social issues," this ob also establishes the boundaries of clinical practice. However, homogenizing patients' social experiences does not lead to better clinical outcomes (Davis 2019), and Dr. Jenkin's case resulted in outsourcing care to either less-credentialed staff or to punitive administrative systems such as CPS.

Sometimes providers struggled to rationalize the kinds of contradictions that arise in response to perinatal substance use. For example, many of the obs I spoke with found the legal response to illegal substance exposure to be unfair, given that several legal chemical exposures are just as, if not more, harmful to fetal development. In the account below, an ob who worked at a teaching hospital supported the notion that substance use is both a form of child abuse and an outcome of structural disadvantage for which individuals should not be held responsible. When I asked this ob, Dr. Ahmed, how she felt about the state's child abuse statute that classifies illicit substance use during pregnancy as child abuse, she responded:

The concept of child neglect—and this is gonna make me sound like a socialist—but the concept of child neglect from my perspective is really a societal issue. And if you're talking about it being a societal issue, then that means that if you truly don't want people to use drugs, or have access to drugs, then you crack down on it in an effective way. That's not actually being done. Right? So if you take your lower socioeconomic status kind of neighborhoods—for example, provide them with access to things like . . . a safe park where people can take their children—rather than. . . I don't know if you've driven down to the Southside of Chicago neighborhoods. But truly they're deserts. They are [food] deserts. And if you're gonna blame an individual for that, that's just wrong. Right? But if you're gonna blame an individual for it, then also put the crackdown on cigarettes and alcohol.

Like it's not . . . to me the state does it in a very narrow-minded way. I'm not saying that it's not child neglect. It is. But so is alcohol use. So is cigarette smoking, 'cause cigarette smoking results in lifetime lung issues. We know that asthma—childhood asthma—is related to cigarette smoking. That's awful. But it's not child neglect to smoke cigarettes. But it's child neglect to smoke marijuana—when the issues come hand in hand. Similarly, if you're not providing the social structure to allow people, and facilitate people, to improve their status in life so they don't need marijuana . . . I mean why do people go to things like marijuana, alcohol, cigarettes, whatever? It's because of the stresses of life, right? 'Cause they can't pay their bill-to-bill, and they're working three jobs to try to afford it. Or because they don't have access to easy birth control. I mean if you decrease social stressors, they won't need to resort to these things.

In Dr. Ahmed's words, we can see how this ob struggles to reconcile the disproportionate responses to illicit in utero substance exposure with the known harms caused by several licit (e.g., alcohol and tobacco) exposures. She seems to conclude that, since there are no easy solutions to address the "societal issues" that may contribute to "social stressors" and thereby the use of illicit substances to cope, policies should at least be consistently applied to *all* potentially harmful substances. Powerless to effect change at the structural level, Dr. Ahmed reasons that some version of fairness may be achieved through standardizing punitive responses. When faced with the undesirable option of blaming individuals for their structural circumstances, she seeks to level the proverbial playing field—not by asserting that perinatal substance use resulting from structural disadvantage should not be legally encoded as child abuse—but instead by holding the position that *all* types of substance use during pregnancy should be regarded as forms of child neglect.

Dr. Ahmed's reasoning demonstrates that, when faced with inconsistencies in policy responses to substance use during pregnancy, some obs may resort to thinking in absolute terms. When engaging in structural-causal thinking, structural problems that are viewed as interlocking and insurmountable can encourage thinking in extremes, wherein anything less than structural overhaul will not suffice to address the enormity of the social problem. What is reasonable, fair, and pragmatic shifts dramatically in the face of a seemingly insurmountable problem.

Proponents of universal drug screening often reflect this logic. The risks associated with drug testing patients, which include child welfare involvement, possible incarceration, and system avoidance, have been shown to outweigh the clinical information that drug tests yield in perinatal care (ACOG 2011). As a result, the American College of Obstetricians and Gynecologists (ACOG) has advocated that providers assess for substance use during pregnancy using verbal screening measures instead of conducting biologic drug testing.

Yet despite efforts by professional organizations like ACOG to discourage biologic testing, some hospitals and jurisdictions have sought to apply testing more widely so as to reduce racial biases in testing. This apparent fairness—"everyone gets tested"—distracts from the more meaningful ways in which drug testing is a form of obstetric violence and of the criminalization of care. Why? Because the results of urine drug testing rarely affect clinical management (ACOG 2011; Dupouy et al. 2014). If drug testing were overwhelmingly associated with better outcomes, improved clinical management, and healthier mothers and babies, then it would be an unproblematic facet of care. But, I argue, the underlying issue is an ethical one: testing constitutes obstetric violence because it is associated with many undesirable social, legal, and health outcomes and risks to the mother-infant dyad that can include the criminalization of obstetric patients with SUDs.

The ob interlocutors also often endorsed connecting with and finding commonalities with their patients. Empathetic approaches, however, were limited by the underlying inability of providers to address the social and environmental causes of substance use. The ob quoted below, Dr. Griffiths, takes an empathetic tack:

I think that the challenges that we have are kind of the same that a lot of people have, and it's a social issue. I do try and find—for me—some commonality. I kinda joke with them. I said, "You know, your heroin is my ice cream. I know that you don't get up every day saying 'Okay, this is what I'm gonna do.' I don't get up every day saying 'Okay, I'm gonna eat two kinds of ice cream.' But whenever stressors or something's going on, and you get overwhelmed, and you can't cope, and you just wanna feel better in that moment, that's where you go. I get that." For me, I can remove myself from the supermarket. With them, how do you remove yourself from your community, from your home environment, from, you know . . . ? And . . . that's where I think . . . the solution really is. But as a society . . . we're not invested in community care. And so, I think . . . we're chasing our tails on this, honestly.

The distal (structural and endemic) situatedness and embeddedness of the social problem makes it difficult for obs to feel equipped to compe-tently address the issues of substance-using pregnant patients. The met-aphor of indulging in ice cream finds its natural limit as this ob concedes that environmental and circumstantial factors powerfully influence addictive behavior. Her astute observation that the lack of investment in community care leaves biomedical providers "chasing their tails" on complex issues like substance dependency during pregnancy points to an underlying flaw in structural competency as a clinical training mo-dality. *Awareness* of the distal causes of addiction and of the forms of socio-political disinvestment that contribute to addiction does not necessarily engender a sense of competence among professionals. Anti-thetically, awareness of structural inequalities may impede productive clinical interactions if providers see the social issues before them as too distal to treat or to cure.

## Discussion

Medical sociologists have called for the biomedical establishment to embrace "progressive health care tactics" (Brown 2011; Metzl and Han-sen 2014; Stonington et al. 2018). The call for biomedical providers to widen the traditional medical gaze to incorporate an understand-ing of illness and disease that is rooted in social relations, structures of inequality, and community environments optimistically re-envisions healthcare providers' abilities to sociologically diagnose illness and dis-ease as effects of inequality and stratified opportunities. My findings reveal that the ob interlocutors already engaged in a process of "social diagnosis" (Brown 2011), in which signs of social precarity and disad-vantage *were* identified and incorporated into clinical decision-making. However, the ability of providers to identify disadvantages did not im-prove patient care; rather, it created a new set of iatrogenic effects. Patients who were believed to be substance users were moved onto a "problematic" clinical track that stymied clinical action and limited therapeutic approaches.

There are several pitfalls and fallacies that arise when maternity care practitioners engage in structural-causal thinking. One surprising outcome is that obs who have some awareness of structural inequality may actually feel *less* competent and less equipped to address the needs of socially and economically marginalized patients. Obs who feel powerless to address the complex needs of patients within their scope of practice may be more willing to hand patients off to coercive and punitive systems that are perceived as better equipped to address patients' needs. My findings suggest that obs who believe that patients lack strong institutional support (familial or community-based) are likely to endorse more surveillant and coercive institutional involvement.

I found that although the ob interlocutors were aware of structural limitations in health care—such as lack of continuity of care, limited time and resources for patient care, and lack of treatment capacity—this biomedical structural awareness did not extend to their own enforcement activities and interactions with patients. For example, the problem of continuity of care in maternal-infant medicine was believed to be resolved by the child welfare system, which can step in and monitor families when providers cannot. One of the obs with whom I spoke did not identify routine reporting to CPS or system involvement via clinical interactions as forms of structural inequality in and of themselves. This finding points to perhaps the biggest blind spot in structural-causal thinking. For the ob interlocutors, "structure" is something that exists outside of biomedicine. They did not perceive biomedicine and biomedical practitioners as perpetuating inequities that may affect health when, for example, they reported families to CPS. Instead, obstetricians who engaged in structural-causal thinking often believed that they were *correcting for structural asymmetries* when they collaborated with child welfare systems.

As previously noted, biomedical deference to outside actors like CPS meaningfully impacts patient care. When providers view substance use through a social problem lens informed by criminal-legal risk, they stop attending to their patients' clinical needs and start engaging as auxiliaries of the state. Norms in care are retracted, for instance when providers non-consensually drug-test patients or refuse to provide health-based resources and counseling for substance-using patients. This biomedical underperformance is enabled by structural-causal thinking that homogenizes patients' complex needs as a chaotic jumble of adversities, risks, and disadvantages.

My findings also highlight that addiction is viewed variously as a biomedical, moral, and structural problem. Because substance use is frequently used as a proxy for other sorts of social risks, and social risk is often extricated from clinical practice (vis-à-vis the construction of a false social-clinical binary), people with substance use disorders are subject to discrimination and criminalization within the clinic. For example, in her analysis of drug courts, Rebecca Tiger (2012) argues that the medical framing of addiction complements criminal-legal approaches. She posits that the disease model of addiction defines substance dependency as chronic, recurring, and incurable; this definition is then cited by state actors to justify more intensive, coercive, and surveillant methods of managing substance users (Tiger 2012). This logic appears to be in play among biomedical professionals as well: if one cannot be "fixed" via traditional biomedical means, then that individual requires closer monitoring and control via other means.

## Conclusion: Beyond Awareness and Toward Competence

I conclude by offering some examples of ways in which obstetricians can go beyond the awareness of structure and toward a model of actionable solutions:

*Reducing structural harm at home.* First, obs must integrate biomedicine as a structure in their personal evaluations of determinants of health. Applying the logics of harm reduction, obs should consider the ways in which they can tackle structural harms that have become a part of routine clinical practice. For guidance, obs need look no further than their own professional organization, the American College of Obstetricians and Gynecologists. In 2020, ACOG released a policy statement in opposition to the criminalization of individuals seeking pregnancy-related care. This policy statement encourages obs to obtain consent for drug testing, to communicate with patients about the risks and harms associated with a positive toxicology result, and to avoid coercion and threats of criminalization in order to gain patient consent to and compliance with their treatment plans. Obs may go a step further by actively engaging in research or in institutional policy reforms that will help to assess the need and institutional capacity to de-implement harmful practices, such as routine toxicology screening in perinatal care.

*Know the lay of the land.* Obs can also reduce harm by becoming informed about federal, local, and institutional responses to substance use during pregnancy. I suggest that obs should research federal and state laws, such as mandated reporting requirements, to understand the reach of the law and their obligations to comply with it. Within their own practices, departments, and units, obs can set about investigating formal institutional responses and policies regarding SUDs and pregnancy. Obs can consider asking questions such as: How are the risks of substance use communicated to patients, how is informed consent for testing obtained, how is patient privacy protected, what happens when you make a hotline call to child welfare, what are patients' experiences with CPS once a report is made, and what is the best way to refer patients to treatment and other resources? While obs are aware of certain structural facets underlying perinatal substance use, that awareness frequently stops short of their own activities and institutions. Researching the full scope of medical, legal, and social responses may instill a sense of competence in an area that was previously wrought with uncertainty and risk.

*Provide care where you can.* Although biomedical staff cannot address the structural factors that impact addiction, it is within their scope of practice to counsel patients who admit to substance use; to refer patients to treatment providers without subjecting them to CPS and its many deficiencies; and to address the health needs of substance users, which include risk of overdose, infection of the heart valves related to injection substance use, inadequate nutrition, cardiovascular problems, risks associated with withdrawal symptoms, and risks of HIV or hepatitis C transmission. Some obs may qualify to obtain a waiver to provide buprenorphine (a synthetic opioid used in a similar fashion to methadone) in their clinical practices. Alternatively, obs can research local integrated care facilities that may be better equipped to care for patients with SUDs.

*Mobilize for political change.* If obs believe that state laws and policies are putting patients at risk of experiencing system involvement or criminalization for seeking care, they should politically mobilize against those laws and policies. In states such as New York, Illinois, and Tennessee, physicians have partnered with state representatives and legal advocacy groups to combat legislative efforts to criminalize pregnant patients, and have sought to codify protections for patients into law. There are several resources available to obs who are interested in groups doing advocacy work on the issue of perinatal drug use, including the National Advocates for Pregnant Women, the Movement for Family Power, the Academy for Perinatal Harm Reduction, the Birth Rights Bar Association, and Interrupting Criminalization, to name a few.

To recap, these are all ways in which obstetricians can go beyond the awareness of structure to address forms of discrimination that emerge in clinical interactions, thereby giving substance-using pregnant women, mothers, and their babies better chances to enjoy healthy lives.

**Katharine McCabe** is a postdoctoral researcher with the John J. Reilly Center for Science, Technology, and Values at the University of Notre Dame. She researches gender, race, and sexuality, the politics of reproduction, and legal and institutional responses to substance use and addiction. Katharine's current research examines medico-legal responses to pregnant substance users. She also examines state policies on child welfare responses to maternal substance use and regional reproductive healthcare responses to the opioid crisis. Katharine's research has been published in the *Journal of Health and Social Behavior, Social Science and Medicine, The Journal of Women's Health, Perspectives on Sexual and Reproductive Health*, and *Sex Roles*.

## Notes

1. I use the terms "substance use disorder" (SUD), "addiction," and "substance use" interchangeably to capture the ways in which illicit substance use during pregnancy has been described historically. For example, pregnant people who use illicit substances during pregnancy are often described as having a substance use disorder, which would suggest that they have been assessed by a health professional and met the diagnostic criteria for a use disorder. However, many pregnant patients are determined to have used substances during pregnancy through urinary drug tests, which, absent diagnostic evaluation, do not indicate a pattern of substance misuse.
2. The "war on drugs" refers to a punitive pattern of responses to drug use surges that defined US drug policy from the end of the Nixon era through the end of the 20th century. Prohibitionary drug policies and criminal-legal measures (such as mandatory sentencing for drug-related offenses) targeted Black communities for surveillance and over-policing. Black women were targeted typically through their reproductive behaviors (see Roberts 2002; Alexander 2010).
3. See SAMHSA guidelines https://www.samhsa.gov/medication-assisted-treat ment/become-buprenorphine-waivered-practitioner.

## References

Alexander M. 2010. *The New Jim Crow: Mass Incarceration in the Age of Color Blindness.* New York: The New Press.

American Bar Association (ABA). 2021. *Case Law Review: Key Legal Issues in Civil Child Protection Cases Involving Prenatal Substance Exposure.* Retrieved 8 November 2022 from https://www.americanbar.org/content/dam/aba/administra tive/child_law/prenatal-substance-use-case-law-brief_full-508.pdf.

American College of Obstetricians and Gynecologists (ACOG). 2011. "Substance Abuse Reporting and Pregnancy: The Role of the Obstetrician. Committee Opinion No. 473." *Obstetrics & Gynecology* 117: 200–201.

————. 2020. "Opposition to Criminalization of Individuals during Pregnancy and the Postpartum Period: Statement of Policy." *ACOG*, December. Retrieved 8 November 2022 from https://www.acog.org/clinical-information/policy-and-position-statements/statements-of-policy/2020/opposition-criminalizati on-of-individuals-pregnancy-and-postpartum-period#:~:text=ACOG%20belie ves%20that%20it%20is,the%20postpartum%20period%20(11).

Brayne S. 2014. "Surveillance and System Avoidance: Criminal Justice Contact and Institutional Attachment." *American Sociological Review* 79(3): 367–391.

Brown P, Lyson M, Jenkins T. 2011. "From Diagnosis to Social Diagnosis." *Social Science and Medicine* 73(6): 939–43.

Britton BV, Nagarajan N, Zogg CK, et al. 2016. "Awareness of Racial/Ethnic Dispar-ities in Surgical Outcomes and Care: Factors Affecting Acknowledgment and Action." *American Journal of Surgery* 212(1): 102–108.

Bridges KM. 2020. "Race, Pregnancy, and the Opioid Epidemic: White Privilege and the Criminalization of Opioid Use during Pregnancy." *Harvard Law Review* 133(3): 770–851.

Campbell N. 2012. "Medicalization and Biomedicalization: Does the Diseasing of Addiction Fit the Frame?" In *Critical Perspectives on Addiction*, ed. Netherland J, 3–25. Bingley: Emerald Group Publishing Limited.

Charmaz K. 2014. *Constructing Grounded Theory*, 2nd edn. London: Sage Publications.

Cleveland LM, McGlothen-Bell K, Scott LA, Recto P. 2020. "A Life-Course Theory Exploration of Opioid-Related Maternal Mortality in the United States." *Addiction* 115(11): 2079–2088.

Davis DA. 2019. "Obstetric Racism: The Racial Politics of Pregnancy, Labor, and Birthing." *Medical Anthropology* 38(7): 560–573.

D'Andrade AC. 2015. "Parents and Court-Ordered Services: A Descriptive Study of Service Use in Child Welfare Reunification." *Families in Society: The Journal of Contemporary Social Services* 96(1): 25–34.

Dupouy J, Mémier V, Catala H, et al. 2014. "Does Urine Drug Abuse Screening Help for Managing Patients? A Systematic Review." *Drug and Alcohol Depen-dence* 136(2014): 11–20.

Faherty LJ, Kranz AM, Russell-Fritch J, et al. 2019. "Association of Punitive and Re-porting State Policies Related to Substance Use in Pregnancy with Rates of Neo-natal Abstinence Syndrome." *JAMA Network Open* 2(11): e1914078–e1914078.

Fong K. 2020. "Getting Eyes in the Home: Child Protective Services Investigations and State Surveillance of Family Life." *American Sociological Review* 85(4): 610–638.

Gowan T, Whetstone S. 2012. "Making the Criminal Addict: Subjectivity and Social Control in a Strong-Arm Rehab." *Punishment & Society* 14(1): 69–93.

Guttmacher Institute. 2021. "Substance Use During Pregnancy." Retrieved De-cember 10 2021 from https://www.guttmacher.org/state-policy/explore/subst ance-use-during-pregnancy.

Harris Interactive. 2011. *2011 Physicians' Daily Life Report*, prepared for the Rob-ert Wood Johnson Foundation. Retrieved 8 November 2022 from https://www .issuelab.org/resources/12550/12550.pdf.

Kurzer-Yashin D, Sue K. 2020. *Pregnancy and Substance Use: A Harm Reduction Toolkit*. New York: National Harm Reduction Coalition and Academy of Perina-

tal Harm Reduction. Retrieved 8 November 2022 from https://www.perinatal
harmreduction.org/toolkit-pregnancy-substance-use.

Kendrick J, Nuccio E, Leiferman JA, Sauaia A. 2015. "Primary Care Providers'. Perceptions of Racial/Ethnic and Socioeconomic Disparities in Hypertension Control." *American Journal of Hypertension* 28(9): 1091–1097.

Kleinman A, Benson, P. 2006. "Anthropology in the Clinic: The Problem of Cultural
Competency and How to Fix It." *PLoS Medicine* 3(10): e294.

Knight KR. 2015. *Addicted. Pregnant. Poor.* Durham NC: Duke University Press.

———. 2020. "Structural Factors that Affect Life Contexts of Pregnant People with
Opioid Use Disorders: The Role of Structural Racism and the Need for Structural Competency." *Women's Reproductive Health* 7(3): 164–171.

Link BG, Phelan J. 1995. "Social Conditions as Fundamental Causes of Disease."
*Journal of Health and Social Behavior* Spec: 80–94.

McCabe K. 2021. "Criminalization of Care: Drug Testing Pregnant Patients." *Journal
of Health and Social Behavior* 63(2): 162–176.

McCorkel JA. 2013. *Breaking Women: Gender, Race, and the New Politics of Imprison-
ment.* New York: New York University Press.

McKim A. 2008. "'Getting Gut-Level': Punishment, Gender, and Therapeutic Governance." *Gender & Society* 22(3): 303–323.

Metzl JM, Hansen H. 2014. "Structural Competency: Theorizing a New Medical
Engagement with Stigma and Inequality." *Social Science & Medicine* 103(2014):
126–133.

Metzl JM, Petty J, and Olowojoba OV. 2018. "Using a Structural Competency
Framework to Teach Structural Racism in Pre-Health Education." *Social Science
& Medicine* 199(2018): 189–201.

Paltrow LM, Flavin J. 2013. "Arrests of and Forced Interventions on Pregnant Women
in the United States, 1973–2005: Implications for Women's Legal Status and
Public Health." *Journal of Health Politics, Policy and Law* 38(2): 299–343.

Pew Research Center. 2014. "America's Changing Drug Policy Landscape." *Pew Research Center,* 2 April. Retrieved 8 November 2022 from https://www.pewre
search.org/politics/2014/04/02/americas-new-drug-policy-landscape/.

Reich JA. 2005. *Fixing Families: Parents, Power, and the Child Welfare System.* New
York: Routledge.

Roberts DE. 2002. *Shattered Bonds: The Color of Child Welfare.* New York: Basic
Civitas Books.

Roberts SC, Pies C. 2011. "Complex Calculations: How Drug Use During Pregnancy
Becomes a Barrier to Prenatal Care." *Maternal and Child Health Journal* 15(3):
333–341.

Sangoi L. 2020. *"Whatever They Do, I'm Her Comfort, I'm Her Protector": How the
Foster System Has Become Ground Zero for the U.S. Drug War.* Movement for
Family Power. Retrieved 8 November 2022 from https://www.movementfor
familypower.org/ground-zero.

Schiff DM, Nielsen TM, Hood M, et al. 2018. "Fatal and Nonfatal Overdose among
Pregnant and Postpartum Women in Massachusetts." *Obstetrics and Gynecology*
132(2): 466–474.

Shepherd SM. 2019. "Cultural Awareness Workshops: Limitations and Practical
Consequences." *BMC Medical Education* 19(1): 1–10.

Stone R. 2015. "Pregnant Women and Substance Use: Fear, Stigma, and Barriers to Care." *Health & Justice* 3(1): 1–15.

Stonington SD, Holmes SM, Hansen H, et al. 2018. "Case Studies in Social Medicine—Attending to Structural Forces in Clinical Practice." *New England Journal of Medicine* 379(20): 1958–1961.

Subbaraman MS, Roberts SC. 2019. "Costs Associated with Policies Regarding Alcohol Use during Pregnancy: Results from 1972–2015 Vital Statistics." *PloS One* 14(5): e0215670.

Substance Abuse and Mental Health Services Administration (US) and Office of the Surgeon General (US) (SAMHSA). 2016. "Health Care Systems and Substance Use Disorders." In *Facing Addiction in America: The Surgeon General's Report on Alcohol, Drugs, and Health*, 6-1–6-71. Washington DC: US Department of Health and Human Services. Retrieved 8 November 2022 from https://addiction.surgeongeneral.gov/sites/default/files/chapter-6-health-care-systems.pdf.

Terplan M, Kennedy-Hendricks A, Chisolm MS. 2015. "Article Commentary: Prenatal Substance Use: Exploring Assumptions of Maternal Unfitness." *Substance Abuse: Research and Treatment* 9: SART-S23328.

Tiger R. 2012. *Judging Addicts: Drug Courts and Coercion in the Justice System*. New York: New York University Press.

# CHAPTER 10

# Contraceptive Provision by Obstetricians/Gynecologists in the United States

## Biases, Misperceptions, and Barriers to an Essential Reproductive Health Service

*Melissa Goldin Evans*

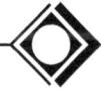

## Introduction:
## Contraception as an Essential Reproductive Health Service

*Unintended Pregnancies and Contraceptive Usage by Method Type*

Most women spend the majority of their reproductive lives avoiding pregnancy. Nearly half (45%) of all pregnancies in the United States are unintended (i.e., mistimed or unwanted), with little improvement over the last 30 years (Finer and Zolna 2016). Unintended pregnancies increase the risk of short interpregnancy intervals (Gemmill and Lindberg 2013; Cheslack Postava and Winter 2015; White, Teal, and Potter 2015), and both unintended pregnancies and short interpregnancy intervals are associated with adverse health and social outcomes for the infant and the mother (Gavin et al. 2014; Ahrens et al. 2019; Hutcheon et al. 2019).

Women who experience an unintended pregnancy are left with two choices: have an abortion or have an unplanned birth. Both options are rife with complex emotional and financial considerations (Roberts, Berglas, and Kimport 2020). Unplanned births are more common among women in poverty than among women with higher income levels (Finer and Zolna 2016), and this may be because of the inability to pay for an abortion, lacking a way get to an abortion provider, or living in a state that restricts abortion access (Roberts et al. 2020; Upadhyay et al. 2021). Given the economic burden of raising a child, it is imperative that women who do not wish to become pregnant be able control their reproductive futures.

The risk of unintended pregnancies is significantly reduced when women use effective methods of contraception (American College of Obstetricians and Gynecologists [ACOG] 2015, 2018). Long-acting reversible contraceptives (LARCs)—intrauterine devices (IUDs) and implants (a small hormone-releasing rod inserted into the skin of the upper arm)—are more effective than non-LARCs such as the pill, patch, ring, diaphragm, and condoms in reducing the risks of unintended pregnancies (ACOG 2017a). There are two main categories of LARCs: progestin-containing LARCs—including implants and most IUDs—and non-hormonal copper IUDs (ACOG 2017a).

Although LARCs are highly efficacious (ACOG 2017a) and are also highly tolerable (low discontinuation rates and high satisfaction rates) (Birgisson et al. 2015; Simmons et al. 2019), they are utilized by less than 14% of US women at risk of unintended pregnancies (IUDs: 12.0%; implants: 2.6%) (Guttmacher Institute 2021). Despite the three-fold increase in LARC use over the past decade (Beshar et al. 2021), among women at risk of unintended pregnancies, permanent female contraceptives—salpingectomies (excisions of the fallopian tube), tubal ligations, and tubal implants—are the most common methods of contraception (28%), followed by the pill (17%) and male condoms (13%); 11% use no method (Guttmacher Institute 2021).

Postpartum LARCs, whether inserted immediately postpartum or during a follow-up visit, are especially effective in reducing the risk of short interpregnancy intervals (Lopez et al. 2015; White et al. 2015; ACOG 2018). However, rates of postpartum LARC uptake are lower than sterilization rates in the immediate postpartum period before hospital discharge, and also lower than sterilization and moderately effective methods by three and 18 months postpartum (White et al. 2015).

### LARC Eligibility and Benefits for Certain Populations

The American College of Obstetricians and Gynecologists (ACOG) and the Centers for Disease Control and Prevention (CDC) state that LARCs are acceptable for use in women regardless of age, parity, history of sexually transmitted infections (STIs), and ectopic pregnancy, and that LARCs provide a rapid return to fertility after removal (Curtis, Jatlaoui et al. 2016; Curtis, Tepper et al. 2016; ACOG 2017a, 2017b).

Furthermore, certain populations of women may benefit more from using a LARC than a non-LARC. For example, the long-term presence of LARCs makes them a good option for adolescents who want to avoid pregnancy but find it difficult to consistently use contraception (Raine et al. 2011; Pazol et al. 2015). LARCs can be safely used by women with certain chronic conditions (e.g., hypertension, diabetes, and obesity), and estrogen-free LARCs (i.e., copper IUDs and implants) are advantageous for women for whom hormone-containing drugs are not well-tolerated (Curtis, Tepper et al. 2016).

Specific to postpartum women, ACOG and the CDC recommend certain contraceptive methods based on breastfeeding status, timing of method initiation for optimal safety, and resumption of sexual activity (Curtis, Tepper et al. 2016; ACOG 2018). For example, some hormonal contraceptive methods are not safe within the first 21 days postpartum, due to their risk associated with venous thromboembolism (a potentially very dangerous blood clotting medical condition), but LARCs, sterilization, and progestin-only contraceptives (i.e., pill or intramuscular injection) can safely be initiated during this time (Curtis, Tepper et al. 2016).

Immediate (i.e., before hospital discharge) postpartum IUD insertions have minimal contraindications (e.g., the presence of intrauterine infection), and despite their higher expulsion rates (Averbach et al. 2020), the CDC and ACOG recommend IUDs for most women immediately postpartum because they are safe and their benefits outweigh their risks (ACOG 2016; Curtis, Tepper et al. 2016). Implants can also be initiated immediately after delivery and do not have a risk of expulsion (ACOG 2016). Furthermore, immediate postpartum or "postplacental" (i.e., while still in the delivery room) LARCs are a logical strategy for postpartum contraceptive use in populations with low rates of postpartum follow-up who could not afford a LARC after pregnancy-related insurance benefits expire or who would otherwise use a less effective method (White, Potter, et al. 2014; White, Teal, and Potter 2015; Lopez et al. 2015; ACOG 2016). Although IUD expulsion rates vary by timing (e.g., immediate or delayed), delivery type, and IUD type (Averbach et al. 2020), many women have them replaced (Chen et al. 2010; Woo et al. 2015).

## LARC Counseling and Provision Practices

Contraceptive services for women of reproductive age and for postpartum women, such as counseling and provision, are standard best practices for obstetrician/gynecologists (ob/gyns) (ACOG 2017a). The vast majority of ob/gyns in national surveys agreed that they had adequate time to counsel (92%) (Luchowski et al. 2014a) and were comfortable counseling about LARCs (>97%) (Davis et al. 2018). Likewise, whereas most ob/gyns residents surveyed in 2015 were largely comfortable inserting LARCs (>90%) (Davis et al. 2018) and most ob/gyns in a national 2020 survey offered IUDs (96%) and implants (84%) (Weigel et al. 2021), immediate postpartum LARC provision is rarer. A 2017 survey among ACOG Fellows found that while 81% placed LARCs during the first postpartum visit, only 27% provided immediate postpartum LARCs (Holden et al. 2018). Similarly, few ACOG members in a 2016/2017 survey offered immediate postpartum IUDs and implants (19% and 21% respectively) (Castleberry et al. 2019).

### Overview of LARC Access Barriers

Patient, provider, and clinic/office-level factors influence the uptake and provision of LARCs. Without access to all methods of contraception, women are more likely to opt for less effective methods and for methods with higher rates of user error (Bergin et al. 2012; Biggs et al. 2012; Potter et al. 2014). However, landmark studies have shown that once access and payment barriers are removed and comprehensive contraceptive counseling occurs, women choose LARCs more than other methods and continue to use LARCs longer than other methods (Ricketts, Klinger, and Schwalberg 2014; Birgisson et al. 2015; Simmons et al. 2019). Two of these programs demonstrated that improved access to LARCs resulted in lower rates of teen pregnancy, teen birth, and abortion (Ricketts et al. 2014; Birgisson et al. 2015).

At the patient level, consideration of LARCs as an option depends on awareness and knowledge of LARCs, personal preferences for LARC features, and accessibility (e.g., LARC availability in the clinic/office) (Bergin et al. 2012; Birgisson et al. 2015; Jackson et al. 2015). Furthermore, although sterilization, like LARCs, is safe for anytime or immediate postpartum use and is highly effective and user-independent, it is a procedure that is permanent, whereas LARCs are reversible (ACOG 2016; Curtis, Tepper et al. 2016). A patient's decision to use either of these methods may be based on her future reproductive goals: older women and women with more children rely more on sterilization, whereas younger women with fewer births rely more on LARCs (Baldwin et al. 2012; Whiteman et al. 2012). However, socioeconomic disparities in LARC use versus sterilization remain, and thus the decision to permanently end childbearing opportunities might have more to do with a lack of access to health care that restricts contraceptive choice or with economic realities such as not being able to afford to have more children (Beshar et al. 2021).

For postpartum women, access to contraceptives also impacts their ability to prevent short interpregnancy intervals. Some inpatient postpartum women who desire an IUD during a follow-up visit don't receive one because they don't return to the clinic for an insertion (e.g., due to scheduling, financial, transportation, or insurance barriers, particularly among those who are low-income or rural), and this failure to obtain a desired IUD resulted in use of less effective methods or no method (Bergin et al. 2012; Salcedo et al. 2015; Zerden et al. 2015). Even among postpartum women who desire sterilization, those with Medicaid are more likely than their privately insured counterparts to have an unfulfilled sterilization request and to subsequently have a short interpregnancy interval (Arora et al. 2018). Thus, the immediate postpartum period, while a woman is still in the hospital, may be the best opportunity for providing LARCs and other contraceptive options (Lopez et al. 2015; ACOG 2016).

The rest of this chapter focuses on LARC barriers and solutions at the clinician and clinic/health system levels, since most patient-level barriers to contraceptive access are logistical (i.e., related to from whom and where they receive contraceptive services). Concentrating on the following modifiable upstream barriers can have a larger impact on making LARC access more universal and equitable: provision of patient-centered routine unbiased contraceptive counseling, ob/gyns' knowledge about appropriate LARC candidates, LARC insertion training, and work environments supportive of same-day insertions.

## Methods

In this literature-based review, I examine how ob/gyns' biases, misperceptions, and barriers reduce reproductive-age women's access to LARCs in the United States. I have structured my review to follow the different provider-level barriers a patient may face when trying to access LARCs, starting with the importance of contraceptive counseling to educate the patient about her method choices. Then, if a LARC is chosen, this review delves into the different reasons why an ob/gyn may be unwilling or unable to provide a LARC. I used the following terms to search for relevant articles published between 2000–2020 in PubMed and Medline (EBSCO) databases: long-acting reversible contraceptives,

LARCs, contraception, family planning, barriers, obstetricians, gynecologists, ob/gyn, access, knowledge, attitudes, behaviors, uptake, provision, patient, provider, relationship, clinic, protocols, and policies.

## Contraceptive Counseling

### The Importance of Contraceptive Counseling

Since, as previously mentioned, most US women try to avoid pregnancy during the majority of their approximately 39 reproductive years (Cleland, Peipert et al. 2011), and given the enormous health, societal, and financial impacts of unintended pregnancies, contraceptive care and counseling are among the most essential preventive health services that healthcare practitioners can provide (Cleland, Conde-Agudelo et al. 2012; ACOG 2015). Patient knowledge, awareness, and likelihood of using moderately and highly effective contraceptive methods improve with receipt of contraceptive counseling and education (Zapata, Tregear, et al. 2015). Similarly, prenatal or postpartum contraceptive counseling increases the odds of postpartum contraceptive use (Zapata, Murtaza et al. 2015).

### Recommendations for Contraceptive Counseling

The CDC and ACOG recommend that all women of reproductive age receive comprehensive contraceptive counseling that is unbiased and evidence-based—i.e., eligibility is not based on women's age, parity, or gynecologic history (Gavin et al. 2014; ACOG 2015). Healthcare providers to reproductive-aged women such as ob/gyns should use every interaction as an opportunity to discuss and review their patients' reproductive health plans, including the patient's articulated goals regarding her reproductive future and how she can achieve those goals (e.g., contraceptive use) (Dehlendorf, Krajewski et al. 2014; Gomez et al. 2014). Ob/gyns should also capitalize on the period of increased healthcare access when women are pregnant and postpartum and should provide these women with comprehensive contraceptive counseling that includes the option of immediate postpartum LARC insertion (Lopez et al. 2015; ACOG 2016, 2018).

Above all, contraceptive counseling should occur within a reproductive justice framework (Luna and Luker 2013; Gubrium et al. 2016; Brandi and Fuentes 2019), which declares, among other things, that all people have the right to equal access to all reproductive technologies and health services (SisterSong 1997; Luna and Luker 2013). When trying to improve access and uptake of LARCs, it is important to consider the historical and present-day coercive contraceptive practices directed toward systematically minoritized women from patient, provider, and policy standpoints (Boonstra et al. 2000; Gold 2014; Harris and Wolfe 2014). From the days of slavery to eugenics and population control at the turn of the 20th century, and forced or coerced sterilizations throughout the 20th and 21st centuries, there have been attempts to control the fertility of marginalized women (e.g., low-income, non-white, and mentally incapacitated women, and female prisoners) (Raine 2012; Harris and Wolfe 2014). These efforts indirectly influence contraceptive provision and use (Thorburn and Bogart 2005; Downing, Laveist, and Bullock 2007; Dehlendorf, Ruskin et al. 2010). Evidence of differential treatment by providers based on patient race and socioeconomic status (SES) is particularly concerning in light of the historical efforts to control the fertility of non-white and poor women (Dehlendorf, Ruskin et al. 2010). Furthermore, compared to their counterparts, low-income and Women of Color report perceiving racial discrimination in obtaining contraceptives and receiving unsolicited contraceptive counseling, such as pressure from their healthcare provider to use contraceptives as a means to control their family size (Jackson et al. 2015; Gomez and Wapman 2017). Moreover, some Women of Color prefer contraceptive characteristics that allow them to control when to start and stop a method; such characteristics are aligned with methods that are inherently less effective and require less frequent or no interactions with their healthcare provider (Jackson et al. 2015). Thus, again, contraceptive counseling should follow the tenets of reproductive justice, meaning that it should take a patient-centered, shared decision-making approach that upholds and preserves patient autonomy (SisterSong 1997; Gomez et al. 2014; Bryson et al. 2021).

The patient-provider relationship influences patient decision-making and contraceptive use (Zapata, Tregear et al. 2015; Dehlendorf, Henderson et al. 2016), and ob/gyns should foster a trusting relationship with their patients by treating all of their patients equally and respectfully (Harris and Wolfe 2014; Kathawa and Arora 2020). Women who are more satisfied with their relationships and interactions with their healthcare providers are more likely to correctly use and continue to use contraceptives, whereas miscommunications and patient mistrust of providers can contribute to dissatisfaction with their care and can lead to contraceptive misuse (Dehlendorf, Henderson et al. 2016).

Contraceptive counseling should occur within the context of the patient's expressed needs and concerns (e.g., preferences for method characteristics beyond effectiveness at preventing pregnancy), rather than judging the patient's risk of unintended pregnancy by their SES risk factors alone (Dehlendorf, Krajewski et al. 2014; Gavin et al. 2014). Ob/gyns should initiate the conversation by eliciting which contraceptive characteristics (e.g., effectiveness, privacy, side effects) are important to the patient (Kathawa and Arora 2020; Bryson et al. 2021). Inquiring about their patients' opinions and past experiences with contraceptives can help ob/gyns to correct any misconceptions and to better understand the reasons why their patients have been dissatisfied with previous methods (Jackson et al. 2015; Kathawa and Arora 2020; Bryson et al. 2021). When discussing contraceptive options, ob/gyns should address the side effects, risks, and benefits of use, method effectiveness, how the contraceptive works, and how to use it correctly (Dehlendorf, Krajewski et al. 2014; Gavin et al. 2014). Once a method is initiated, a patient's adherence and continuation may be improved if her ob/gyn routinely evaluates her concerns and experiences with the method (Dehlendorf, Krajewski et al. 2014; Gavin et al. 2014).

Like all contraceptive use, postpartum use is associated with the ability to fulfill one's own reproductive desires, yet some US women do not receive prenatal or postpartum contraceptive counseling (Hernandez et al. 2012; Zapata, Murtaza et al. 2015). While counseling should ensure patient autonomy, there are unique medical contraceptive considerations and recommendations for postpartum women due to the lactation and ovulation changes following pregnancy (as described above in the section on "LARC Eligibility and Benefits for Certain Populations").

## Provider-Level Barriers to LARC Provision

### LARC Knowledge, Biases, and Misperceptions

LARC education and training are associated with LARC insertions (Madden et al. 2010; Luchowski et al. 2014a, 2014b). Some ob/gyns incorrectly believe that certain patient populations (e.g., nulliparous [having never given birth], adolescent, or postpartum women) are inappropriate LARC candidates; these beliefs vary by ob/gyns' residency training, age, patient load, insertion volume, same-day insertion protocols, and geographic location (Luchowski et al. 2014a, 2014b; Castleberry et al. 2019). Consequently, biases and misperceptions about LARC safety and patient eligibility can prevent LARC provision.

ACOG and the CDC state that LARCs are safe and effective for women who are nulliparous, in adolescence, postpartum, or have a history of STIs, ectopic pregnancy, or pelvic inflammatory disease (PID) (Curtis, Jatlaoui et al. 2016; Curtis, Tepper et al. 2016). However, biases and misperceptions about LARCs persist, and the sources of misinformation may be traced back to damages caused to the reputation of IUDs decades ago by the unsafe Dalkon Shield, which caused septic abortions and pelvic infections (Boonstra et al. 2000; Cheng 2000). The Federal Drug Administration (FDA) advised its removal from the market in 1974 and its removal from women in 1983, but the Dalkon Shield's tarnished reputation affected utilization of other, safe IUDs (Cheng 2000). IUD uptake in the United States plummeted from about 8% of contraceptive users in 1973 to less than 1% in 1998 (Cheng 2000). By the late 1980s and throughout the 1990s, there were only two IUDs on the US market—ParaGard and Progestasert. ParaGard was more widely used and is still available today. Progestasert required annual removals and was not popular (Cheng 2000); it was discontinued in 2001 and was replaced with Mirena (also still available) in the same year (Lethaby et al. 2015).

Moreover, it was not until 2005 that ACOG first stated that IUDs do not increase the risk of pelvic inflammatory disease, are not associated with subsequent infertility, and are safe to use in women with a history of ectopic pregnancy (ACOG 2017a). Also in 2005, the FDA changed the labeling on ParaGard Copper 380A IUDs (Cu-IUD) to include wording stating that insertions are safe for nulliparous, postpartum, and post-abortion women, despite their higher risk for expulsions (FDA 2005). Of contraceptive users, 13% now rely on an IUD (Guttmacher Institute 2021). There are currently five IUDs on the US market: the copper-containing IUD (Paragard) and four levonorgestrel (a synthetic progestin)-releasing intrauterine devices—Mirena, Kyleena, Liletta, and Skyla (ACOG 2017b).

However, enduring misperceptions about these methods may prevent their use among women for whom they would be a good contraceptive fit. Although the majority of ob/gyns believe that IUDs are generally safe, some have selective beliefs about safety and eligibility (Luchowski et al. 2014a, 2014b; Castleberry et al. 2019). For example, Alicia Luchowski and colleagues (2014b) surveyed members of ACOG in 2008/2009 and found that only 13% of ob/gyns correctly agreed that patients in all five commonly misunderstood categories of eligibility—nulliparous, adolescent, history of STI, history of PID, and history of ectopic pregnancy—were appropriate candidates for IUDs. In this 2008/2009 survey among ACOG members, only 43% believed that LARCs were a good first option for nulliparous and parous adolescents (Luchowski et al. 2014b).

In 2011, ACOG released a Committee Opinion stating that LARCs are an appropriate option for adolescents (ACOG 2011); and in 2015, a national survey among senior ob/gyn residents found that 92% would recommend LARCs to adolescent and nulliparous patients (Davis et al. 2018). Thus, beliefs among ob/gyns about adolescent LARC eligibility seem to have improved, which may be due to findings from the

2007–2011 Contraceptive CHOICE project (Secura et al. 2014; Birgis-son 2015)—a large prospective cohort study designed to promote the use of LARCs to reduce unintended pregnancies in the St. Louis region via educating adolescents about LARCs. This education was successful: of the 1,404 teenage girls and young women enrolled in CHOICE, 72% chose a LARC method; the remaining 28% chose another method (Se-cura et al. 2014).

A survey among ACOG members in 2016/2017 also found that nearly all (92%) offered IUDs to women under 21 (and it can be reason-ably assumed that most women under 21 are nulliparous) (Castleberry et al. 2019). However, misguided beliefs and lack of provision of LARCs to postpartum women continue. In the 2008/2009 ACOG member sur-vey on beliefs, only 43% of ACOG members believed that LARCs could be placed immediately postpartum (Luchowski et al. 2014b), and in the 2016/2017 survey about LARC practices, only approximately 20% offered immediate postpartum LARCs (Castleberry et al. 2019).

### LARC Insertion Training

Training also influences LARC insertion practices. In the 2008/2009 survey among ACOG Fellows (Luchowski et al. 2014b), the majority (92%) received IUD insertion training during residency but fewer re-ceived implant training (51%) (Luchowski et al. 2014a). Lack of im-plant insertion training prevented a third (32%) from inserting implants. However, implant insertions were five times more likely among those who had received continuing medical education (CME) within the last year compared to those who had not (60% vs. 12%) (Luchowski et al. 2014a). More recently, a 2015 national survey among ob/gyn residents found that more than 80% had received some form of LARC didactic or insertion training (Davis et al. 2018), and a 2016 survey found that most (85%) senior residents had some LARC insertion experience (Maples et al. 2020). LARC training and insertion experiences were lowest in the US West, in community-based (versus university-based) programs, and among ob/gyns of a race/ethnicity other than non-Hispanic white (Ma-ples et al. 2020). Furthermore, approximately three out of five (59%) ob/gyn residents received training in programs that did not offer training in immediate postpartum LARCs (Maples et al. 2020).

## System-Level Barriers that Restrict LARC Provision and Access

In addition to knowledge and training, LARC provision is influenced by clinic/office site factors, such as LARC availability on-site and same-day insertion protocols. ACOG and the CDC recommend same-day insertions (ACOG 2015; Curtis, Tepper et al. 2016), which are possible if LARCs are purchased directly by the clinic and stored on-site (Parks and Peipert 2016). These researchers further recommend that barriers to immediate postpartum LARCs (e.g., inadequate reimbursement) should be removed (ACOG 2016). Lack of LARCs' on-site availability may impede their uptake by necessitating the need for referrals or a two-visit protocol to order the method and to insert the method (Bergin et al. 2012; Biggs et al. 2013; Zerden et al. 2015). Additional visits are burdensome for patients and may put some patients at risk of an unintended pregnancy by creating gaps in contraceptive use, use of a less effective method in the interim, and losing patients via lack of follow-up (Bergin et al. 2012; Thiel de Bocanegra et al. 2014). Additional visits would compound other clinic-level logistical barriers (e.g., difficulty of making an appointment), particularly for women in rural areas where there may be limited availability of clinicians (Biggs et al. 2012; Stuart et al. 2013; Beeson et al. 2014; Martins et al. 2016).

Although a prerequisite for same-day insertions, on-site availability of LARCs does not necessarily translate into same-day provision. Whereas most of the ob/gyns in national surveys stored LARCs on-site (73–79%), same-day practices were uncommon, yet improving (Biggs et al. 2013; Luchowski et al. 2014a; Weigel et al. 2021). In 2008/2009, just 13% of ob/gyns offered same-day IUD insertions (Luchowski et al. 2014a). A 2016/2017 survey (Castleberry et al. 2019) found that same-day IUD insertion practices had doubled to 29% (LARC on-site storage was not assessed), and a 2020 survey found that 40% of ob/gyns offered same-day LARC insertions (Weigel et al. 2021). Same-day insertions were more likely among obs who were younger, in large practices, or practiced in a university setting, whereas they were least likely among those in solo private practices or in the US South (Castleberry et al. 2019; Weigel et al. 2021).

Despite the ACOG's and the CDC's recommendations for same-day insertions (ACOG 2015; Curtis, Tepper et al. 2016), some providers prefer a two-visit protocol because they believe that it allows adequate time to provide contraceptive counseling, STI screening, and IUD insertion (Biggs et al. 2013; Kavanaugh et al. 2013; Luchowski et al. 2014a), or they first test for pregnancy and then, if negative, the LARC is provided at follow-up (Reproductive Health Access Project 2020). However, some ob/gyns may have financial disincentives for same-day protocols if their patient's insurance requires prior authorization for LARCs or prohibits billing for more than one service per visit (e.g., an annual exam or an IUD insertion) (Weigel et al. 2021); similar barriers exist for copper IUDs when used as emergency contraception (Pagano et al. 2021).

For some women, postpartum LARC intentions were not fulfilled because their demand for a LARC was unmet. The unmet demand is partially explained by women not returning for their postpartum visit, which, for some women, is due to burdensome multi-visit protocols, expiration of pregnancy-related Medicaid coverage, gaps in insurance coverage, distance to clinic, and the costs of the LARCs (Bergin et al. 2012; White et al. 2014; Salcedo et al. 2015; Zerden et al. 2015). Such access issues may contribute to the greater postpartum reliance on sterilizations over LARCs (Baldwin, Rodriguez, and Edelman 2012; Whiteman et al. 2012; White et al. 2015).

Access is also restricted by the availability of immediate postpartum LARCs. Among the 73% of ACOG Fellows who reported not offering immediate postpartum LARCs, the most commonly cited barrier was LARC availability (70%), followed by cost of reimbursement (56%), and lack of training (48%) (Holden et al. 2018). The higher immediate postpartum IUD uptake and provision at teaching hospitals (Whiteman et al. 2012) may reflect those hospitals' advocacy for and ob/gyn training in immediate postpartum IUDs (Whiteman et al. 2012; Holden et al. 2018).

Similarly, insurance policies may financially disincentivize immediate postpartum LARCs, and thus create a barrier for postpartum women who desire one. The typical bundled global fee for maternity care (i.e., a single fee for a predetermined list of obstetric prenatal, delivery, and postpartum services) does not reimburse hospitals or providers for the additional costs associated with immediate insertion of LARCs, but postpartum insertions rates might increase if hospitals were allowed to bill separately for LARCs and get reimbursed for their additional costs (Moniz et al. 2015; Holden et al. 2018; Kroelinger et al. 2019; Lacy et al. 2020). Indeed, one national survey found that insertions were more likely among ob/gyns who work in US states where Medicaid polices reimburse for LARCs separately from the global delivery fee (Castleberry et al. 2019).

## Recommendations for Overcoming Barriers and Increasing Patient Access to LARCs

The risks of unintended pregnancy and short interpregnancy intervals could be reduced by increasing access to LARCs and minimizing barriers to LARC uptake and provision at patient, provider, and health systems levels. At the patient level, women should receive comprehensive patient-centered contraceptive counseling, and then can choose the method they desire. Given that more women have insurance since the

Affordable Care Act (2010) expanded Medicaid coverage (Jones and Sonfield 2016; Sonfield 2021) and that contraceptive costs are rarely a reason for inconsistent or discontinued use (Daniels and Mosher 2013; Pazol et al. 2015), access issues related to contraceptive use will likely continue to be logistical (e.g., making an appointment, attending the appointment, obtaining a prescription, and filling a prescripttion), particularly for women who live in rural areas (Biggs et al. 2012; Stuart et al. 2013; Beeson et al. 2014; Martins et al. 2016).

At the provider level, barriers to LARC provision could be reduced by increasing ob/gyn awareness of LARC safety guidelines, training more ob/gyns in patient-centered counseling and LARC insertion practices, and offering LARCs on-site for same-day insertions. Two-visit protocols are commonly cited reasons why many women do not return for a desired IUD (Bergin et al. 2012; Salcedo et al. 2015; Zerden et al. 2015), yet the majority of ob/gyns still require at least two visits and thereby maintain this substantial barrier to care (Luchowski et al. 2014a; Castleberry et al. 2019; Weigel et al. 2021). Same-day protocols are possible if LARCs are purchased directly by the clinic and stored on-site, and a checklist is used to rule out pregnancy (Parks and Peipert 2016). Additionally, insurers should discontinue prior authorization policies and allow for more than one service to be billed per visit. The University of California San Francisco maintains a guide to LARC reimbursement by public and private insurance coverage and how to navigate stocking, reimbursement, and other barriers to same-day insertions (Armstrong et al. 2016).

Despite ACOG's (2016) recommendations, immediate postpartum LARC uptake in the United States has been underutilized (Whiteman et al. 2012; White, Potter et al. 2014; White, Teal 2015; Zapata, Murtaza et al. 2015). Postpartum contraceptive access and uptake during this time of increased interactions with the healthcare system are especially important for women with Medicaid to ensure that their preferred method is obtained before their pregnancy-related Medicaid coverage expires 60 days postpartum. Due to the permanence of sterilization, all women should have equitable access to LARCs, so that their choices in method and their ability to control their future reproductive capacities are not limited.

Inadequate immediate postpartum LARC insertion training and reimbursement policies create provider- and system-level barriers to uptake. It is the responsibility of ob/gyn residency training programs across the country to ensure that residents are trained and gain experience in providing LARCs so they can offer this essential reproductive healthcare service to their patients. The 2017 survey of ACOG Fellows found that among the 73% not providing immediate postpartum LARCs, most would like to or would consider offering them in the future (78%) and would like or would consider training to do so (86%) (Holden et al. 2018). In addition, ACOG (2016) recommends supportive processes and infrastructure to promote the availability of immediate postpartum LARC insertions. This includes insurance policies that allow immediate postpartum LARCs to be billed separately from the bundled global delivery fee (ACOG 2016). Statewide quality improvement projects to increase access to immediate postpartum LARCs have been successful in part due to unbundling LARC devices from the global delivery fee (Kroelinger et al. 2019). These projects also credit their successes to having provider champions who engage state and facility stakeholders (Kroelinger et al. 2019).

In closing, I stress that contraceptive access and provision are cornerstones of high-quality reproductive health care. If a woman is not receiving the healthcare information and services she needs, then she may be inadequately equipped to fulfill her own reproductive desires. Ob/gyns are critical in their patients' contraceptive decision-making processes. However, it bears repeating that in efforts to increase access to LARCs, extreme care must be taken to ensure that *all* methods of contraception are available to *everyone*, method coercion does not occur, and contraceptive choices are made by the patients based on their desires. Equitable access to LARCs is possible through systemic healthcare and policy changes that train the ob/gyn workforce and support same-day insertions. Ob/gyns and the healthcare systems within which they work are vital to ensuring equitable access to contraceptive care so that women can achieve their reproductive goals.

**Melissa Goldin Evans** is a researcher at the Mary Amelia Center for Women's Health Equity Research within Tulane's School of Public Health and Tropical Medicine (SPHTM). She earned her MsPH from SPTHM in 2006 and her PhD in Community Health Sciences from Louisiana State University Health Sciences Center, School of Public Health in 2017. Her work spans the life course, from early childhood through postpartum care, but her primary interest is in reducing inequities in maternal and child health through improved access to contraceptives.

### References

Ahrens K, Nelson H, Stidd R, et al. 2019. "Short Interpregnancy Intervals and Adverse Perinatal Outcomes in High-Resource Settings: An Updated Systematic Review." *Paediatric and Perinatal Epidemiology* 33: O25–O47.

American College of Obstetricians and Gynecologists. 2011. "Practice Bulletin No. 121: Long-Acting Reversible Contraception: Implants and Intrauterine Devices." *Obstetrics & Gynecology* 118(1): 184–196.

———. 2015. "Committee Opinion No. 642: Increasing Access to Contraceptive Implants and Intrauterine Devices to Reduce Unintended Pregnancy (reaffirmed 2018)." *Obstetrics & Gynecology* 126: e44–48.

———. 2016. (Reaffirmed 2020). "Committee on Obstetric Practice, Committee Opinion Number 670: Immediate Postpartum Long-Acting Reversible Contraception." *Obstetrics & Gynecology* 128(2): 332–337.

———. 2017a. (Reaffirmed 2021). "ACOG Practice Bulletin No. 186: Long-Acting Reversible Contraception: Implants and Intrauterine Devices." *Obstetrics & Gynecology* 118: 184–196.

———. 2017b. "Practice Bulletin No. 186. "Summary: Long-Acting Reversible Contraception: Implants and Intrauterine Devices." *Obstetrics & Gynecology* 130: 1173–1175.

———. 2018. "ACOG Committee Opinion No. 736: Optimizing Postpartum Care." *Obstetrics & Gynecology* 131: e140–e150.

Armstrong E, Mckee C, Gandal-Powers M, et al. 2016. "Intrauterine Devices & Implants: A Guide to Reimbursements" *University of California, San Francisco*, 6 April. Retrieved 8 November 2022 from https://larcprogram.ucsf.edu/.

Arora K, Wilkinson B, Verbus E, et al. 2018. "Medicaid and Fulfillment of Desired Postpartum Sterilization." *Contraception* 97: 559–564.

Averbach S, Ermias Y, Jeng G, et al. 2020. "Expulsion of Intrauterine Devices after Postpartum Placement by Timing of Placement, Delivery Type, and Intrauterine Device Type: A Systematic Review and Meta-Analysis." *American Journal of Obstetrics & Gynecology* 223: 177–188.

Baldwin M, Rodriguez M, Edelman A. 2012. "Lack of Insurance and Parity Influence Choice between Long-Acting Reversible Contraception and Sterilization in Women Postpregnancy." *Contraception* 86: 42–47.

Beeson T, Wood S, Bruen B, et al. 2014. "Accessibility of Long-Acting Reversible Contraceptives (LARCs) in Federally Qualified Health Centers (FQHCs)." *Contraception* 89: 91–96.

Bergin A, Tristan S, Terplan M, et al. 2012. "A Missed Opportunity for Care: Two-Visit IUD Insertion Protocols Inhibit Placement." *Contraception* 86: 694–697.

Beshar I, So J, Chelvakumar M, et al. 2021. "Socioeconomic Differences Persist in Use of Permanent vs Long-Acting Reversible Contraception: An Analysis of the National Survey of Family Growth, 2006 to 2010 vs 2015 to 2017." *Contraception* 103: 246–254.

Biggs M, Arons A, Turner R, et al. 2013. "Same-Day LARC Insertion Attitudes and Practices." *Contraception* 88: 629–635.

Biggs M, Karasek D, Foster D. 2012. "Unprotected Intercourse among Women Wanting to Avoid Pregnancy: Attitudes, Behaviors, and Beliefs." *Womens Health Issues* 22: e311–318.

Birgisson N, Zhao Q, Secura G, et al. 2015. "Preventing Unintended Pregnancy: The Contraceptive CHOICE Project in Review." *Journal of Women's Health* 24: 349–353.

Boonstra H, Duran V, Northington Gamble V. et al. 2000. "The 'Boom and Bust Phenomenon': The Hopes, Dreams, and Broken Promises of the Contraceptive Revolution." *Contraception* 61: 9–25.

Brandi K, Fuentes L. 2019. "The History of Tiered-Effectiveness Contraceptive Counseling and the Importance of Patient-Centered Family Planning Care." *American Journal of Obstetrics & Gynecology* 222(4S): S873–S877.

Bryson A, Koyama A, Hassan A. 2021. "Addressing Long-Acting Reversible Contraception Access, Bias, and Coercion: Supporting Adolescent and Young Adult Reproductive Autonomy." *Current Opinion in Pediatrics* 33(4): 345–353.

Castleberry N, Stark L, Schulkin J, et al. 2019. "Implementing Best Practices for the Provision of Long-Acting Reversible Contraception: A Survey of Obstetrician-Gynecologists." *Contraception* 100: 123–127.

Chen B, Reeves M, Hayes J, et al. 2010. "Postplacental or Delayed Insertion of the Levonorgestrel Intrauterine Device after Vaginal Delivery: A Randomized Controlled Trial." *Obstetrics & Gynecology* 116: 1079–1087.

Cheng D. 2000. "The Intrauterine Device: Still Misunderstood after All These Years." *Southern Medical Journal* 93: 859–864.

Cheslack Postava K, Winter A. 2015. "Short and Long Interpregnancy Intervals: Correlates and Variations by Pregnancy Timing among U.S. Women." *Perspectives on Sexual and Reproductive Health* 47: 19–26.

Cleland J, Conde-Agudelo A, Peterson H, et al. 2012. "Contraception and Health." *Lancet* 380: 149–156.

Cleland K, Peipert J, Westhoff C, et al. 2011. "Family Planning as a Cost-Saving Preventive Health Service." *New England Journal of Medicine* 364: e37.

Curtis K, Jatlaoui T, Tepper N, et al. 2016. "U.S. Selected Practice Recommendations for Contraceptive Use, 2016." *MMWR Recommendations and Reports* 65(4): 1–66.

Curtis K, Tepper N, Jatlaoui T, et al. 2016. "U.S. Medical Eligibility Criteria for Contraceptive Use, 2016." *MMWR Recommendations and Reports* 65(3): 1–103.

Daniels K, Mosher W. 2013. "Contraceptive Methods Women Have Ever Used: United States, 1982–2010." *National Health Statistics Reports* 62: 1–15.

Davis S, Braykov N, Lathrop E, et al. 2018. "Familiarity with Long-Acting Reversible Contraceptives among Obstetrics and Gynecology, Family Medicine, and Pediatrics Residents: Results of a 2015 National Survey and Implications for Contraceptive Provision for Adolescents." *Journal of Pediatric and Adolescent Gynecology* 31: 40–44.

Dehlendorf C, Henderson J, Vittinghoff E, et al. 2016. "Association of the Quality of Interpersonal Care during Family Planning Counseling with Contraceptive Use." *American Journal of Obstetrics & Gynecology* 215(1): 78.e109

Dehlendorf C, Krajewski C, Borrero S. 2014. "Contraceptive Counseling: Best Practices to Ensure Quality Communication and Enable Effective Contraceptive Use." *Clinical Obstetrics and Gynecology* 57: 659–73.

Dehlendorf C, Ruskin R, Grumbach K, et al. 2010. "Recommendations for Intrauterine Contraception: A Randomized Trial of the Effects of Patients' Race/Ethnicity and Socioeconomic Status." *American Journal of Obstetrics & Gynecology* 203: 319 e1–8.

Downing R, Laveist T, Bullock H. 2007. "Intersections of Ethnicity and Social Class in Provider Advice Regarding Reproductive Health." *American Journal of Public Health* 97: 1803–1807.

Federal Drug Administration (FDA). 2005. "Paragard Prescribing Information." Retrieved 8 November 2022 from http://www.accessdata.fda.gov/drugsatfda_docs/label/2005/018680s060lbl.pdf.

Finer L, Zolna M. 2016. "Declines in Unintended Pregnancy in the United States, 2008–2011." *New England Journal of Medicine* 374: 843–852.

Gavin L, Moskosky S, Carter M, et al. 2014. "Providing Quality Family Planning Services: Recommendations of CDC and the U.S. Office Of Population Affairs." *MMWR Recommendations and Reports* 63: 1–54.

Gemmill A, Lindberg L. 2013. "Short Interpregnancy Intervals in the United States." *Obstetrics & Gynecology* 122: 64–71.

Gold R. 2014. "Guarding Against Coercion While Ensuring Access: A Delicate Balance." *Guttmacher Institute, Guttmacher Policy Review* 17: 3. Retrieved 8 November 2022 from https://www.guttmacher.org/gpr/2014/09/guarding-against-coercion-while-ensuring-access-delicate-balance.

Gomez A, Fuentes L, Allina A. 2014. "Women or LARC First? Reproductive Autonomy and the Promotion of Long-Acting Reversible Contraceptive Methods." *Perspectives on Sexual and Reproductive Health* 46: 171–175.

Gomez A, Wapman M. 2017. "Under (Implicit) Pressure: Young Black and Latina Women's Perceptions of Contraceptive Care." *Contraception* 96: 221–226.

Gubrium A, Mann E, Borrero S, et al. 2016. "Realizing Reproductive Health Equity Needs More Than Long-Acting Reversible Contraception (LARC)." *American Journal of Public Health* 106: 18–19.

Guttmacher Institute 2021. "Fact Sheet: Contraceptive Use in the United States by Method." *Guttmacher Institute.* Retrieved 8 November 2022 from https://www.guttmacher.org/fact-sheet/contraceptive-method-use-united-states.

Harris L, Wolfe T. 2014. "Stratified Reproduction, Family Planning Care and the Double Edge of History." *Current Opinion in Obstetrics & Gynecology* 26: 539–544.

Hernandez L, Sappenfield W, Goodman D, et al. 2012. "Is Effective Contraceptive Use Conceived Prenatally in Florida? The Association between Prenatal Contraceptive Counseling and Postpartum Contraceptive Use." *Maternal and Child Health Journal* 16: 423–429.

Holden E, Lai E, Morelli S, et al. 2018. "Ongoing Barriers to Immediate Postpartum Long-Acting Reversible Contraception: A Physician Survey." *Contraception and Reproductive Medicne* 3: 23.

Hutcheon J, Nelson H, Stidd R, et al. 2019. "Short Interpregnancy Intervals and Adverse Maternal Outcomes in High-Resource Settings: An Updated Systematic Review." *Paediatric and Perinatal Epidemiology* 33: O48–O59.

Jackson A, Karasek D, Dehlendorf C, et al. 2015. "Racial and Ethnic Differences in Women's Preferences for Features of Contraceptive Methods." *Contraception* 93(5): 406–411.

Jones R, Sonfield A. 2016. "Health Insurance Coverage among Women of Reproductive Age before and after Implementation of the Affordable Care Act." *Contraception* 93: 386–391.

Kathawa C, Arora K. 2020. "Implicit Bias in Counseling for Permanent Contraception: Historical Context and Recommendations for Counseling." *Health Equity* 4: 326–329.

Kavanaugh M, Frohwirth L, Jerman J, et al. 2013. "Long-Acting Reversible Contraception for Adolescents and Young Adults: Patient and Provider Perspectives." *Journal of Pediatric and Adolescent Gynecology* 26: 86–95.

Kroelinger C, Morgan I, Desisto C, et al. 2019. "State-Identified Implementation Strategies to Increase Uptake of Immediate Postpartum Long-Acting Reversible Contraception Policies." *Journal of Women's Health* 28: 346–356.

Lacy M, Mcmurtry Baird S, Scott T, et al. 2020. "Statewide Quality Improvement Initiative to Implement Immediate Postpartum Long-Acting Reversible Contraception." *American Journal of Obstetrics & Gynecology* 222: S910 e1–S910 e8.

Lethaby A, Hussain M, Rishworth JR, Rees MC. 2015. "Progesterone or Progestogen-Releasing Intrauterine Systems for Heavy Menstrual Bleeding." *Cochrane Database of Systematic Reviews* 4: CD002126.

Lopez L, Bernholc A, Hubacher D, et al. 2015. "Immediate Postpartum Insertion of Intrauterine Device for Contraception." *Cochrane Database of Systematic Reviews* 6: CD003036.

Luchowski A, Anderson B, Power M, et al. 2014a. "Obstetrician-Gynecologists and Contraception: Long-Acting Reversible Contraception Practices and Education." *Contraception* 89(6): 578–583.

———. 2014b. "Obstetrician-Gynecologists and Contraception: Practice and Opinions about the Use of IUDs in Nulliparous Women, Adolescents and Other Patient Populations." *Contraception* 89(6): 572–577.

Luna Z, Luker K. 2013. "Reproductive Justice." *The Annual Review of Law and Social Science* 9: 327–352.

Madden T, Allsworth J, Hladky K, et al. 2010. "Intrauterine Contraception in Saint Louis: A Survey of Obstetrician and Gynecologists' Knowledge and Attitudes." *Contraception* 81: 112–116.

Maples J, Espey E, Evans M, et al. 2020. "Obstetrics-Gynecology Resident Long-Acting Reversible Contraception Training: The Role of Resident and Program Characteristics." *American Journal of Obstetrics & Gynecology* 222: S923 e1–S923 e8.

Martins S, Starr K, Hellerstedt W, et al. 2016. "Differences in Family Planning Services by Rural-Urban Geography: Survey of Title X-Supported Clinics in Great Plains and Midwestern States." *Perspectives on Sexual and Reproductive Health* 48(1): 9–16.

Moniz M, Dalton V, Davis M, et al. 2015. "Characterization of Medicaid Policy for Immediate Postpartum Contraception." *Contraception* 92: 523–531.

Pagano H, Zapata L, Curtis K, et al. 2021. "Changes in U.S. Healthcare Provider Practices Related to Emergency Contraception." *Womens Health Issues* 31(6): 560–566.

Parks C, Peipert J. 2016. "Eliminating Health Disparities in Unintended Pregnancy with Long-Acting Reversible Contraception (LARC)." *American Journal of Obstetrics & Gynecology* 214: 681–688.

Pazol K, Whiteman M, Folger S, et al. 2015. "Sporadic Contraceptive Use and Non-use: Age-Specific Prevalence and Associated Factors." *American Journal of Obstetrics & Gynecology* 212: 324 e1–8.

Potter J, Hopkins K, Aiken A, et al. 2014. "Unmet Demand for Highly Effective Postpartum Contraception in Texas." *Contraception* 90: 488–495.

Raine S. 2012. "Federal Sterilization Policy: Unintended Consequences." *Virtual Mentor* 14: 152–157.

Raine T, Foster-Rosales A, Upadhyay U, et al. 2011. "One-Year Contraceptive Continuation and Pregnancy in Adolescent Girls and Women Initiating Hormonal Contraceptives." *Obstetrics & Gynecology* 117: 363–371.

Reproductive Health Access Project. 2020. "Quick Start Algorithm for Hormonal Contraception." *Reproductive Health Access Project*, 7 March. Retrieved 8 November 2022 from https://www.reproductiveaccess.org/resource/quick-start-algorithm/quickstartalgorithm/.

Ricketts S, Klingler G, Schwalberg R. 2014. "Game Change in Colorado: Widespread Use of Long-Acting Reversible Contraceptives and Rapid Decline in Births Among Young, Low-Income Women." *Perspectives on Sexual and Reproductive Health* 46: 125–132.

Roberts S, Berglas N, Kimport K. 2020. "Complex Situations: Economic Insecurity, Mental Health, and Substance Use among Pregnant Women Who Consider—But Do Not Have—Abortions." *PLoS One* 15: e0226004.

Salcedo J, Moniaga N, Harken T. 2015. "Limited Uptake of Planned Intrauterine Devices during the Postpartum Period." *Southern Medical Journal* 108: 463–468.

Secura GM, Madden T, McNicholas C, Mullersman C, et al. 2014. "Provision of No-Cost, Long-Acting Contraception and Teenage Pregnancy." *New England Journal of Medicine* 371: 1316–1323.

Simmons R, Sanders J, Geist C, et al. 2019. "Predictors of Contraceptive Switching and Discontinuation within the First 6 Months of Use among Highly Effective Reversible Contraceptive Initiative Salt Lake Study Participants." *American Journal of Obstetrics & Gynecology* 220: 376 e1–376 e12.

SisterSong. 1997. "Reproductive Justice." Retrieved 8 November 2022 from https://www.sistersong.net/reproductive-justice.

Sonfield A. 2021. "Uninsured Rate for People of Reproductive Age Ticked Up between 2016 and 2019." *Guttmacher Institute, Policy Analysis*, 1 April. Retrieved 8 November 2022 from https://www.guttmacher.org/article/2021/04/uninsured-rate-people-reproductive-age-ticked-between-2016-and-2019.

Stuart J, Secura G, Zhao Q, et al. 2013. "Factors Associated with 12-Month Discontinuation Among Contraceptive Pill, Patch, and Ring Users." *Obstetrics & Gynecology* 121: 330–336.

Thiel de Bocanegra H, Cross Riedel J, Menz M, et al. 2014. "Onsite Provision of Specialized Contraceptive Services: Does Title X Funding Enhance Access?" *Journal of Women's Health* 23: 428–433.

Thorburn S, Bogart L. 2005. "African American Women and Family Planning Services: Perceptions of Discrimination." *Women and Health* 42: 23–39.

Upadhyay U, Mccook A, Bennett A, et al. 2021. "State Abortion Policies and Medicaid Coverage of Abortion Are Associated with Pregnancy Outcomes among

Individuals Seeking Abortion Recruited Using Google Ads: A National Cohort Study." *Social Science and Medicine* 274: 113747.

Weigel G, Frederiksen B, Ranji U, et al. 2021. "OBGYNs and the Provision of Sexual and Reproductive Health Care: Key Findings from a National Survey." *Women's Health Policy, Kaiser Family Foundation*, 25 February. Retrieved 8 November 2022 from https://www.kff.org/womens-health-policy/report/obgyns-and-the-provision-of-sexual-and-reproductive-health-care-key-findings-from-a-national-survey/.

White K, Potter J, Hopkins K, et al. 2014. "Variation in Postpartum Contraceptive Method Use: Results from the Pregnancy Risk Assessment Monitoring System (PRAMS)." *Contraception* 89: 57–62.

White K, Teal S, Potter J. 2015. "Contraception after Delivery and Short Interpregnancy Intervals among Women in the United States." *Obstetrics & Gynecology* 125: 1471–1477.

Whiteman M, Cox S, Tepper N, et al. 2012. "Postpartum Intrauterine Device Insertion and Postpartum Tubal Sterilization in the United States." *American Journal of Obstetrics & Gynecology* 206: 127 e1–7.

Woo I, Seifert S, Hendricks D, et al. 2015. "Six-Month and 1-Year Continuation Rates Following Postpartum Insertion of Implants and Intrauterine Devices." *Contraception* 92: 532–535.

Zapata L, Murtaza S, Whiteman M, et al. 2015. "Contraceptive Counseling and Postpartum Contraceptive Use." *American Journal of Obstetrics & Gynecology* 212: 171 e1–8.

Zapata L, Tregear S, Curtis K, et al. 2015. "Impact of Contraceptive Counseling in Clinical Settings: A Systematic Review." *American Journal of Preventive Medicine* 49: S31–45.

Zerden M, Tang J, Stuart G, et al. 2015. "Barriers to Receiving Long-acting Reversible Contraception in the Postpartum Period." *Women's Health Issues* 25: 616–621.

# CHAPTER 11

# Cognition, Risk, and Responsibility

## Home Birth and Why Obstetricians Fear It

*Amali U. Lokugamage and Claire Feeley*

## Introduction

Planned, midwife-attended home births are, in general, natural and physiologic with good outcomes (in high-resource countries with easy access to higher-level centers of care) for low-risk mothers and babies (Birthplace 2011). Worldwide, great advances have been made in the safety of birth, but wide disparities exist among countries, and the United Nation's Millennium Development Goal for maternal health (MDG 5) has not been achieved. However, work from the World Health Organization (WHO 2018) has recommitted to an agenda supporting physiologic births and reducing cesarean birth rates (WHO 2018). One of the authors of this chapter, Amali Lokugamage, is an obstetrician who gave birth at home in England; she understands full well obstetricians' fears and even antipathy to home birth as encoded in the documents produced by the American College of Obstetricians and Gynecologists (ACOG) Committee on Obstetric Practice (2011).

However, the United Kingdom's National Institute for Health and Care Excellence (NICE)—the national body concerned with improving health outcomes for the nation—also produced maternity care guidelines that include home birth as a viable option (NICE 2014). This chapter discusses contrasting models of care, the politics of home birth, its place in well-resourced countries, and obstetricians' fears and anxieties around births—especially home births.

## Contrasting Models of Care:
## A Brush with Death Versus Enlivenment, Life-Giving, and Life-Enhancing Experiences and Opportunities

Contemporary life in risk-averse societies fosters the fear-based technocratic model of birth and health care, described in the Introduction to this volume. Reducing the hazards of rare, severe complications for a small number of childbearers carries the inevitable costs of interfering with the normal physiology of labor and birth, thereby causing iatrogenic harm, in what Melissa Cheyney and Robbie Davis-Floyd (2019:8) have called the "obstetric paradox": intervene in birth to keep it safe, thereby causing harm.

The overdiagnosis and overtreatment of pathologies during pregnancy and labor—the "too much medicine" (Miller et al. 2016) so prevalent in maternity care in high-resource countries—can cause significant harm to the mother-baby dyad, despite intentions otherwise. Interventions or practices that cause individual psychobiological harm can eventually interact and affect societal health; these effects are particularly difficult to track because of the complexities of their interactions. In pregnancy and birth, mind–body interactions are extremely important to the proper physiologic functions of the body via hormones such as natural oxytocin, which also plays a part in societal behavior (Uvnäs-Moberg 1998; Kantrowitz-Gordon 2005; Baumgartner et al. 2008; Olza, Uvnäs-Moberg et al. 2020), as we will further discuss later on in this chapter.

In the UK, where professional midwives care for most normal births, obstetricians mainly see only problem pregnancies and sudden, life-threatening emergencies. Their perceptions of the greater numbers of women who have normal pregnancies and non-medicalized births are thus biased. Obstetric students and practicing obstetricians rarely witness the joyous, even ecstatic state that some women experience during uncomplicated, low-tech deliveries (Olza, Uvnäs-Moberg et al. 2020). Unsurprisingly, obstetricians have a deep-seated belief that all pregnancies are potentially problematic until proven otherwise by a good outcome. In contrast, the midwifery model of care (described in Davis-Floyd 2018c) promotes childbearing as a normal life event and not a medical event whereby in healthy women, most pregnancies and births proceed without complications. Problems that could occur in pregnancy can be due to pre-existing medical conditions (e.g., poorly controlled diabetes mellitus); some may be due to new conditions occurring in pregnancy; and some can be created through iatrogenic harm—the latter is the focus of our chapter. The biomedical versus social models of childbirth—or, in Davis-Floyd's terms (see the Introduction to this volume), the technocratic versus the humanistic and holistic models of birth that prevail in home births (see Cheyney 2011; Davis-Floyd 2022) are cultural views that certainly contrast but can also be synergistic when practitioners adopt approaches based on respect and "mutual accommodation" (Jordan 1997:73).

All models of health care are also heavily culturally influenced, even those supposedly based on science. Medical anthropologist and psychiatrist Arthur Kleinman pointed out that:

> Healing efficacy is not a straightforward resultant, but rather determined by evaluations which are tied to the beliefs and values of different sectors of healthcare systems, and which therefore might be (and often are) discrepant. Healing is viewed differently across cultures and in different sectors of healthcare. It is not the same thing for practitioner and patient. This is an argument to the effect that all healthcare explanatory models, including those of modern professional medicine and psychiatry, are culture-laden and freighted with particular social interests. And so is our present standard of healing. (Kleinman and Sung 1979:8)

Natural birth is the evolutionary norm (see Cheyney and Davis-Floyd 2020a, 2020b, 2021). Therefore, any biomedicalization should be justified. Helping people overcome illness is a strong motivator for those who choose to study biomedicine, but in the desire to deal with pathologies, doctors often lose—or never develop—faith in the normality of childbirth. The simplicity of birth for the majority of women, and women's innate abilities to let their bodies use nature's programming to deliver a child (especially if they are well nurtured and nourished during pregnancy), are only rarely observed by obstetricians in day-to-day clinical life. While 300,000 women die every year from problems related to childbirth (WHO 2019), the global burden is in low-income countries without the resources to detect or manage the leading causes of maternal deaths, such as hemorrhage and hypertensive disorders of pregnancy (WHO 2019). While this number is 35% lower than in 2000, and rare in England (MMR 9/100,000), from such statistics stems a belief that birth is a "brush with death."

## Home Birth as a Political Issue

Midwifery is a strong and respected profession in the United Kingdom, and more powerful still in the Netherlands (see Cheyney, Goodarzi et al. 2019) and New Zealand (see Georges and Daellenbach 2019; Daellenbach et al. 2023), but has far less respectability and influence in the United States, where midwives attend only around 10% of births.[1] In the UK, market forces and delivery fees were curtailed by the inception of the National Health Service in Britain in 1948. However, in the United States, where private healthcare delivery is the norm, the power of the midwifery profession was eroded during the 20th century, losing the competition for the birth market to the biomedical profession, which expounded the view that hospital birth was the "safest" way to have a baby. Since the 1970s, there has been a slight revival in US community midwifery (midwives who attend births in homes or freestanding birth centers), buoyed by the influence of the "natural childbirth" and the midwifery movements. But market forces still retard its growth, currently swayed by the fee-paying structures of insurance companies and the domination of the technocratic obstetric profession (Teijilingen et al. 2004). The American College of Obstetrician and Gynecologists (ACOG) has historically stood against home birth (ACOG Committee on Obstetric Practice 2011), though:

> in 2016, with homebirth on the rise [in the US] and increasing pressure to evaluate the literature, the *ACOG Planned Homebirth Statement* acknowledged for the first time that good outcomes at homebirths can occur in other countries with well-trained midwives and an integrated health care system with safe and timely transport to nearby hospitals. (Anderson, Daviss, and Johnson 2021:220)

The Royal College of Obstetricians and Gynaecologists in Britain at present (2022) does not object to home birth as an option for low-risk mothers, and total midwifery care of uncomplicated pregnancies is seen as quite normal. Historically (prior to two decades ago), the paucity of evidence on midwifery practices such as those used in home births had been the ammunition of anti-homebirth campaigners because of the cultural perception that obstetric and gynecologic clinical practice is rigorously evidence-based. Robust arguments beyond the scope of this chapter challenge the hierarchy of evidence that supervalues[2] the randomized controlled trial (RCT) (Berg 2000; Howick 2011; Greenhalgh, Howick, and Maskrey 2014). However, given the obstetric and biomedical reliance upon such scientific methods as the "gold standard" of research to inform clinical guidelines, and the fact that an evaluation of the ACOG clinical guidelines revealed that only one-third of the recommendations put forth by the College in its practice bulletins are based on high quality RCT evidence, suggests contradictory messaging

(Wright et al. 2011). Furthermore, this pattern of low-quality evidence underpinning clinical guidelines is seen in analyses of the Royal College of Obstetricians and Gynaecologists (RCOG) as well as the Society for Gynecologists and Obstetricians of Canada (SOGC) guidance (Prusova et al. 2014; Ghui et al. 2016). Nevertheless, obstetrics wields great sociocultural power and influence in knowledge generation and dissemination.

Dutch midwifery has enjoyed considerable state support, including legislation to protect midwives against competition from doctors for normal deliveries, no doubt contributing to the facts that 75% of Dutch midwives are independent, and 13.1% of Dutch women give birth at home (Cheney, Goodarzi et al. 2019). Social attitudes influence this relatively high homebirth rate—the highest in high-resource countries—as the Dutch tend to consider birth as more of a social than a medical event. However, until the 1980s, the Dutch homebirth rate was around 70%, then fell to 30%, where it stayed for many years; then, for a variety of reasons (see below), fell to its present 13% (KNOV 2017; Cheney, Goodarzi et al. 2019).

As we inferred previously, prior to a decade ago, evidence for homebirth outcomes was slim, but now much more safety evidence has amassed via a large-scale good quality cohort studies. In 2009, cohort data from the Netherlands suggested that for healthy women, home and hospital births were equally safe for the baby where there is the infrastructure to transfer the mother to hospital should the need arise. However, the Dutch perinatal mortality rates were higher than elsewhere in Europe (de Jonge, van der Goes et al. 2009)—a situation that was first attributed to home births, yet later and more comprehensive data analysis showed that the higher mortality rates were not due to home births, but rather to the lower nutrition and health of the immigrant population, as almost all of these deaths took place in hospitals. However, the too-early press reports on these studies blamed home births for the higher perinatal mortality rates, and the damage was done—the Dutch homebirth rate plummeted from 30% to 13% as both midwives and mothers lost confidence in home birth (Cheney et al. 2019). At that time, there was no consensus on perinatal safety in any other pre-existing smaller homebirth observational studies (Duran 1992; Olsen, and Jewell 1998; Janssen, Reime et al. 2004; Mori, Dougherty, and Whittle 2008; Gyte, Dodwell et al. 2009; Janssen, Saxell et al. 2009; Kennare et al. 2010).

Yet in a prospective[3] study on the statistical outcomes of births attended in the United States by certified professional midwives (CPMs), in which all CPMs were required to participate, Kenneth C. Johnson and Betty-Anne Daviss (2005) showed that around 90% of planned home births attended by CPMs took place safely and successfully at home, while around 10% required hospital transport. Of these 10 out of 100 transports, only 3 took place in emergency situations; the rest were preventative. The overall cesarean rate was around 4%, and the perinatal mortality rate was 2/1000—the same as for low-risk hospital births in the United States, showing that home birth with a CPM carries no additional risk. The results of this Johnson and Daviss study, which was based on the outcomes of 7,000 courses of care, were greatly reinforced by a follow-up study on almost 17,000 courses of self-reported CPM care, which showed nearly identical results (Cheyney, Bovbjerg et al. 2014). The database on which this study was based now contains prospectively entered data on the outcomes of over 175,000 courses of CPM home and birth center care; publications on this data are pending (Melissa Cheyney, personal communication with Robbie Davis-Floyd, September 2022).

The same group of studies cited above also showed that the medical intervention rates, operative delivery rates, and associated risks to the mother were lower in planned home births of low-risk mothers. This is in marked contrast to the position of the American College of Obstetricians and Gynecologists, which in 2010 concluded that all home birth are unsafe, based on an American meta-analysis (Wax et al. 2010) that showed better maternal outcomes in home births, yet a three times higher perinatal mortality rate (still very low). This study has since been thoroughly discredited (see Anderson, Daviss, and Johnson 2021 for full descriptions) and the quality and flawed nature of this study's data has been subsequently highlighted (Horton 2010; Gyte, Dodwell, and Macfarlane 2011; Sandall, Bewley, and Newburn 2011; Zohar and De Vries 2011). In short, *no such tripling exists in the corrected data*, and in fact, both perinatal and neonatal mortality were similar for planned home births versus planned hospital births (de Jonge, Geerts et al. 2015). In a rare move, international investigators called for this study's retraction by the journal in which it was published (the *American Journal of Obstetrics & Gynecology*), to no avail. This refusal yet again reveals the tenacity with which some US obstetricians—who often still cite the discredited Wax study to "prove" the "dangers" of home birth—cling to evidence that seems to support their views—in this case, that home birth carries more risk and danger than hospital birth despite the much more compelling evidence to the contrary.

Another study that discredited home births (Snowden et al. 2017), and which US obstetricians also frequently cite, unfortunately looked only at community births (births at home and in freestanding birth centers) outcomes in the state of Oregon, where around a third of the births are attended by unlicensed midwives, naturopaths, and other uncertified practitioners; thus this study could conclude nothing definitive about births attended by CPMs.

Planned home birth in high-resource countries is usually an ideological choice (see Klassen 2001; Cheyney 2011; Davis-Floyd 2022); hence it would be extremely difficult to recruit pregnant women for a randomized controlled trial (i.e., randomizing a woman who wanted a home birth to a hospital birth or vice versa) to answer the question of safety definitively. However, in 2011, in the United Kingdom, a prospective cohort study of 64,538 low-risk mothers showed that nulliparous women who intended to have a home birth at the beginning of labor had a very slight increased risk (0.1%) of perinatal complications on a composite measure of all morbidity when compared to those who started care of labor at an obstetric unit (Birthplace in England Collaborative Group 2011). This study did not have the ability to detect any differences in maternal mortality because maternal deaths are so rare in high-resource nations. There were no significant differences in the perinatal complication rate for multiparous patients in all places of birth. This study confirmed that the medical intervention rate was much higher in low-risk women who delivered in obstetric units as compared with midwifery units or at home. The Birthplace study also revealed an economic advantage to home birth and to midwifery care of low-risk mothers. For example, Anderson, Daviss, and Johnson (2021) have shown that if only 10% more births in the United States took place in homes or freestanding birth centers, 11 billion USD could be saved annually—321 million USD for each percentage point increase. These savings would be passed on to consumers in the form of lowered insurance premiums.

Two systematic reviews (Hutton et al. 2019; Reitsma et al. 2020) assessed the outcomes of 500,000 mother-baby dyads of those intending to birth at home. The findings revealed that those within well-integrated settings (between primary and secondary care/community and hospital settings) were less likely to experience biomedical interventions, with no adverse outcomes for neonates. There are clear scientific and social benefits to midwifery care (Sandall et al. 2016). However, many national governments still do not invest financially in midwives, nor do they support midwives in their vital roles in the care of normal pregnancies. This lack of support for midwives is highlighted in the *State of the World's Midwifery* report (UNFPA, ICM, and WHO 2021), which has called for urgent global investment in midwifery to meet the reproductive and sexual health needs of women and babies, noting that 350,000 skilled midwives are needed to meet the world's needs for maternity care. Large-scale successful midwifery and home birth depend on governmental backing, as seen in the British and Dutch examples provided above.

## Home Birth in Well-Resourced Countries

In high-resource countries, the move of birth from home to hospital for low-risk mothers was never backed by evidence (Olsen and Jewell 1998). As previously mentioned, there are no randomized controlled trials on the absolute safety of home birth; however, as also previously noted, there are meta-analyses that provide large reviews of observational data (Hutton et al. 2019; Reitsma et al. 2020). Arguably, observational data in "real world settings" that focus on the planned (not actual) place of birth offer the most useful findings that practitioners can apply to "real world" clinical practice. The review authors were careful to differentiate between well-integrated settings (like the UK and the Netherlands), to those less well-integrated in other contexts where less positive neonatal outcomes were found (Hutton et al. 2019). There is some controversy regarding home birth in "high-risk" mothers, and while it is generally recommended that they birth in hospitals, the parameters of "high risk" are also changing as new evidence comes to light and women increasingly make autonomous decisions (Holten and Miranda 2016; Feeley, Thomson, and Downe 2020; Davis-Floyd 2022).

Planned term home births with professionally trained midwives well equipped for immediate maternal and fetal resuscitation are distinct from unplanned emergency home births, in which rates of problematic outcomes are much higher. Some complications may (rarely) occur at any birth, but some *cannot* occur in out-of-hospital settings, such as increased maternal pain from artificial labor augmentation; stalled labors resulting from the stress of the hospital environment; problems in pushing due to the lithotomy position (which greatly reduces the size of the pelvic outlet, in contrast to upright or all-fours positions that maximize pelvic opening); anaphylaxis related to drug allergies; and total spinal block related to epidurals. In planned home births, continuity of care by a known midwife ensures continuous physical and emotional support, and systematic reviews show that these factors improve birth outcomes (see, e.g., Sandall et al. 2016).

## The Benefits of Home Birth:
## Physiology and the Price of Interventions

Normal, physiologic birth is an important aspect of public health, and home births are physiologic births. Normal labor and birth accelerate fetal maturity, leading to improved physiologic functions in the baby, such as endocrine, immune system, thyroid function, respiration, neurology, and temperature regulation (Otamiri et al. 1991; Bird, Spencer, and Mould 1996; Vogl et al. 2006); greater mother and baby bonding; and higher breastfeeding rates, which in turn lead to better lifelong emotional and physical health for babies (Kim et al. 2011; Olza, Uvnäs-Moberg et al. 2020). Moreover, research has found that the gut flora of babies born at home are significantly more diverse than in babies born in hospitals (Combellick et al. 2018), adding to the growing awareness of the importance of infant gut seeding at the time of birth and the potential longer-term influences on the microbiome (and later health outcomes). Normal birth, in particular home birth, affirms health, promotes empowerment in mothers (Downe 2008; Lokugamage 2011; Cheyney 2011; Olza, Leahy-Warren et al. 2018), and is a social event that has been linked to fostering positive emotional qualities in society via the birthing hormone oxytocin (Uvnäs-Moberg 1998).

A study by Anna Ransjo-Arvidson and colleagues (2001) showed that babies whose mothers receive epidurals and/or systemic opioids (which can include pethidine, morphine, fentanyl, butorphanol tartrate, and nalbuphine) during labor as compared to unmedicated babies exhibited reduced breast-seeking and breastfeeding behaviors, were less likely to breastfeed within 150 minutes of birth, and cried more, whereas 90%–100% of newborns not exposed to these medications exhibited all six measured breastfeeding behaviors. Epidurals have also been associated with the persistence of the occiput-posterior malposition of the fetus, which is linked with more interventions and operative delivery (delivery by forceps, vacuum extractor, or cesarean) (Lieberman et al. 2005). Biomedical interventions decrease the likelihood of establishing breastfeeding (Nissen et al. 1996; Forster and McLachlan 2007). The health risks to the child of not breastfeeding for at least six months include an elevated chance of developing Type 1 and Type 2 diabetes, obesity, recurrent ear infections, leukemia, diarrhea, and hospitalization for lower respiratory tract infections. For mothers, not breastfeeding their babies is associated with an increased incidence of premenopausal breast cancer, ovarian cancer, retained gestational weight gain, Type 2 diabetes, myocardial infarction, and the metabolic syndrome[4] (Stuebe 2009).

Women who consider home birth are not "selfish" nor resigned to a ghastly painful experience of labor without medical interventions. There is an endogenous system of pain relief provided by endorphins. Supportive companionship, laboring and/or birthing in water, massage, hypnosis, yoga, and acupuncture all have some evidence of supporting the normal physiology of birth and reducing distress, anxiety, and desires for pain relief (Lokugamage and Barbira-Freedman 2016; Smith et al.

2018; Thomson et al. 2019; Lokugamage et al. 2020; Feeley, Cooper, and Burns 2021; Kara and Miller 2021).

## So Why Do Doctors Fear Home Birth?

Obstetricians are rare on-lookers to the emotional power, ensuing bonding, breastfeeding, nurturing, and long-term benefits of home birth, and are not able to experientially contrast this with a woman who feels disempowered by a "cascade of interventions," less bonded with her baby, and less capable of breastfeeding.

Obstetricians only look after a woman until she has delivered, and they are mostly unaware of how the experience of birth affects women in the long term and influences the meaning of their lives, because it is a major life event that women tend to remember vividly for the rest of their lives, as fully explained by our series lead editor Robbie Davis-Floyd in the third edition of *Birth as an American Rite of Passage* (2022).

There is a lack of biomedical training about home birth and the handling of uncertainty, as well as a lack of training on how best to deal with homebirth transfers to hospitals (see Cheyney, Everson, and Burcher [2014] and Davis-Floyd [2003, 2018a]). In addition to fearing home births and homebirth transfers, obstetricians often base their practices on fearful and traumatic birth attendance experiences; all obstetricians sooner or later experience a fetal death, and from then on, their fear of birth increases, as does the defensive nature of their practices (Davis-Floyd 1987, 2018b). Thus, obstetricians' conceptualizations of safety and risk tend to hinge on acute situations that carry a high emotional charge, rather than on a broader and longer-term perspective. Lack of awareness of the positive evidence surrounding planned, midwife-attended home births, and not understanding that, in the obstetric paradox, standard obstetric procedures cause unintentional iatrogenic harm (see Liese et al. 2021) can perpetuate obstetricians' fears of home birth. Obstetricians are continually immersed in crisis medicine rather than in the normal physiology of birth; this immersion promotes an ethos of the frailty of birthing bodies and can generate post-traumatic stress disorder (PTSD) (Kruper et al. 2019). A meta-analysis (de Boer et al. 2011) reviewed existing data on the impacts of work-related critical incidents in hospital-based healthcare practitioners. It showed that work-related critical incidents may induce post-traumatic stress symptoms of anxiety, depression, and even PTSD itself.

Obstetricians fear that they may be implicated in a bad outcome that could have been prevented, fanning their ever-present fear of litigation, as well as fear for their professional survival and the impacts on their families should their careers be threatened. Obstetricians also fear the lack of facilities and familiar tools if something goes wrong at home, but without understanding homebirth midwives' transfer policies and protocols, the infrequency of complications, or midwives' capabilities for dealing with, for examples, postpartum hemorrhage, retained placentas, and neonatal resuscitation (Cheyney, Everson, and Burcher 2014; Davis-Floyd 2018a). It is hard for obstetricians to realize that, as noted above, many avoidable or ameliorable complications occurring in hospitals *cannot happen at home.* In addition to the examples provided above of complications that can't happen at home, further examples include hyperstimulation due to drugs; incorrect obtainment or interpretation of laboratory-based test; delays, poor communication, and prescribing errors among members of large teams; and hospital-acquired disorders such as infections and thrombosis.

The oxytocin behavioral system is the opposite of the "fight, flight, or freeze" response to stress and fear. Professor Uvnäs-Moberg, an oxytocin physiologist, asserts that the human oxytocic behavioral system promotes positive emotions, and that normal birth amplifies this system within childbearers and promotes higher habitual oxytocin secretion (Uvnäs-Moberg 1998; Olza, Uvnäs-Moberg et al. 2020). These findings validate the social neurobiological theory that oxytocin encourages calmness, trust, generosity, compassion, and social cohesion through the neurobiology of maternal and pair bonding—thus also conversely providing insights into the origins of human anxiety and violence (Pedersen 2004). Professor Kosfeld's (2007) neurobiological research points to oxytocin helping humans to overcome their natural aversion to uncertainty regarding the behaviors of others. Could it be that obstetricians, who base decisions about birth, in part, on their prior experiences with traumatic births, become habitually low oxytocin secretors? Could it be that low levels of oxytocin make it more difficult for them to deal with uncertainty—hence a preference for biomedicalized birth, which they perceive as offering more control and certainty? Home birth involves trusting a woman's body to do its physiologic best, and oxytocin is a mediator of trust (Van IJzendoorn and Bakermans-Kranenburg 2012). Could doctors be better trained or helped to deal with fear and uncertainty, as homebirth midwives are?

Contemporary women's fears of loss of control, insecurity, and failure resonate with the same fears in obstetricians, pitting both against the homebirth ethos. Obstetrics clearly has a crucial role to play when there are actual biomedical problems, but to view all pregnancies through the lens of risk-averse biomedical culture does a disservice to those women who are capable of discovering the benefits of natural birth. Fear of childbirth prevents women from discovering their intuitive wisdom and capabilities. As most new mothers find, "control" is at best temporary and at worst illusory. Perhaps a better strategy might be to understand those who have resilience in the face of uncertainty, who have strong coping mechanisms, and who can "embrace loss of control" and face their fears, as homebirthing women/birthing people do. In a passage from her book *Insecure at Last: Losing It in Our Security-Obsessed World*, Eve Ensler (2006:2) writes:

> Is it possible to live surrendering to the reality of insecurity, embracing it, allowing it to open us and transform us and be our teacher? What would we need in order to stop panicking, clinging, consuming, and start opening, giving—becoming more ourselves the less secure we realize we actually are?

## A Way Forward? Overcoming Fear

Yet perhaps the tide is turning. While the Royal College of Obstetricians and Gynaecologists (RCOG) in the UK has long supported home births, accounts from obstetricians themselves had been sparse. However, through the visibility of social media and blog posts, a growing number of obstetricians are sharing their experiences of home birth; some share their own homebirth experience, while others share about attending a home birth. Many mirror the reflective article by a UK obstetrician who attended a home birth with midwives (Wilcox and Pitcher 2019). In her words, we see this obstetrician's self-awareness that her professional experiences were "skewed by . . . women transferred during labor or newly postpartum, due to complications" (2019:21). However, through a willingness to take an opportunity to attend a home birth with experienced midwives, she first noticed the liminal differences between home and hospital birth:

> I was struck by the aura of calm in the room and the fact that we were all intensely focused on the woman and supporting her. In contrast to the hospital, there were no distractions and no other women requiring our attention: our common purpose was her and her baby and family. This was total privacy with no interruption . . . we were guests at their home and their birth, so the permission and relationship between us and the couple felt subtly different to me from a hospital birth.

Furthermore, this doctor's reflections offer optimism that obstetricians' fears can be overcome:

> As I was leaving, the grandmothers collected the older two boys from the nursery [day care center] and brought them home to meet their new baby brother. I felt I had experienced something very special. Although I have witnessed many midwifery-led births [in hospitals], this birth had an aura of calm and a different intimacy I had not experienced before. It left me asking myself why you wouldn't want this type of care provided in the familiar surroundings and comfort of your own home if it was your safest option. (Quoted in Wilcox and Pitcher 2019:21)

## Conclusion:
## The Need to Address Obstetricians' Fears Surrounding Home Birth

The COVID-19 pandemic has highlighted the urgency of addressing obstetric fears surrounding home birth, as hospitals were centers of increased infection spread. In the UK, pandemic responses varied widely, with some Hospital Trusts (which are organizations responsible for delivering local health services across hospitals and community settings) increasing their homebirth services, responding to an increased demand by women keen to stay away from contagious hospital settings. However, in other places, homebirth services were cancelled and birthing services re-centralized. This disparity in responses mirrors the issues we have highlighted herein, whereby the pandemic has served to magnify existing organizational beliefs and attitudes. Therefore, we must learn from those organizations in which obstetricians and midwives are united within a humanistic philosophy grounded both in physiology and in evidence-based practice, in which home births are protected, supported, and celebrated.

## Acknowledgment

This chapter is updated and adapted from Lokugamage A. 2011. "Fear of Home Birth in Doctors and Obstetric Iatrogenesis." *International Journal of Childbirth* 1(4): 263–272. We thank IJC for providing permission to draw on this article herein.

**Amali Lokugamage** is a consultant obstetrician and gynecologist involved in medical education in London, UK. She has more than 30 years of experience in the specialty. Her main clinical interests lie in medical gynecology and general obstetrics, with expertise in normalizing birth. She has published in the fields of human rights in childbirth, healthcare inequalities, and decolonization.

**Claire Feeley** is a midwife, researcher, and educator. She has more than ten years of experience across all areas of midwifery that includes home-birth settings. Her clinical and research practice has focused on women's health inequalities, namely around the issues of childbirth choice, autonomy, rights, and care provision, with a focus on normal physiological birth and full-scope midwifery. She has published extensively in these fields.

## Notes

1. This information was retrieved 21 November 2022 from: www.birthbythenumbers.org/midwifery/.
2. "Supervalue" is a term coined by series editor Robbie Davis-Floyd in her first book, *Birth as an American Rite of Passage* (1992, 2003, 2022).
3. The term "prospective" is important here; it means that when a midwife takes on a client, she must enter that client in the database, and then must account for the outcome of that birth. This prospective entry prevents midwives who enter their data from hiding any deaths.
4. "Metabolic syndrome" consists of a group of conditions that put individuals at higher risk for heart disease and diabetes. It includes high blood pressure, high blood sugar, excess body fat around the waist, and abnormal cholesterol or triglyceride levels.

## References

ACOG (American College of Obstetricians and Gynecologists) Committee on Obstetric Practice. 2011. "ACOG Committee Opinion No. 476: Planned Home Birth." *Obstetrics and Gynecology* 11: 425–428.

Anderson DA, Daviss BA, Johnson KC. 2021. "What If Another 10% of Deliveries in the United States Took Place at Home or in a Birth Center? Safety, Economics, and Politics." In *Birthing Models on the Human Rights Frontier: Speaking Truth to Power*, eds. Daviss BA, Davis-Floyd R, 205–228. Abingdon, Oxon: Routledge.

Baumgartner T, Heinrichs M, Vonlanthen A, Fischbacher U, Fehr E. 2008. "Oxytocin Shapes the Neural Circuitry of Trust and Trust Adaptation in Humans." *Neuron* 58(4): 639–650.

Berg, M. 2000. *Guidelines, Professionals and the Production of Objectivity: Standardisation and the Professionalism of Insurance Medicine.* Oxford: Blackwell Publishers.

Bird JA, Spencer T, Mould ME. 1996. "Endocrine and Metabolic Adaptation Following Caesarean Section or Vaginal Delivery." *Archives of Disease in Childhood. Fetal and Neonatal Edition* 74(2): F132–134.

Birthplace in England Collaborative Group. 2011. "Perinatal and Maternal Outcomes by Planned Place of Birth for Healthy Women with Low Risk Pregnancies: The Birthplace in England National Prospective Cohort Study." *British Medical Journal* 343: d7400.

Cheyney M. 2011. "Homebirth as Ritual Performance." *Medical Anthropology Quarterly* 25(4): 519–542.

Cheyney M, Bovbjerg M, Everson C, et al. 2014. "Outcomes of Care for 16,924 Planned Homebirths in the United States: The Midwives Alliance of North America Statistics Project, 2004 to 2009." *Journal of Midwifery & Women's Health* 59(1): 17–27.

Cheyney M, Davis-Floyd R. 2019. "Birth as Culturally Marked and Shaped." In *Birth in Eight Cultures*, eds. Davis-Floyd R, Cheyney M, 1–16. Long Grove IL: Waveland Press.

Cheyney M, Davis-Floyd R. 2020a. "Birth and the Big Bad Wolf: A Biocultural, Co-Evolutionary Perspective, Part 1." *International Journal of Childbirth* 09(4): 177–192.

———. 2020b. "Birth and the Big Bad Wolf: A Biocultural, Co-Evolutionary Perspective, Part 2." *International Journal of Childbirth* 10(2): 66–78.

———. 2021. "Birth and the Big Bad Wolf: Biocultural Evolution and Human Childbirth." In *Birthing Techno-Sapiens: Human-Technology Co-Evolution and the Future of Reproduction*, ed. Davis-Floyd R, 15-46. Abingdon, Oxon: Routledge.

Cheyney M, Everson C, Burcher P. 2014. "Homebirth Transfers in the United States: Narratives of Risk, Fear, and Mutual Accommodation." *Qualitative Health Research* 24(4): 443–456.

Cheyney M, Goodarzi B, Wiegers T, et al. 2019. "Giving Birth in the United States and the Netherlands: Midwifery as Integrated Option or Contested Privilege?" In *Birth in Eight Cultures*, eds. Davis-Floyd R, Cheyney M, 165–202. Long Grove IL: Waveland Press.

Combellick J, Shin H, Shin D, Cai Y, et al. 2018. "Differences in the Fecal Microbiota of Neonates Born at Home or in the Hospital." *Scientific Reports* 8: 15660.

Daellenbach R, Davies L, Meeks M, et al. 2023. "Interprofessional Education for Medical and Midwifery Students in Aotearoa/New Zealand." In *Obstetric Violence and Systemic Disparities: Can Obstetrics Be Humanized and Decolonized?* eds. Davis-Floyd R, Premkumar A, Chapter 11. New York: Berghahn Books.

Davis-Floyd R. 1987. "Obstetric Training as a Rite of Passage." *Medical Anthropology Quarterly* 1(3): 288–318.

———. 2003. "Home Birth Emergencies in the U.S. and Mexico: The Trouble with Transport." *Social Science and Medicine* 56(9): 1913–1931.

———. 2018a. "Home Birth Emergencies in the US and Mexico: The Trouble with Transport." In *Ways of Knowing about Birth: Mothers, Midwives, Medicine, and Birth Activism*, Davis-Floyd R and Colleagues, 283–322. Long Grove IL: Waveland Press.

———. 2018b. "Medical Training as Technocratic Initiation." In *Ways of Knowing about Birth: Mothers, Midwives, Medicine, and Birth Activism*, Davis-Floyd R and Colleagues, 107–140. Long Grove IL: Waveland Press.

———. 2018c. "The Midwifery Model of Care: Anthropological Perspectives." In *Ways of Knowing about Birth: Mothers, Midwives, Medicine, and Birth Activism*, Davis-Floyd R and Colleagues, 323–338. Long Grove IL: Waveland Press.

———. 2022. *Birth as an American Rite of Passage*, 3rd edn. Berkeley: University of California Press.

de Boer JM, Lok A, Verlaat EV, Duivenvoorden HJ, Bakker AB, Smit BJ. 2011. "Work-Related Critical Incidents in Hospital-based Health Care Providers and the Risk of Post-traumatic Stress Symptoms, Anxiety, and Depression: A Meta-Analysis." *Social Science & Medicine* 73(2): 316–326.

de Jonge A, Geerts CC, van der Goes BY, Mol BW, Buitendijk SE, Nijhuis JG. 2015. "Perinatal Mortality and Morbidity up to 28 Days after Birth among 743,070 Low-Risk Planned Home and Hospital Births: A Cohort Study Based on Three Merged National Perinatal Databases." *BJOG: An International Journal of Obstetrics and Gynecology* 122(5): 720–728.

de Jonge A, van der Goes BY, Ravelli, ACJ, Amelink-Verburg BW, Mol W, Nijhuis JG, Gravenhorst JB, Buitendijk SE. 2009. "Perinatal Morality and Morbidity in a Nationwide Cohort of 529,688 Low-risk Planned Home and Hospital Births." *BJOG: An International Journal of Obstetrics & Gynecology* 116(9): 1177–1184.

Downe S. 2008. *Normal Childbirth: Evidence and Debate*, 2nd ed. Edinburgh: Churchill Livingstone Elsevier.

Duran AM. 1992. "The Safety of Home Birth: The Farm Study." *American Journal of Public Health* 82(3): 450–453.

Ensler E. 2006. *Insecure at Last: Losing It in Our Security Obsessed World*. New York: Villard.

Feeley C, Cooper M, and Burns E. 2021. "A Systematic Meta-Thematic Synthesis to Examine the Views and Experiences of Women Following Water Immersion during Labour and Waterbirth." *Journal of Advanced Nursing* 77(7): 2942–2956.

Feeley C, Thomson G, Downe S. 2020. "Understanding How Midwives Employed by the National Health Service Facilitate Women's Alternative Birthing Choices: Findings from a Feminist Pragmatist Study." *Plos One* 15(11): e0242508.

Forster D, McLachlan H. 2007. "Breastfeeding Initiation and Birth Setting Practices: A Review of the Literature." *Journal of Midwifery & Women's Health* 52(3): 273–280.

Georges N, Daellenbach R. 2019. "Divergent Meanings and Practices of Childbirth in Greece and New Zealand." In *Birth in Eight Cultures*, eds. Davis-Floyd R, Cheyney M, 129–164. Long Grove IL: Waveland Press.

Ghui R, Bansal JK, McLaughlin C, Kotaska A, Lokugamage A. 2016. "An Evaluation of the Guidelines of the Society of Obstetricians and Gynaecologists of Canada." *Journal of Obstetrics and Gynaecology* 36(5): 658–662.

Greenhalgh T, Howick J, Maskrey N. 2014. "Evidence-Based Medicine: A Movement in Crisis?" *British Medical Journal* 348: g3725.

Gyte G, Dodwell MJ, Macfarlane A. 2011. "Home Birth Meta-Analysis: Does It Meet AJOG's Reporting Requirements?" *American Journal of Obstetrics and Gynecology* 204(4): e15.

Gyte G, Dodwell M, Newburn M, et al. 2009. "Estimating Intrapartum-Related Perinatal Mortality Rates for Booked Home Births: When the 'Best' Available Data

Are Not Good Enough." *BJOG: An International Journal of Obstetrics & Gynecology* 116(7): 933–942.

Holten L, Miranda E. 2016. "Women's Motivations for Having Unassisted Childbirth or High-Risk Homebirth: An Exploration of the Literature on 'Birthing Outside the System.'" *Midwifery* 38: 55–62.

Horton R. 2010. "Urgency and Concern About Home Births." *Lancet* 376(9755): 1812.

Howick J. 2011. *The Philosophy of Evidence-Based Medicine.* Chichester, UK: Wiley-Blackwell BMJ Books.

Hutton E, Reitsma A, Simioni G, et al. 2019. "Perinatal or Neonatal Mortality among Women Who Intend at the Onset of Labour to Give Birth at Home Compared to Women of Low Obstetrical Risk Who Intend to Give Birth in Hospital: A Systematic Review and Meta-Analyses." *EClinicalMedicine* 14: 59–70.

Janssen P, Reime B, Ryan ER, Etches DJ. 2004. "Outcomes of Planned Hospital Birth Attended by Midwives vs Physicians in British Columbia." *Journal of Midwifery & Women's Health* 49(5): 462–463.

Janssen PA, Saxell L, Page L, et al. 2009. "Outcomes of Planned Home Birth with Registered Midwife versus Planned Hospital Birth with Midwife or Physician." *Canadian Medical Association Journal = Journal De L'Association Medicale Canadienne* 181(6–7): 377–383.

Johnson KC, Daviss BA. 2005. "Outcomes of Planned Homebirths with Certified Professional Midwives: Large Prospective Study in North America." *British Medical Journal* 330(7505): 1416–1423.

Jordan B. 1997. "Authoritative Knowledge and Its Construction." In *Childbirth and Authoritative Knowledge: Cross-Cultural Perspectives*, eds. Davis-Floyd R, Sargent C, 55–79. Berkeley: University of California Press.

Kantrowitz-Gordon I. 2005. "The Oxytocin Factor: Tapping the Hormone of Calm, Love, and Healing." *Journal of Midwifery & Women's Health* 50(1): e6.

Kara K, Miller S. 2021. "Water as a Technology to Support Embodied Autonomous Birthing." In *Birthing Techno-Sapiens: Human-Technology Co-Evolution and the Future of Reproduction*, ed. Davis-Floyd R, 179–192. Abingdon, Oxon: Routledge.

Kennare RM, Keirse M, Graeme R. Tucker GR, Chan AC. 2010. "Planned Home and Hospital Births in South Australia, 1991–2006: Differences in Outcomes." *Medical Journal of Australia* 192(2): 76–80.

Kim P, Feldman R, Mayes LC, Eicher V, Thompson NT, Leckman JF, Swain JE. 2011. "Breastfeeding, Brain Activation to Own Infant Cry, and Maternity Sensitivity." *Journal of Child Psychology and Psychiatry and Allied Disciplines* 52(8): 907–915.

Klassen PE. 2001. *Blessed Events: Religion and Homebirth in America.* Princeton NJ: Princeton University Press.

Kleinman A, Sung LH. 1979. "Why Do Indigenous Practitioners Successfully Heal?" *Social Science and Medicine Part B: Medical Anthropology* 13 B(1): 7–26.

Kosfeld M. 2007. "Trust in the Brain: Neurobiological Determinants of Human Social Behaviour." *EMBO Reports* 8: S44–S47.

Kruper A, Kristina K, Kristina P, Robert T, Domeyer-Klenske AE. 2019. "Secondary Traumatic Stress in Obstetrics & Gynecology: Provider Experience and Programmatic Needs." *Obstetrics & Gynecology* 133: 182S.

Lieberman E, Davidson K, Lee-Parritz A, Elizabeth S. 2005. "Changes in Fetal Position During Labor and Their Association with Epidural Analgesia." *Obstetrics & Gynecology* 105(5): 974–982.

Liese K, Davis-Floyd R, Stewart K, Cheyney M. 2021. "Obstetric Iatrogenesis in the United States: The Spectrum of Unintentional Harm, Disrespect, Violence, and Abuse." *Anthropology & Medicine* 28(2): 1–17.

Lokugamage A. 2011. *The Heart in the Womb: An Exploration of the Roots of Love and Social Cohesion.* London: Docamali Ltd.

Lokugamage A, Barbira-Freedman F. 2016. "The Pyschobiological Revival of the 'Three P's' in an Integrated Antenatal Education Model." *International Journal of Birth and Parenting Education* 3: 7–9.

Lokugamage A, Eftime A, Porter D, et al. 2020. "Birth Preparation Acupuncture for Normalising Birth: An Analysis of NHS Service Routine Data and Proof of Concept." *Journal of Obstetrics and Gynecology: The Journal of the Institute of Obstetrics and Gynecology* 40(8): 1096–1101.

Miller E, Abalos M, Chamillard A, et al. 2016. "Beyond Too Little, Too Late and Too Much Too Soon: A Pathway Towards Evidence-Based, Respectful Maternity Care Worldwide." *Lancet* 388(10056): 2176–2192.

Mori RM, Dougherty M, Whittle M. 2008. "An Estimation of Intrapartum-Related Perinatal Mortality Rates for Booked Home Births in England and Wales between 1994 and 2003." *BJOG: An International Journal of Obstetrics & Gynecology* 115(5): 554–559.

NICE. 2014. "Intrapartum Care for Health Women and Babies." *National Institute for Health and Care Excellence.* Retrieved 8 November 2022 from https://www.nice.org.uk/guidance/cg190.

Nissen E, Uvnäs-Moberg K, Svensson K, Stock S, Widström AM, Winberg J. 1996. "Different Patterns of Oxytocin, Prolactin but Not Cortisol Release During Breastfeeding in Women Delivered by Caesarean Section or by the Vaginal Route." *Early Human Development* 45(1–2): 103–118.

KNOV. 2017. "Midwifery in the Netherlands." Retrieved 10th January 2022 from https://www.europeanmidwives.com/.

Olsen O, Jewell MD. 1998. "Home Versus Hospital Birth." *Cochrane Database of Systematic Reviews* 2: CD000352.

Olza IP, Leahy-Warren P, Benyamini Y, et al. 2018. "Women's Psychological Experiences of Physiological Childbirth: A Meta-Synthesis." *BMJ Open* 8(10): e020347.

Olza I, Uvnäs-Moberg K, Ekström-Bergström A, et al. 2020. "Birth as a Neuro-Psycho-Social-Event: An Integrative Model of Maternity Experiences and Their Relation to Neurohormonal Events During Childbirth." *PloS One* 15(7): e0230992.

Otamiri G, Göran G, Ledin T, Leijon I, Lagercrantz H. 1991. "Delayed Neurological Adaptation in Infants Delivered by Elective Caesarean and the Relation to Catecholamine Levels." *Early Human Development* 26(1): 51–60.

Pedersen CA. 2004. "Biological Aspects of Social Bonding and the Roots of Human Violence." *Annals of the New York Academy of Sciences* 1036: 106–127.

Prusova K, Churcher L, Tyler A, Lokugamage AU. 2014. "Royal College of Obstetricians and Gynaecologists Guidelines: How Evidence-Based Are They?" *Journal of Obstetrics and Gynaecology* 34(8): 706–711.

Ransjo-Arvidson A, Matthiesen A, Lilja G, Nissen E, Widstrom A, Uvnas-Moberg K. 2001. "Maternal Analgesia during Labor Disturbs Newborn Behavior: Effects on Breastfeeding, Temperature, and Crying." *Birth.* 28(1): 5–12.

Reitsma A, Simioni J, Brunton G, Kaufman K, Hutton EK. 2020. "Maternal Outcomes and Birth Interventions among Women Who Begin Labour Intending to Give Birth at Home Compared to Women of Low Obstetrical Risk Who Intend to Give Birth in Hospital: A Systematic Review and Meta-Analyses." *Lancet* 21(100319).

Sandall J, Bewley S, Newburn N. 2011. "'Home Birth Triples the Neonatal Death Rate': Public Communication of Bad Science?" *American Journal of Obstetrics and Gynecology* 204(4): e17–18.

Sandall J, Soltani H, Gates S, Shennan A, Devane D. 2016. "Midwife-Led Continuity Models Versus Other Models of Care for Childbearing Women." *Cochrane Database of Systematic Reviews* 4: CD004667.

Smith CA, Levett KM, Collins CT, et al. 2018. "Relaxation Techniques for Pain Management in Labour." *Cochrane Database of Systematic Reviews* 3: CD009514.

Snowden JM, Tilden EL, Snyder J, Quigley B, Caughey AB, Cheng YW. 2015. "Planned Out-of-Hospital Birth and Birth Outcomes." *New England Journal of Medicine* 373: 2642–2653.

Stuebe A. 2009. "The Risks of Not Breastfeeding for Mothers and Infants." *Reviews in Obstetrics and Gynecology* 2(4): 222–231.

Teijilingen E, Lowis G, McCaffery P, Porter M, eds. 2004. *Midwifery and the Medicalization of Childbirth: Comparative Perspectives.* Hauppauge NY: Nova Science Publishers.

Thomson G, Feeley F, Hall Moran V, et al. 2019. "Women's Experiences of Pharmacological and Non-Pharmacological Pain Relief Methods for Labour and Childbirth: A Qualitative Systematic Review." *Reproductive Health* 16(71): 1–20.

UNFPA, ICM, and WHO. 2021. "The State of the Worlds' Midwifery: 2021." *UNFPA,* 5 May. Retrieved 8 November 2022 from https://www.unfpa.org/publications/sowmy-2021.

Uvnäs-Moberg K. 1998. "Oxytocin May Mediate the Benefits of Positive Social Interaction and Emotions." *Psychoneuroendocrinology* 23(8): 819–835.

Van IJzendoorn MH, Bakermans-Kranenburg M. 2012. "A Sniff of Trust: Meta-Analysis of the Effects of Intranasal Oxytocin Administration on Face Recognition, Trust to In-Group, and Trust to Out-Group." *Psychoneuroendocrinology* 37(3): 438–443.

Vogl SE, Worda C, Egarter C, et al. 2006. "Mode of Delivery Is Associated with Maternal and Fetal Endocrine Stress Response." *BJOG: An International Journal of Obstetrics and Gynecology* 113(4): 441–445.

Wax J, Lucas RFL, Lamont M, Pinette P, Cartin A, Blackstone J. 2010. "Maternal and Newborn Outcomes in Planned Home Birth vs Planned Hospital Births: A Meta-Analysis." *American Journal of Obstetrics and Gynecology* 203(3): 243.e1–8.

WHO. 2019. *Maternal Mortality: Levels and Trends 2000 to 2017.* World Health Organization: Sexual and Reproductive Health and Research. Retrieved 26 November 2022 from https://apps.who.int/iris/handle/10665/327596.

———. 2018. *WHO Recommendations Non-Clinical Interventions to Reduce Unnecessary Caesarean Sections.* Geneva: World Health Organisation. Retrieved 8 November 2022 from http://apps.who.int/iris/bitstream/handle/10665/275377/9 789241550338-eng.pdf?ua=1.

Wilcox F, Pitcher P. 2019. "Home Birth: Can Midwives and Obstetricians Work Together to Provide True Choice and Support?" *The Practising Midwife* 22(2). Retrieved 8 November 2022 from https://www.all4maternity.com/home-birth-can-midwives-and-obstetricians-work-together-to-provide-true-choice-and-support/.

Wright JD, Pawar N, Gonzalez JSR, et al. 2011. "Scientific Evidence Underlying the American College of Obstetricians and Gynecologists' Practice Bulletins." *Obstetrics & Gynecology* 118(3): 505–512.

Zohar N, De Vries R. 2011. "Study Validity Questioned." *American Journal of Obstetrics and Gynecology* 204(4): e14.

# Conclusions
## Concepts, Conceptual Frameworks, and Lessons Learned

*Robbie Davis-Floyd and Ashish Premkumar*

In these Conclusions, as we have done in the Conclusions to Volume I (Davis-Floyd and Premkumar 2023a) of this three-volume book series—and also in the Conclusions to Volume III (Davis-Floyd and Premkumar 2023b)—we present some of the concepts, conceptual frameworks, and theories that our chapter authors found useful in their analyses in the hope that others might find them useful as well. We also describe some of the most important lessons that these chapters provide for practitioners, social scientists, and policy makers. The trope of the importance of *listening to obstetricians* runs throughout these chapters, because positive, humanistic changes cannot be effected unless obstetricians' perspectives are understood. As some our chapters in this volume suggest, such understandings can lead to the development of programs to "re-socialize" obs into practicing evidence-based, humanistic care. (Unless otherwise indicated, all direct quotes and all italics in them are from the chapters themselves.)

## The Theoretical Concepts and Frameworks That Our Chapter Authors Found Useful

Robbie Davis-Floyd's Chapter 1 on "Open and Closed Knowledge Systems, the 4 Stages of Cognition, and the Cultural Management of Birth" is a conceptual framework itself. To briefly recap, Robbie called attention to the differences between "open" and "closed" knowledge systems, and presented "4 Stages of Cognition" (a schema originated by Harold Schroder, Michael Driver, and Siegfried Streufert [1967]), correlating each Stage with one or more anthropological concepts. She correlated closed, Stage 1 thinking with naïve realism ("Our way is the only way or the only way that matters"); fundamentalism ("Our way is the only *right* way"); and fanaticism ("Our way is so right that all who disagree with it should be assimilated or eliminated"). She coded Stage 2 thinking as ethnocentrism ("Other ways may be ok for others, but our way is best"), and Stage 3, open thinking as cultural relativism ("All ways have value; individual behaviors should be understood within their sociocultural contexts"). Noting the limitations of cultural relativism, she moved to Stage 4, globally humanistic thinking ("We must search for better ways that honor the human rights of all individuals"), and stated that global humanists are anathemas to Stage 1 fundamentalist and fanatical thinkers, which is why Stage 4 humanistic obstetricians are so often persecuted by Stage 1 members of what Barbara Katz Rothman (2021) calls the "Biomedical Empire"—as profoundly illustrated in many of the chapters (all of which are written by obstetricians) in Volume I of this series (Davis-Floyd and Premkumar 2023a).

Defining rituals as "patterned, repetitive, and symbolic enactments of cultural or individual beliefs and values" (Davis-Floyd [1992] 2003, 2018b, 2022), Robbie showed how rituals can be used to enact the values and beliefs of people at all 4 Stages of Cognition, and to move people out of "Substage"—a condition of intense irritability, anxiety, anger, burnout, breakdown, hysteria, panic—otherwise known as "losing it." Because, as Robbie described, ritual "stands as a barrier between cognition and chaos," anyone can use it to make their way out of chaos and back into cognition. Robbie also made good use of ritual researcher Dimitris Xygalatas's concepts of rituals as "mechanisms of resilience" and "life-hacks," as we further discuss below.

Co-authors Margaret Dunlea, Martina Hynan, Jo Murphy-Lawless, Magdalena Ohaja, Malgorzata Stach, and Jeannine Webster were among those chapter authors who found this "4 Stages of Cognition" schema useful; for examples, they stressed that Irish obstetrics, which they called "an obstetric fraternity," is a tightly closed knowledge system that shuts out all conflicting evidence, and stated, "All contemporary evidence supporting midwifery-led services such as planned home birth, or birth in an alongside or freestanding midwifery unit . . . is rejected out of hand by the members of this Stage 1, fundamentalist obstetric system." Additionally, these authors pointed to the critical concerns of:

> staff burnout, poor morale, and severe recruitment and retention challenges—all of which are a direct result of stressful working conditions that can put practitioners into what . . . Davis-Floyd calls

"Substage" . . . In this condition, practitioners cannot feel empathy for others and may treat them with disrespect and even violence and abuse, especially those below them in the obstetric hierarchy, such as laboring women.

Anthropologists Vania Smith-Oka and Lydia Dixon also found this "4 Stages of Cognition" schema useful; for example, they noted that even though some of the practices in the Mexican hospitals they studied are outdated:

> many of them remain due to a combination of socialization and inertia (for example, obstetricians say things like, "This is how I was trained and how things are done") . . . In her chapter in this volume, Davis-Floyd refers to the effects of these attitudes as "Stage 1 naïve realism"—a position from which obstetricians come to view their way as the only possible way. This naïve realism helps to explain why practitioners . . . who were deeply concerned with changing the practices within their hospitals, would often find themselves having to justify why they were *not* engaging in these routine practices. Davis-Floyd . . . would label such doctors "Stage 4 humanistic practitioners," as they are among those proposing that "there must be better ways that honor everyone's human rights."

Nicholas (Nick) Rubashkin too found Davis-Floyd's theoretical framework useful: citing Jo Murpy-Lawless, one of our volume authors, he analyzed obstetrics as a closed knowledge system:

> Using history as an example, Jo Murphy-Lawless (1998) dated the obstetric tendency toward closed system thinking to the very origins of the profession in 17th-century Ireland (see also Chapter 2 in this volume). Murphy-Lawless (1998:157) went so far as to project the closed nature of obstetrics into the future, writing that "knowledge formation within obstetrics will always be premised on a closed form of rationality that excludes women yet operates at the expense of women." The fact that obstetric researchers invented a rational object like the VBAC calculator without soliciting input from birthing individuals neither into the design nor into the application of the calculator is testimony to the dynamics of closed system thinking.

Importantly, Nick stressed that the calculator failed to consider women's levels of commitment to having a VBAC, given that such commitments play a primary role in women's decisions to go for a VBAC and in their successes in achieving one, if they do. Thus we (Robbie and Ashish) argue here that "patient's level of commitment" should have been one of the variables that the calculator took into account:

> The calculator's early statistical prediction did not address the role of confidence in one's capacity to birth. By forcing an early decision, the calculator neglected the possibility that a woman [with a previous cesarean] might need to rebuild her confidence over the course of her pregnancy ... By demanding an early decision to schedule a repeat cesarean, the VBAC calculator sliced through other, more qualitative approaches to the uncertainty of planning a VBAC.

Another risk that the calculator did not consider "was the psychological risk to the woman who deeply desired a TOLAC [trial of labor after cesarean] but was forbidden to have one. As Davis-Floyd (2022) and others have shown, postpartum depression and even PTSD can result from such denial of deep desire." In efforts to use the calculator more appropriately, "the group of providers who ultimately used the calculator in select cases *started* with women's preferences and would only apply the calculator if the woman had some level of indecision about her options."

Nick went on to note a contradiction in the ACOG guidelines and in the policies that counseled (or forbade) women with low scores from attempting a VBAC, on which only a few of the ob interlocutors in his study had commented:

> Namely, no similar policies came into effect to counsel (or force) women with "high" scores to attempt a VBAC. A . . . perinatologist pointed out this contradiction: "Because the standard of care at this point, at least in the US, is if somebody wants a repeat section, they can have one. . . . Even if they predict success scores over 90, they can still have a repeat section if they want, which is funny." The contradiction is "funny" because a woman's autonomous decision to have a VBAC is circumscribed around those who are good candidates for vaginal birth, but even good candidates for vaginal birth can elect to have a cesarean. While I am of course not advocating that women with high scores should be forced into vaginal births they don't desire, I am saying that the contradictory approaches to "good" and "bad" VBAC candidates demonstrate that the protected form of autonomy in obstetrics is when a patient "elects" for a cesarean birth, and not the other way around.

We editors note that this is typical of ob Stage 1 closed system funda-mentalist thinking, in which patient "choice" is too often constrained by what the obstetric establishment wants the patient to do (see Davis-Floyd 2022). Nick highlighted that: "A *preference-sensitive* approach to counseling would say that a good VBAC candidate is anyone who wants to have a VBAC."

Returning to the chapter by Margaret Dunlea, Martina Hynan, Jo Murphy-Lawless, Magdalena Ohaja, Malgorzata Stach, and Jeannine Webster on the culture of obstetrics in Ireland, we note that they began with sociologist Pat O'Connor's (2000) characterization of Irish soci-ety "as one where the 'patriarchal dividend' continues to underpin a widespread cultural acceptance of male-oriented authority as entirely appropriate. Nowhere is this dominance more vividly to the fore than in relation to the institutions, policies, and practices surrounding childbirth in Ireland." These authors emphasized the international influence of the famous (or notorious, depending on one's point of view) textbook writ-ten by members of the "obstetric fraternity": *Active Management of La-bour* (1980) by Kieran O'Driscoll and Declan Meagher of the National Maternity Hospital, Dublin:

> That text went through three more editions . . . and cemented the international reputation of Irish obstetrics for strictly time-managed labor and birth according to a series of templates to be applied to each woman, along with recourse to augmentation with oxytocin, administered intravenously to any labor that deviated from norms laid down by the templates. These templates for active management were and are rigorously applied to first-time mothers in particu-lar and are referred to in the textbook as "one of the fundamental truths of clinical obstetrics."

In Ireland, as opposed to Northern Ireland, Scotland, the UK, and other European countries (excluding Greece; see below), maternity care is fully obstetric-led, with midwives being entirely subjugated to obste-tricians' control, to the great detriment of Irish childbearers, who are themselves entirely subjugated to obstetric control. Finding useful the work of Michel Foucault, co-authors Dunlea, Hynan, Murphy-Lawless, Ohaja, Stach, and Webster noted that:

> In the sciences, structures of formal language are classically em-ployed to establish jurisdiction. They do so by seeking to delimit knowledges that strengthen any given field of power while exclud-

ing what they find troublesome or challenging. "What they sanction, what they exclude in order to function" (Foucault 1974:294) entails building a grammar that effectively becomes the sole legitimated mode of speaking. They also seek to secure that lodestone of seeming "objectivity" to underwrite their assertion of maintaining universal principles, but as Foucault observed, "the universality of our knowledge has been acquired at the cost of exclusions." (1974:294)

What is excluded in Ireland is the woman herself. "Whatever she may have to say about her body, her pregnancy, or her labor is to be disregarded. The woman facing these iron laws of regulated labor should have not only no voice but her very conduct in the delivery room as laid down in all four editions of *Active Management* must be under obstetric direction and her actions censured when needed." Also excluded is the midwife, who is "relegated to the offstage role of . . . companion, with her work being defined by obstetric rationales . . . The midwife must fit into the obstetric authority . . . hence the outright refusal to even incorporate the term 'midwifery-led care'" into the foundational documents of Irish obstetrics. Dunlea and colleagues quoted consultant ob Peter Boylan, co-author of the 3rd edition of *Active Management of Labour*, as saying "We do not want to repeat the mistakes of separating out midwifery and obstetric care. They are both the same. All obstetricians are midwives and are proud to be midwives, but they are also looking after more complicated cases." Said the authors: "In this way, Irish obstetric discourse obliterates midwives by coding obstetricians *as* midwives."

Using Martina Hynan's identification of "the male obstetric gaze" and Melissa Cheyney and Robbie Davis-Floyd's definition of the "obstetric paradox," these authors stated that:

Martina Hynan (2018) has shown how the "male obstetric gaze" has flourished from the 18th century onward, lying at the core of the Mastership system and imposing its "effective deletion of the mother's body" from a presumed scientific knowledge of how labor and birth occur, while simultaneously valorizing the technologies in the hands of the obstetricians that are supposedly used to make birth safe (Hynan 2018:126). This is what Melissa Cheyney and Robbie Davis-Floyd (2019:8) have called "the obstetric paradox": "intervene to keep birth safe, thereby causing harm."

Turning now to our chapter authors extensive use of acronyms, we note that acronyms can be helpful in naming problems, and naming problems can make them more salient by generating wider awareness of them. Acronyms can construct theoretical concepts in and of themselves. Thus, here we present some of the theoretical constructs/acronyms that our chapter authors found useful. Anthropologist Michelle Sadler and midwife Gonzalo Leiva, along with anthropologists Vania Smith-Oka and Lydia Zacher Dixon, found helpful Suellen Miller and colleagues' (2016) identification of the TMTS (too much too soon) overperformance of interventions, including cesareans, and the TLTL (too little too late) under-performance of care. These authors also cited Cheyney and Davis-Floyd's (2020) insistence that both TMTS and TLTL maternity care should be replaced by RARTRW care—the right amount at the right time in the right way, and some authors cited Kylea Liese and colleagues' UHDVA acronym for the obstetric iatrogenic spectrum of "unintentional harm, disrespect, violence, and abuse." In his chapter, Nick Rubashkin reconceptualized the name of the "Maternal Fetal Medicine University (MFMU) Network VBAC Success Calculator" by simply calling it "the MFMU VBAC calculator" to emphasize the fact that this calculator is more often used to predict VBAC failure, rather than success. He also noted his dislike of the acronym TOLAC (trial of labor after cesarean), which makes it sound as if a woman who wants to have a VBAC must sit in front of a judge and jury while she labors. Thus instead, when not directly quoting an interlocutor, Nick replaces TOLAC with "labor after a cesarean" or "planned VBAC."

Moving away from acronyms and returning to other concepts and constructs that our chapter authors found useful, we note that Michelle Sadler and Gonzalo Leiva found helpful the Latin concept of obstetrics' *lex artis*, which, as they showed, is being profoundly compromised in today's obstetric practices:

> This Latin concept, mainly used in the legal domain, refers to the set of rules that professionals should honor when exercising their skill or art, to the true guarantee of good medical practice (Arimany-Manso 2012). "Let us continue practicing obstetrics as art, without forgetting it as science," was a warning given in 1949 by Dr. Avendaño, a Chilean ob/gyn who was concerned about the development of the discipline. The dimensions of care that need to be recovered in Chilean birth—indeed, in birth everywhere—are the art of the skills of facilitating physiologic births and the recovering of humanistic values in childbirth care. . . .
>
> It is time to use biomedical power for the benefit of humankind by providing the best birth experiences that we can, in line with the *lexis artis* and with the art of caring.

We couldn't agree more! And we note that Sadler and Leiva also found helpful Davis-Floyd's delineations of and distinctions among "the technocratic, superficially humanistic, deeply humanistic, and holistic paradigms of birth and health care" (see the Introduction to this volume for descriptions of these paradigms); they noted that "a paradigmatic shift is no small thing, and complex problems need complex solutions. Only a set of measures that address the cultural imaginaries of childbirth and the incentives that are driving the extreme medicalization of birth can lead us to a 'deep humanism' (Davis-Floyd 2018a, 2022)." Many of our chapter authors have used the term "technocratic" to describe contemporary obstetric practices. For example, in her chapter on Greek obstetricians, Eugenia (Nia) Georges stated:

> Whereas before [World War II], Greeks had looked to Europe for models of the most advanced and modern medical practice and training, by the 1960s and 1970s, many young Greek doctors . . . preferred to do their specialized training in the United States. Eventually, US influence on the development of Greek obstetric practice became decisive and remains so. Thus, in contrast to much of the rest of Europe, maternity care in Greece more closely resembles the technocratic model of US birth as classically described by Davis-Floyd in *Birth as an American Rite of Passage* ([1992] 2003, 2022). As in the United States, all births are generally understood to be pathological or potentially pathological events that should properly take place in hospitals under the surveillance of physicians and routinely subjected to a similar array of technological interventions.

Georges identified the distinctively Greek adaptations of this technocratic model:

> These include not only Greece's extremely high CB rate, but also the scheduled deliveries of thousands of preterm babies—which do not occur in the United States, where labors are not induced and CBs are not scheduled until 39 weeks, in compliance with the guidelines set out by the American College of Obstetricians and Gynecologists . . . which are specifically designed to avoid preterm births. Other distinctively Greek adaptations of the technocratic model include using general anesthesia for CBs; the informal payments given to their obs by "their" patients; and the close relationships established between obstetricians and patients.

These close relationships, as Georges pointed out, consist of obstetricians being available to their patients 24/7 to keep those patients, as there is an excess of obs in Greece and competition for patients is high. And those "informal payments" that their patients give to their obs in return can amount to as much as 1,000 EUR.

Moving now to the chapter by Vania Smith-Oka and Lydia Dixon on Mexican obs, we note that they framed their chapter in terms of the concepts of "risk" and "responsibility," stating that:

A growing topic of interest to anthropologists of reproduction is how reproductive risk is framed as something that is scientifically measurable and that can be mitigated through technology and behavioral modification—a perspective that reinforces risk as a consequence of patient choices (Fordyce and Maraesa 2012). Scholars have begun to point out how obstetricians also fall into regimes of risk management and responsibilization. That is, it is not just patients' choices, but rather, "all decision-making in maternity care is deeply embedded in social and cultural narratives of risk" (Hallgrimsdottir et al. 2017:617).

Smith-Oka and Dixon, along with Nick Rubashkin and the multiple authors of our chapter on Irish obstetrics (as noted above), found helpful Cheyney and Davis-Floyd's (2019:8) identification of the "obstetric paradox." According to Rubashkin, "The application of statistical instruments in obstetrics has expanded the terrain for surgical intervention into normal pregnancies and births . . . in what Melissa Cheyney and Robbie Davis-Floyd (2019:8) have called the 'obstetric paradox': 'intervene to keep birth safe, thereby causing harm.'" Smith-Oka and Dixon noted: "In an odd reversal to the 'obstetric paradox'. . . the doctors could cause harm by respecting patient requests; they could find themselves performing unnecessary procedures (which are considered obstetrically violent) while acquiescing to patient requests (and aiming to reduce obstetric violence)." The trope of "obstetric violence" runs throughout most of the chapters in this volume in varying ways and from obstetricians' perspectives, although it is more salient in Volume III of this series (Davis-Floyd and Premkumar 2023b), in which Part I is devoted to "Obstetric Violence and Systemic Racial, Ethnic, Gendered, and Socio-Structural Disparities in Obstetricians' Practices."

In their chapter on "How Class, Ethnic, and Gender Differences Are Reproduced in Obstetric Training in Mexico," Vania Smith-Oka, co-author of the preceding chapter, and Megan K. Marshalla addressed the concept of "boundary crossings" in Mexican obstetrics, asking: "How are social, intimate, and physical boundaries crossed during certain interactions? What factors structure the ways in which these boundaries can be crossed and by whom? . . . And how do bodies interact to create and reconfigure knowledge about boundaries and their crossings?" To analyze these issues, and citing multiple studies, Vania and Megan drew on frameworks of "embodied learning" and of "sensory skills in training" to "unpack how, among Mexican biomedical obstetric practitioners and students, knowing and being known, seeing and being seen, touching and being touched, and feeling and being felt are stratified in particular ways by the broader political economy." Vania and Megan also drew on Emma Cohen's (2010:S194) concept of "grounded cognition" to index "the development, maintenance, and refinement of [obstetric residents'] ability to use their bodies to touch, examine, probe, or cut the bodies of their patients." And these authors used Sheila Kitzinger's (1997) concept of "authoritative touch" to note that "touch in childbirth can be classified according to its social function, whether that is instrumental or affective."

Smith-Oka and Marshalla developed their own concept of "somatic translation":

Abstract medical knowledge is internalized through what we have termed *somatic translation,* meaning the embodied processes of learning, repeating, and making the body (of both patient and physician) legible. This "embodiment approach" emphasizes the bidirectionality of the material, neural, and physical realms with the conceptual, behavioral, and perceptual realms ... As bodies are trained to know and perceive, they change and are shaped by this knowledge and these perceptions.

To deepen their scholarly analysis of embodied practice, Vania and Megan additionally built on Rachel Prentice's (2005) work on "mutual articulation," Byron Good's (1994) analysis of how medicine constructs its objects, and Anna Harris's (2016) study of how bodies are configured through multisensory practice. These authors used their concept of "the medical body" to examine "the boundaries that body is allowed to cross":

As we discovered during our interviews, body parts, such as hands, fingers, or ears, become instruments that allow medical practitioners to move across boundaries—a surgeon's hands can move an assistant's hands while cutting a patient's body; a first-year obstetrics resident's fingers can do a pelvic exam on a woman in labor; an intern's hands can palpate a patient's pregnant belly to determine fetal position while their ears can hear the fetal heartbeat. But not just any bodies can cross these boundaries; only medical bodies can do so, because of social conventions and because clinicians are experts who have the requisite skills and are socially expected to touch their patients.

These "requisite skills" have to do with what the trainees interviewed by the authors called *hacer manitas* (being hands-on, using their hands to touch their patients and to perform certain maneuvers). Through *manitas*, "the bodies of obstetric practitioners traverse conventional skin and social boundaries, as well as structural boundaries of gender, race, and class. They also cross boundaries through what we term *somatic translation* in order to see, feel, and sense others' bodies with their own." Thus *hacer manitas* is much easier to do in public as opposed to private hospitals, because the lower socioeconomic status of the "poor and darker-skinned" people who attend public hospitals makes it impossible for them to refuse to be touched. Smith-Oka and Marshalla find "an interesting dynamic between two forms of care":

careful and careless. The "careful" practice in private hospitals suggests a physical distance in which the patient body is not touched by just anyone, evidencing a form of tactile respect. There is a simultaneous social closeness that is marked by politeness and respect for a certain amount of bodily autonomy. The "careless" practice in public hospitals. . . is almost the reverse: a physical closeness between patients and clinicians resulting from being touched by more people, where patients' boundaries are breached more easily and where the lack of patient bodily autonomy reflects a social distance between the patients and the clinicians.

Smith-Oka and Marshalla also developed their own theories of "the violence of knowing" and of "surfacing the body's social interior"; they stated:

The processes of *manitas* and *tacto* that we have described mirror a disconnection between what we term the *violence of knowing* (how knowledge about the body can come at the expense of someone's dignity) on the one hand, and the importance of touch as a legitimate mode of care on the other. This tension matters, because this form of tactile and sensorial learning entails not only a form of boundary crossing that is medically useful, but also a form of boundary crossing that "surfaces" various social inequalities in Mexico by taking advantage of them. We can think of this process as *surfacing the social body's interior*, which unveils and makes visible the various frameworks and structures of society. The ways in which the boundaries are crossed become indicators for the structure of a population that are reproduced within a hospital space.

Moving now to the chapter on the "gentle" cesarean in Switzerland, which is primarily based on an interview with Alexandre Farin—one of the two obstetricians who introduced that procedure to their country, we note that co-authors Caroline Chautems and Irene Maffi made theoretical use of Robbie Davis-Floyd's and Gloria St. John's book title *From Doctor to Healer: The Transformative Journey*, stating that:

> We decided to write this chapter in the form of an interview because we wanted to give voice to an obstetrician who has made a reflexive journey transforming him "from doctor to healer" (Davis-Floyd and St. John 1998)—meaning that he transformed several aspects of his training and previous clinical practices in accordance with a humanized conception of surgical birth and his moral concern for parents' and newborns' experiences of childbirth.

Alexandre Farin called what we would call "technocratic obstetrics" a "cold obstetrics," stating that "I sometimes think that many of my colleagues have lost their sense of what childbirth involves because the interventions they perform disrupt the process. In many hospitals, you find what I would call a 'cold obstetrics.' I think many things we do are useless or even deleterious." Alexandre was facilitated in his paradigm shift from this "cold obstetrics" to a humanized approach when he:

> had the opportunity to attend a special training in patient safety coordination and another one in quality of care. I then realized that healthcare professionals are the third most important cause of death for patients ... I started to think that it was important to discuss couples' wishes and the possibility of birth attendants being less paternalistic. When you start this kind of reflection, you open your eyes to many things ... In sum, I started to think from a clinical point of view, but I later switched to consider the patients' point of view.

Alexandre went on to explain that:

> When it comes to gentle cesareans, the idea came from Christian Valla, the former head of the department at the hospital Le Samaritain in Vevey. One day, he told me about a technique that we could introduce in our service. He proposed: "What if we had gentle

(*douce*)—as it is usually called in French—cesareans?" I wanted to laugh at him, but I said to myself, "Go see what this is first." I read the article from 2008 [Smith, Plaat, and Fisk 2008]. It's far from everything you are taught during your training. You have to rethink your convictions and be open to change.

Once the idea of the "gentle" cesarean was introduced to him, Alexandre soon realized that it is a much better way to perform cesareans than the standardized way he had been using, because it "highlights that this event is a birth, not a surgery. The patients . . . want to give birth to their child. We must not forget that." When Alexandre became Head of the obstetrics unit in his hospital, he found it much easier to make these "gentle" cesareans" the "default protocol" in that hospital. He stated that he was "bored" with standard cesareans, but:

> When I started doing gentle cesareans, what I saw touched me. Parents' reactions, the expressions on their faces affected me. This is what made it possible to transform the cesarean section into childbirth. Furthermore, this is contagious—you can see it when you attend this kind of birth—everybody is happy! Gentle cesareans are different also for the medical team. For cesarean sections to become childbirths requires a shift in the team culture—that is, [to see birth as] an important event and not a technical routine. It brings humanity to the operating room, because otherwise, it is technical. It is surgery: we are cutting meat. And, based on my experiences, I can say that the humanization of the operating room has a positive impact on the morbidity rate and the patients' recovery.

Alexandre went on to note:

> I believe that gentle cesareans are primarily based on respect for the child's birth: it is a newborn, a little human who comes to life, and we have to respect this moment. It is a matter of humanity—or rather humanism. It is also a question of respect toward parents, for whom this birth is an extremely important moment. There is an inconsistency between the way we consider the baby before birth as an extractable fetus and what it eventually becomes—a lovely baby.

Even though it has no effect on the baby's extraction (which is shown on the cover of this book), Alexandre encourages his patients to push a little while he is performing the cesarean because:

I had positive feedback from several patients who said, "Thank you for letting me push!" They told me it was super important for them. So, I keep doing it . . . Some patients thank me and tell me, "You healed me from my previous delivery." They also said, "It's so great to have my baby skin-to-skin right after birth!" I know that for them, seeing the birth or having their baby immediately, skin-to-skin, are fundamental elements. I have much more positive feedback with gentle compared to standard cesareans.

In her chapter on contraceptive provision by US ob/gyns, Melissa Goldin Evans spoke of "reproductive justice" and cited various scholars who have written on that topic, stating: "Above all, contraceptive counseling should occur within a reproductive justice framework . . . which declares, among other things, that all people have the right to equal access to all reproductive technologies and health services." Evans also stressed the importance of the patient–provider relationship, which "influences patient decision-making and contraceptive use," and insisted that "ob/gyns should foster a trusting relationship with their patients by treating all of their patients equally and respectfully." Citing Christine Dehlendorf et al. (2016), Evans noted that "women who are more satisfied with their relationships and interactions with their healthcare providers are more likely to correctly use and continue to use contraceptives, whereas miscommunications and patient mistrust of providers can contribute to dissatisfaction with their care and can lead to contraceptive misuse."

In her chapter on obstetricians' accounts of caring for patients with substance use disorders (SUDs), Katherine McCabe used a number of rich theoretical concepts. She noted that:

Problematic substance use is often categorized in one of two ways. Addiction is typically viewed either through a disease lens as a chronic, recurring medical condition, or through a personal responsibility lens, wherein problem substance use reflects poor decision-making, moral weakness, and/or a proclivity toward criminality. Social scientists have argued that practitioners' opinions about substance use disorder tend to fall between these two approaches—neither completely medicalized as a disease, nor entirely viewed as a moral failing . . . What researchers often do not examine are the ways in which addiction is understood and viewed as a "structurally embedded" or "structurally determined" social problem.

McCabe's analysis critiqued theories of "structural competency," wherein clinicians are expected "to incorporate into clinical practices knowledge of socio-structural inequities faced by patients." Through developing her own theory of "structural-causal thinking," McCabe further demonstrated how structural competency can be used to justify certain forms of clinical care that maintain inequity, at best, or perpetuate harm, at worst:

addiction is often framed as a socio-structural problem that exists among a web of other complex situations and adversities. Counter to the ways in which social scientists think about "structural competency"—an approach that seeks to instill awareness of "upstream" structural causes of health in clinicians—my study results reveal that structural understanding does not always result in more compassionate or patient-centered care. In fact, what I refer to as *structural-causal thinking* may result in providers adopting attitudes or strategies that *negatively* affect the health and wellbeing of pregnant and postpartum people with complex needs.

In a section called "Too Distal to Treat," McCabe described "distal causes" as meaning systematic, endemic, and structural causes "that shape the social, economic, and political context." She noted that these distal causes "are too often neglected, resulting in an inability to adequately address enduring morbidities":

The distal . . . situatedness and embeddedness of the social problem makes it difficult for obs to feel equipped to competently address the issues of substance-using pregnant patients . . . *Awareness* of the distal causes of addiction and of the forms of socio-political disinvestment that contribute to addiction does not necessarily engender a sense of competence among professionals. Antithetically, awareness of structural inequalities may impede productive clinical interactions if providers see the social issues before them as too distal to treat or to cure. . . .
There are several pitfalls and fallacies that arise when maternity care practitioners engage in structural-causal thinking. One surprising outcome is that obs who have some awareness of structural inequality may actually feel *less* competent and less equipped to address the needs of socially and economically marginalized patients. Obs who feel powerless to address the complex needs of patients within their scope of practice may be more willing to hand patients off to coercive and punitive systems that are perceived as better equipped to address patients' needs.

In the chapter by Amali Lokugamage and Claire Feeley, these authors explained the benefits of home birth and the reasons why obstetricians fear it. Citing Arthur Kleinman and Lilias Sung (1979), Amali and Claire underscored the previously noted fact that "all models of health care are . . . heavily culturally influenced, even those supposedly based on science." And certainly, as these authors showed, this insight applies to contemporary obstetrics, the practitioners of which are indeed "heavily culturally influenced" by the culture and traditions of technocratic obstetrics.

Like most of our chapter authors (see below), Amali and Claire pointed to obstetricians' discomfort with physiologic vaginal birth as a primary reason why obs over-intervene: "in the desire to deal with pathologies, doctors often lose—or never develop—faith in the normality of childbirth. The simplicity of birth for the majority of women, and women's innate abilities to let their bodies use nature's programming to deliver a child . . . are only rarely observed by obstetricians in day-to-day clinical life." We (Robbie and Ashish) add to this that, given that few ob/gyns are trained in how to understand and support normal physiologic births, it is hardly surprising that they find their comfort zones in intervention rather than facilitation. For as Robbie has long insisted (Davis-Floyd [1992] 2003, 2018b, 2022), standard obstetric routines and procedures are also *rituals* designed to enact and transmit technocratic core values into the bodies and minds of both care providers and care receivers. The rituals of hospital birth, like many other rituals, provide a sense of safety by generating the feeling that all is under control; as Robbie Davis-Floyd and Charles D. Laughlin (2022:12) put it, "ritual stands as a barrier between cognition and chaos." And even when those rituals/standard procedures cause harm (in the obstetric paradox), their practitioners nevertheless cling to them for the sense of safety and control that rituals can provide. In other words, despite the glaring lack of an evidence base, these rituals/standard obstetric procedures of hospital birth continue to be performed because they make *cultural and emotional*, not *scientific*, sense. Given that "obstetricians are continually immersed in crisis medicine rather than in the normal physiology of birth," Lokugamage and Feeley pointed out that this immersion can generate PTSD: "A meta-analysis (de Boer et al. 2011) reviewed existing data on the impacts of work-related critical incidents in hospital-based healthcare practitioners. It showed that work-related critical incidents may induce post-traumatic stress symptoms of anxiety, depression, and even PTSD itself."

In their efforts to explain why most obstetricians feel so insecure in relation to home birth, and thus are so adamantly opposed to it, Amali and Claire found helpful Eve Ensler's book *Insecure at Last: Losing It in Our Security-Obsessed World*, quoting her as asking (2006:2): "Is it possible to live surrendering to the reality of insecurity, embracing it, allowing it to open us and transform us and be our teacher? What would we need in order to stop panicking, clinging, consuming, and start opening, giving—becoming more ourselves the less secure we realize we actually are?" And then Lokugamage and Feeley asked this poignant question, "Could doctors be better trained or helped to deal with fear, uncertainty, and insecurity, as homebirth midwives are?"

Having provided this overview of some of the concepts and theoretical constructs that our chapter authors in this volume found useful—the "Cognition" in our book title—we turn now to the tropes of "Risk and Responsibility"—also embedded in the title of this book—as they relate to the fundamental question of *why* so many obs in the countries that our chapters address provide TMTS overly interventive care.

## On Risk and Responsibility: Why Do Obstetricians in Multiple Countries Over-Perform Cesareans and Other Interventions?

As Vania Smith-Oka and Lydia Z. Dixon contextualized practices among Mexican obstetricians, they noted that "Mexican obstetricians justify cesareans and obstetrically violent practices with discourses of *risk* and *responsibility*." Arguing that "we must take obstetricians' perspectives and the realities of their medical practices into account" when trying to understand their motivations for over-intervening in births, Vania and Lydia stated that "obstetricians frequently see cesareans as necessary to combat what they understand to be risky bodies and pregnancies in a context of resource scarcity," which "shaped both the justifications for their routine use and the ways in which they were done." It is clear that Vania and Lydia's Mexican ob interlocutors were well aware of the concept of obstetric violence and the activists' demands that they stop it, yet "many of them also had mixed feelings about obstetric violence, considering it an important concern, but also feeling paralyzed by the potential risk to their careers of being accused of violence by intervening too much or too little."

Earlier on in this chapter, Lydia noted that:

> Doctor Valdez . . . scoffed when I mentioned the term "obstetric violence," arguing that:
> The definition is too broad, which is dangerous for patients and doctors. Everything is obstetric violence now: if the patient cannot eat, is left in bed, gets an episiotomy, has a uterine cavity *revisión* without anesthesia, if we leave them there

too long, if we give them Pitocin, if we ask them about birth control too much . . . It's all considered obstetric violence. It's like they want us to leave them to lie there and not do anything! But if we don't do anything, they are like, "Why didn't you help me?" So it's like we cannot win.

We volume editors (Ashish and Robbie) note that of course they can win—simply by asking laboring women about their desires and then doing their best to meet those desires—but that simple concept of *listening to women* does not seem to have occurred to these Mexican ob interlocutors. Another ob interlocutor explained that his colleagues did not all follow the same guidelines when it came to *revisiones* or episiotomies, "even when the evidence exists, the studies exist, it is hard to change minds. The doctors still say: 'That's how I learned, that's how they taught me.'" This is an example of what, in her chapter in this volume, Robbie called "Stage 1 fundamentalism"—the idea that "Our way is the only right way."

In addition to obs' motivations, which also include financial incentives, fears of malpractice lawsuits, and physician convenience, Smith-Oka and Dixon showed that other factors contribute to rising CB rates "including rising maternal age, socioeconomic factors . . . and women's choice"—although this latter reason accounts for only a small percentage of the CBs performed in Mexico and elsewhere. These factors also include the lack of epidural analgesia. The labors of most Mexican women in public hospitals are almost always artificially augmented with the synthetic hormone Pitocin, which causes contractions to be stronger, closer together, and more painful, leaving women to "scream for a cesarean" within a scenario in which the (unnecessary) Pitocin-induced pain often eliminates any previous desire for a vaginal birth. Thus, as these authors demonstrate, the choice for a cesarean can *appear to be made* by the laboring woman, thereby allowing the ob to place the blame for an unnecessary CB on the woman, within a context in which the national government is trying to get obs to reduce their CB rates and epidurals are rarely available for anything besides cesarean births.

Regarding risk, Smith-Oka and Dixon explained that:

Risk takes many forms for the obstetricians with whom we worked; these include:
1. Their concern with risky patients who, doctors believed, engaged in risky practices, such as improper antenatal care or family planning, or whose social conditions, such as living in remote areas, placed them at greater risk;

2. Their belief that all pregnancies and births are underscored by risk . . . [and that] a normal situation could [quickly] turn dangerous;
3. The concern with risk reduction and preventing future risks through timely obstetric interventions, such as CBs, cord tractions, or uterine *revisiones*;
4. Risk from patients themselves, specifically the risk of being sued by them.

We can see that these obstetricians' actions were motivated by ideas of risk and responsibility that frequently did not align with the medical literature and guidelines for maternal care, but rather . . . were uncritically passed on from teacher to student.

In their Chapter 4, Michelle Sadler and Gonzalo Leiva explained that "physiologic birth implies economic damage" for Chilean obs, which is one of the primary reasons why obs in Chile do too many CBs, for a national rate of 53% in 2017. These reasons, which make perfect sense from obs' perspectives, have to do with money, the efficient scheduling of their time, their fear of lawsuits, and their fear of and ignorance about vaginal births. Sadler and Leiva noted that "As cesareans allow ob/gyns to schedule their time efficiently, the more cesareans, the more money, to the extreme of vaginal birth being described as 'economic damage.'" And cesareans are well within Chilean obstetricians' comfort zones, whereas vaginal births are not—as is also true for many obs in countries with high CB rates, such as Greece.

In her chapter, Eugenia (Nia) Georges highlighted the fact that Greece has, and has long had, the highest CB rate in the world, at around 65%. Devoting an entire section to the reasons why, Nia first noted that, unlike obs elsewhere, Greek obstetricians do not make more money by doing cesareans *per se*, but, as one of her humanistic ob interlocutors, who noted that "Time is money," pointed out, scheduling cesareans provides Greek obs with the convenience to also schedule other surgeries and to keep their appointments with their pregnant and postpartum patients, thereby allowing these obs to make more money—as Sadler and Leiva also pointed out. In contrast, Nia's "mainstream" ob interlocutors pointed to "women's demands for the operation prompted by their fears of childbirth"; one ob explained:

"Greek women suffer from tokophobia"—a technical term derived from the Greek for "fear of birth" that began to circulate in the global medical literature in the 1990s, "and so they ask for or even demand the operation" to avoid the pain and trauma of vaginal birth. According to this logic, in responding to a woman's request, obstetricians are respecting her right to choose how she wants to give birth.

Georges continued by describing obstetricians' and families' perceptions that labor is too hard on the baby, which is "squeezed and stressed" as it moves through the birth canal:

> The perception that CBs represent a safer option is widespread in Greece, and even women who initially preferred to give birth vaginally accepted their obs' recommendation to undergo the operation once the suggestion of risk to the baby was introduced. Reflecting at least in part the intersection of a liberal discourse of "choice" with the maternal moral responsibility for their children's health, the cesarean has come to be seen by women (as well as their partners, mothers, and others) as one more among the many modern reproductive technologies that prudent women must consider to reduce potential risks and ensure an optimal outcome, in what I have called "the symbolic domination of modernity" (Georges 2008).

Another reason described by Georges for Greece's high CB rate is that Greek obstetricians have become so accustomed to doing CBs that, as Sadler and Leiva also pointed out, they have become de-skilled in attending vaginal births. *Not attending vaginal births leads to not knowing how to attend vaginal births.* In this particularly Greek tautological phenomenon, in which more than half of expecting mothers have a CB, this de-skilling actually makes CBs the safer option.

Yet another reason that Nia's interlocutors gave for the high CB rate was that in Greece, the "Once a cesarean, always a cesarean" rule still applies, because Greek obstetricians have no training in attending VBACs, and those few who do learn to attend them in other European countries often stay in those countries instead of bringing their humanistic knowledge and expertise back to Greece. This "brain drain" works to ensure the continuance of the hegemonic technocratic model in Greece; new ideas rarely get introduced, and when they do, they don't go far. Thus Georges concluded her chapter by predicting that the CB rate in Greece is likely to remain unremittingly high.

Dunlea and colleagues did not delve deeply into why Irish obs consistently over-intervene in labor and birth, as some of these chapter authors have done that in detail in other works (see, for example, Murphy-Lawless 1998). Instead, they simply pointed out that the influential text *Active Management of Labour* is all about interventions, most especially artificial inductions and augmentations of labor, and that the "obstetric fraternity" insists on total surveillance and control of women's laboring processes. They did mention the "whispered promise of maximum safety in private obstetric-led care" and the realities of a patriarchal maternity care system, the cost of which to pregnant and birthing women in Ireland has been considerable:

> In this firmly patriarchal society . . . efforts at controlling birth extend back to the origins of the Irish Mastership system in the 18th century . . . Patriarchy, paternalism, and the obstetric exercise of power within a rigid hierarchy are foundational for the three great Dublin "lying-in hospitals," which also date back to the 18th century. This weight of historical reputation has exercised a formidable influence, with the presumed universality of obstetric thinking extending to the local policies of every single maternity unit in Ireland since that time.

In their chapter on the benefits of home birth and why obstetricians fear it, Amali Lokugamage and Claire Feeley emphasized the fact that obs in general are unprepared to facilitate normal physiologic birth, and very importantly pointed to the impacts of:

> fearful and traumatic birth attendance experiences; all obstetricians sooner or later experience a fetal death, and from then on, their fear of birth increases, as does the defensive nature of their practices . . . Thus, obstetricians' conceptualizations of safety and risk tend to hinge on acute situations that carry a high emotional charge, rather than on a broader and longer-term perspective.

Indeed, as many have pointed out, including obstetricians themselves (see Volume I [Davis-Floyd and Premkumar 2023a] of this series, in which all chapters are written by obs), obstetrics in general is a fear-based profession. In explaining the reasons for obs' multiple fears of home births, Lokugamage and Feeley highlighted "lack of awareness of the positive evidence surrounding planned, midwife-attended home births" as one of those reasons, and noted that:

> Obstetricians also fear the lack of facilities and familiar tools if something goes wrong at home, but without understanding home-birth midwives' transfer policies and protocols, the infrequency of complications, or midwives' capabilities for dealing with, for examples, postpartum hemorrhage, retained placentas, and neonatal

resuscitation . . . It is hard for obstetricians to realize that many avoidable or ameliorable complications occurring in hospitals *cannot happen at home*.

We too feel it important to emphasize that complications that "cannot happen at home" include, as Amali and Claire explained (we are paraphrasing and summarizing here from their chapter):

hyperstimulation due to drugs; increased maternal pain from artificial labor augmentation; stalled labors resulting from the stress of the hospital environment; problems in pushing due to the lithotomy position; total spinal block related to epidurals; anaphylaxis related to drug allergies; incorrect obtainment or interpretation of laboratory-based tests; delays, poor communication and prescribing errors among members of large teams; and hospital-acquired disorders such as infections and thrombosis.

Having described some of the answers our chapter authors provided to the question of why so many obs in so many different countries consistently over-intervene in birth and fear attending normal physiologic births, we now turn to our chapter authors' suggestions for future humanistic changes in obstetric practices.

## Directions for Future Change: Listening to Care Providers and Care Receivers

In her chapter in this volume, Robbie noted that obstetricians can reduce burnout and both revitalize and re-socialize themselves by learning about, getting to know, and working with midwives who practice the deeply humanistic and holistic "midwifery model of care" (fully described in Davis-Floyd 2018d)—which is easiest to do when attending midwifery conferences where they have the time and energy to assimilate new information; by reading the many books written by midwives about their own personal midwifery journeys; by becoming familiar with the scientific literature that supports normal physiologic births and assimilating that information into their practices; and by, again, listening to women. As is clear from all chapters in this volume, *social scientists need to listen both to women and to their care providers*. Robbie also strongly suggested that stressed-out practitioners about to degenerate into Substage—or who need to bring themselves out of Substage—can use rituals as "life-hacks"—a useful concept she gleaned from ritual researcher Dimitris Xygalatas, who has called rituals both "mechanisms of resilience" and "life-hacks," "meaning that people use them to relieve stress and anxiety and create a sense of calm." Xygalatas noted that rituals actively work in the human brain to achieve those goals, explaining "The mechanism that we think is operating here is that ritual helps reduce anxiety by providing the brain with a sense of structure, regularity, and predictability," noting that ritual is a powerful "mental technology" that we can use "to trick ourselves into [calming down]" (quoted in the *University of Connecticut Science News* 2020:1).

In looking to the future, co-authors Margaret Dunlea, Martina Hynan, Jo Murphy-Lawless, Magdalena Ohaja, Malgorzata Stach, and Jeannine Webster stressed that:

> There is urgent need for thorough reconfiguration of Irish maternity services, increasing the numbers of midwives, the establishment of more midwifery-led units, and the development of community midwifery services across the country. We have the alternative knowledges—authoritative knowledges . . . grounded in women's and midwives' experiences—and a constituency for wide political action . . . We *can* overturn archaic notions of Mastership and obstetric control. Our goal is a strengthened *Midwifeship*—that is, midwives enabled to practice to the full extent of their knowledge and skills.

As they looked to the future, Sadler and Leiva too suggested a much greater utilization of midwives, who, if their training has not been too medicalized, are the experts in facilitating normal physiologic birth, and of "laborists":

> Recognizing ob/gyns' insufficient training in physiologic birth, we should advance in models based on autonomous midwifery for physiologic birth such as midwifery-led birthing units (Long et al. 2016; Sandall et al. 2016). Promising models for private health care are those that reduce the scheduling/economic incentives, such as a collaborative midwifery-obstetrician program based on care provided primarily by midwives, with 24-hour backup from an obstetrician who provides in-house labor and birth coverage without other competing clinical duties . . . (called a "hospitalist" or "laborist" in the United States).

Such laborists may indeed solve many of the problems of TMTS interventions, as they mostly deal with one birth at a time and are not in a hurry to get a birth over so they can move on to the next one or go to an office to see private patients—although they cannot provide continuity of care. (Yet neither can many women's private obstetricians, who often do not actually attend the births of the childbearers under their care.)

Following that humanizing trope, Smith-Oka and Dixon stated: "Many obstetricians across Mexico agree with the need for broad, humanistic reforms to hospital-based care and . . . recognize that many of their colleagues are not willing to change how they practice obstetrics." Yet, as these authors went on to say:

> Blaming individual doctors or trying to change behavior at the individual level will not work. . . . To reduce high rates of CBs and incidences of obstetric violence, change must happen on a systemic level.
>
> For systemic changes to occur, we must understand doctors' decision-making rationales and take their fear-based perspectives about risk and responsibility into account, while also paying attention to the concerns raised by scholars and activists . . .
>
> Bridges must be built between the evidence and obstetricians' and scholar/activists' perspectives and goals. Activists and scholars have increasingly called on obstetricians to reduce CBs, to take concerns about obstetric violence seriously, and to change their practices to create more humane treatment. Given obstetrician participants' awareness of the movement for humanized birth and against obstetric violence . . . it is clear that these calls to action have been heard—and yet the ob interlocutors felt themselves stuck between "a rock and a hard place"—between their perceptions of risk and women's and the government's desires for them to engage in what they perceive as risky behaviors, such as lowering CB rates and stopping the performance of *revisiones*. Linking these broader concerns is a call for obstetrics to get with the times: to recognize the evidence linking humanistic obstetric care to better quantitative and qualitative outcomes.

Vania and Lydia suggested some practical and easily implementable humanistic changes to Mexican maternity wards in public hospitals:

> For example, despite cramped quarters on the ward, privacy curtains could be drawn to allow patients to bring in partners or family members who can support them. Adding that support would reduce patient stress, and potentially also reduce the constant monitoring and interventions performed. Reporting protocols could be

changed so that doctors who conduct *revisiónes* have to justify *why* they did so, rather than having to justify why they do *not* do them. Hospitals could incorporate CB monitoring systems (such as the Robson Classification, supported by the WHO . . . ) into their practices to track not only the number of CBs, but also which patients receive them and why. . . These are just a few minor changes that could have major impacts on patients and on medical interns and residents learning in the wards.

As Davis-Floyd also stressed in her chapter, Smith-Oka and Dixon noted that "re-socialization" courses are essential to train obstetricians in how to facilitate normal physiologic births. "By including their buy-in and input, they can be central to attempts to ensure much-needed systemic changes." Again looking toward the future, Sadler and Leiva expanded the reach of humanism to include:

comprehensive sexual education from early childhood; educational curricula in schools and universities that thoroughly integrate the psychosocial dimensions of health; training, updating, and re-socializing practicing clinicians; childbirth education programs for pregnant families; and stronger regulations to implement the humanistic model of childbirth.

Nick Rubashkin emphasized the racialized/ethnicized nature of the original VBAC calculator, stating that "Because the VBAC calculator explicitly factored in race/ethnicity (as opposed to racism), as an intrinsic risk factor for poor individual health, the calculator put VBAC-interested Black and Hispanic women at risk for cesareans they didn't desire or need." In looking toward the future of the VBAC calculator, Rubashkin explained that "It wasn't until the social movement to abolish race-based medicine emerged that the MFMU was compelled to revise the calculator's use of race/ethnicity as a non-modifiable and essential variable." Thus the members of the MFMU have developed a new calculator that does not include race or ethnicity as variables. Nevertheless, as Nick saliently pointed out:

*any* VBAC prediction tool that exclusively relies on individual risk factors, including the new VBAC calculator, will potentially be used to circumscribe mode-of-birth decisions, especially if one prediction model dominates clinical care. The dominance of one *prenatal* VBAC prediction model narrowed the terrain of counseling, and the new calculator continues to rely only on prenatal factors.

This reliance on prenatal VBAC prediction models matters, because it excludes the possibility of predicting VBAC success by taking into account factors such as women's physical conditions when labor begins. Again looking to the future, Rubashkin strongly suggested that women's desires for a VBAC should be taken into account in *any* VBAC calculator—in other words, that VBAC calculators should be "preference-sensitive," and that:

> For those VBAC candidates who desire a numeric estimate of their probability for a successful VBAC, providers should delve into a robust conversation about the multiple hospital, provider, and individual factors that influence successful VBACs. Providers should also discuss what can be done to potentially increase the probability for success . . . Women who have low probabilities for success should be afforded a range of birth options, not just a cesarean.
>
> Finally, *no VBAC-interested person should be denied a VBAC based on what providers perceive to be a low score.*

Moving from the VBAC calculator to the future of "gentle cesareans" in Switzerland, we note that Alexandre Farin and his like-minded colleagues have been encouraging other obstetricians to watch a gentle cesarean and then spread that procedure to their respective hospitals. In addition, Alexandre noted that gentle cesareans are having effects outside of obstetrics:

> There are changes occurring. Some anesthetists use hypnosis. They speak to patients; they prepare them. Before gentle cesareans, few anesthetists were interested in obstetric patients' experiences. Now they all look at them and interact with them during surgery. They are more present in general. One surgeon told me that gentle cesareans have changed his approach to other surgeries under epidural anesthesia. He wants to lower the surgical drape to keep eye contact with the patients. I believe that gentle cesareans can help build a new culture of the relationship between the medical team and patients.

In Katherine McCabe's chapter on US obs' treatments of substance-using patients, she concluded "by offering some examples of ways in which obstetricians can go beyond the awareness of structure and toward a model of actionable solutions." Briefly, these include advocating for the decriminalization of illicit substance use during pregnancy; researching federal and state laws such as mandated reporting requirements to understand the reach of the law and their obligations to comply with it; learning what happens when they involve child welfare and what the best ways are to refer patients to treatment and other resources; and others. As McCabe explained, "These are all ways in which obstetricians can go beyond the awareness of structure to address forms of discrimination that emerge in clinical interactions, thereby giving substance-using pregnant women, mothers, and their babies better chances to enjoy healthy lives."

In looking to the future of ob/gyn contraceptive counseling, Melissa Goldin Evans suggested that it should occur:

> within the context of the patient's expressed needs and concerns (e.g., preferences for method characteristics beyond effectiveness at preventing pregnancy) . . . When discussing contraceptive options, ob/gyns should address the side effects, risks, and benefits of use, method effectiveness, how the contraceptive works, and how to use it correctly . . . Once a method is initiated, a patient's adherence and continuation may be improved if her ob/gyn routinely evaluates her concerns and experiences with the method . . .
>
> . . . extreme care must be taken to ensure that *all* methods of contraception are available to *everyone*, method coercion does not occur, and contraceptive choice is made by the patient based on her desires.

In their chapter Conclusion, Amali Lokugamage and Claire Feeley stressed that "The COVID-19 pandemic has highlighted the urgency of addressing obstetricians' fears surrounding home birth." Many families in various high-resource countries have opted for planned, midwife-attended home births or for births in freestanding, midwife-led birth centers (wherever these are available) to avoid possible hospital contagion and the possibilities of being separated from their support people and their newborns (see Davis-Floyd, Gutschow, and Schwartz 2020; Gutschow and Davis-Floyd 2021). Thus homebirth rates have been rising in various countries, and community midwives have been doing their best to meet the demand (Davis-Floyd, Gutschow, and Schwartz 2020; Gutschow and Davis-Floyd 2021). But they need supportive obstetricians as backups for transfers, and that is one reason why we (Ashish and Robbie) believe that it is essential for obs to learn about the evidence showing the safety of home births in high-resource countries and to stop fearing that all such transfers will be "train wrecks." Thus Lokugamage and Feeley concluded their chapter by futuristically insisting that "we must learn from those organizations in which obstetricians and midwives are united within a humanistic philosophy grounded both in physiology and in evidence-based practice, in which home births are protected, supported, and celebrated."

## Conclusion: Our Readers' Next Step?

In these Conclusions to Volume II of this three-volume series, we have presented concepts used and reasons given by our chapter authors in this volume for obs' overperformance of interventions, including cesareans, and have also presented these authors' suggestions for future directions away from obstetric violence and toward humanistic changes. We hope that these suggestions will be taken up by those looking to effect policy and protocol changes in obstetrics in many countries. Again looking to the future, we hope that our readers will now turn to Volume III of this series, *Obstetric Violence and Systemic Disparities: Can Obstetrics Be Humanized and Decolonized?* (Davis-Floyd and Premkumar 2023b).

As Davis-Floyd (1987, 2018c) and others have shown, obstetric training is a lengthy and intensive rite of passage that heavily socializes its initiates into the core value and belief system of their profession and the rituals that consistently enact them, making change extremely difficult: "That's how I learned; that's how they taught me." Yet change is indeed possible, as is shown in the chapters in Part 2 of Volume III on humanizing and de-colonizing obstetrics, and also by the obstetricians who wrote the chapters that constitute Volume I, *Obstetricians Speak: On Training, Practice, Fear, and Transformation* (Davis-Floyd and Premkumar 2023a). Several of these ob authors made paradigm shifts from technocratic to humanistic or even holistic practice, receiving rich rewards in the forms of both provider and patient satisfaction while being subject to bullying and persecutions by their Stage 1, fundamentalist and fanatical colleagues—as are also described in some of the chapters in Volume III. We, your editors, have conceived and designed this three-volume series as an integrated whole, and we sincerely hope that you will read it as such!

**Robbie Davis-Floyd,** Adjunct Professor, Dept. of Anthropology, Rice University, Houston, Fellow of the Society for Applied Anthropology, and Senior Advisor to the Council on Anthropology and Reproduction is a cultural/medical/reproductive anthropologist interested in transformational models of maternity care, and an international speaker. She is author of more than 80 peer-reviewed articles and book chapters; 24 encyclopedia entries; and three books; and lead- or co-editor of 17 collections, the latest of which is the solo-edited *Birthing Techno-Sapiens: Human-Technology Co-Evolution and the Future of Reproduction* (2021) Email: davis-floyd@outlook.com

**Ashish Premkumar** is an Assistant Professor of Obstetrics and Gynecology at the Pritzker School of Medicine at The University of Chicago and a doctoral candidate in the Department of Anthropology at The Graduate School at Northwestern University. He is a practicing maternal-fetal medicine subspecialist. His research focus is on the intersections of the social sciences and obstetric practices, particularly surrounding the issues of risk, stigma, and quality of health care during the perinatal opioid use disorder epidemic of the 21st century. E-mail: premkumara@bsd.uchicago.edu.

## References

Arimany-Manso J. 2012. "Professional Liability in Cardiology." *Revista Española de Cardiología* 65(9): 788–790.

Cheyney M, Davis-Floyd R. 2019. "Birth as Culturally Marked and Shaped." In *Birth in Eight Cultures*, eds. Davis-Floyd R, Cheyney M, 1–16. Long Grove IL: Waveland Press.

———. 2020. "Birth and the Big Bad Wolf: A Biocultural, Co-Evolutionary Perspective, Part 2." *International Journal of Childbirth* 10(2): 66–78.

Cohen E. 2010. "Anthropology of Knowledge." *Journal of the Royal Anthropological Institute* 16: S193–202.

Davis-Floyd R. 1987. "Obstetric Training as a Rite of Passage." *Medical Anthropology Quarterly* 1(3): 288–318.

———. (1992) 2003. *Birth as an American Rite of Passage*, 2nd ed. Berkeley: University of California Press.

———. 2003. "Home Birth Emergencies in the U.S. and Mexico: The Trouble with Transport." *Social Science and Medicine* 56(9): 1913–1931.

———. 2018a. "The Technocratic, Humanistic, and Holistic Models of Birth and Health Care." In *Ways of Knowing about Birth: Mothers, Midwives, Medicine, and Birth Activism*, Davis-Floyd R and Colleagues, 3–44. Long Grove IL: Waveland Press.

———. 2018b. "The Rituals of Hospital Birth: Enacting and Transmitting the Technocratic Model." In *Ways of Knowing about Birth: Mothers, Midwives, Medicine, and Birth Activism*, Davis-Floyd R and Colleagues, 45–70. Long Grove IL: Waveland Press.

———. 2018c. "Medical Training as Technocratic Initiation." In *Ways of Knowing about Birth: Mothers, Midwives, Medicine, and Birth Activism*, Davis-Floyd R and Colleagues, 107–140. Long Grove IL: Waveland Press.

———. 2018d. "The Midwifery Model of Care: Anthropological Perspectives." In *Ways of Knowing about Birth: Mothers, Midwives, Medicine, and Birth Activism*, Davis-Floyd R and Colleagues, 323–338. Long Grove IL: Waveland Press

————. 2022. *Birth as an American Rite of Passage*, 3rd ed. Abingdon, Oxon: Routledge.

Davis-Floyd R, Gutschow K, Schwartz D. 2020. "Pregnancy, Birth, and the COVID-19 Pandemic in the United States." *Medical Anthropology* 39(5): 413–427.

Davis-Floyd R, Laughlin CD. 2022. *Ritual: What It Is, How It Works, and Why*. New York: Berghahn Books.

Davis-Floyd R, Premkumar A., eds. 2023a. *Obstetricians Speak: On Training, Practice, Fear, and Transformation*. New York: Berghahn Books.

————, eds. 2023b. *Obstetric Violence and Systemic Disparities: Can Obstetrics Be Humanized and Decolonized?* New York: Berghahn Books.

Davis-Floyd R, St. John G. 1998. *From Doctor to Healer: The Transformative Journey*. New Brunswick NJ: Rutgers University Press.

de Boer JM, Lok A, Verlaat EV, et al. 2011. "Work-related Critical Incidents in Hospital-based Health Care Providers and the Risk of Post-traumatic Stress Symptoms, Anxiety, and Depression: A Meta-Analysis." *Social Science & Medicine* 73(2): 316–326.

Dehlendorf C, Ruskin R, Grumbach K, et al. 2010. "Recommendations for Intrauterine Contraception: A Randomized Trial of the Effects of Patients' Race/Ethnicity and Socioeconomic Status." *American Journal of Obstetrics & Gynecology* 203: 319 e1–8.

Ensler E. 2006. *Insecure at Last: Losing it in our Security Obsessed World*. New York: Villard.

Fordyce L, Maraesa A. 2012. "Introduction: The Development of Discourses Surrounding Reproductive Risks." In *Risk, Responsibility, and Narratives of Experience*, eds. Fordyce L, Maraesa A, 1–13. Nashville TN: Vanderbilt University Press.

Foucault M. 1974. *The Order of Things: An Archaeology of the Human Sciences*. London: Tavistock Publications.

Georges E. 2008. *Bodies of Knowledge: The Medicalization of Reproduction in Greece*. Nashville TN: Vanderbilt University Press.

Good BJ. 1994. *Medicine, Rationality, and Experience*. Cambridge: Cambridge University Press.

Gutschow K, Davis-Floyd R. 2021. "The Impacts of COVID-19 on US Maternity Care Practitioners: A Follow-up Study." *Frontiers in Sociology* 6: 1–18.

Hallgrimsdottir H, Shumka L, Althaus C, Benoit C. 2017. "Fear, Risk, and the Responsible Choice: Risk Narratives and Lowering the Rate of Caesarean Sections in High-Income Countries." *AIMS Public Health* 4(6): 615–632.

Harris A. 2016. "Listening-Touch, Affect and the Crafting of Medical Bodies through Percussion." *Body & Society* 22(1): 31–61.

Hynan M. 2018. "Hidden in Plain Sight: Mapping the Erasure of the Maternal Body from Visual Culture." In *Untangling the Maternity Crisis*, eds. Edwards N, Mander R, Murphy-Lawless J, 124–132. London: Routledge.

Kitzinger S. 1997. "Authoritative Touch in Childbirth: A Cross-Cultural Approach." In *Childbirth and Authoritative Knowledge: Cross-Cultural Perspectives*. eds. Davis-Floyd R, Sargent, CF, 209–232. Berkeley: University of California Press.

Kleinman A, Sung LH. 1979. "Why Do Indigenous Practitioners Successfully Heal? *Social Science and Medicine Part B: Medical Anthropology* 13 B(1): 7–26.

Kosfeld M. 2007. "Trust in the Brain. Neurobiological Determinants of Human Social Behaviour." *EMBO Reports* 8: S44–S47.

Liese K, Davis-Floyd R, Stewart K, Cheyney M. 2021. "Obstetric Iatrogenesis in the
United States: The Spectrum of Unintentional Harm, Disrespect, Violence, and
Abuse." *Anthropology & Medicine* 28(2): 1–17.

Long Q, Allanson ER, Pontre J, et al. 2016. "Onsite Midwife-Led Birth Units
(OMBUs) for Care around the Time of Childbirth: A Systematic Review." *BMJ
Global Health* 1: e000096.

Miller S, Abalos E, Chamillard M, et al. 2016. "Beyond Too Little, Too Late and Too
Much, Too Soon: A Pathway Towards Evidence-Based, Respectful Maternity
Care Worldwide." *Lancet* 388(10056): 2176–2192.

Murphy-Lawless J. 1998. *Reading Birth and Death: A History of Obstetric Thinking.*
Bloomington: Indiana University Press.

O'Connor P. 2000. "Ireland: A Man's World." *Economic and Social Review* 31(1):
81–102.

O'Driscoll K, Meagher D. 1980. *Active Management of Labour: The Dublin Experience.* St. Annes, Sussex: W.B. Saunders.

Prentice R. 2005. "The Anatomy of a Surgical Simulation: The Mutual Articulation
of Bodies in and through the Machine." *Social Studies of Science* 35(6): 837–866.

Rothman BK. 2021. *The Biomedical Empire: Lessons Learned from the COVID-19
Pandemic.* Stanford: Stanford University Press.

Sandall J, Soltani H, Gates S, et al. 2016. "Midwife-Led Continuity Models Versus
Other Models of Care for Childbearing Women." *Cochrane Database of Systematic Reviews* 4, CD004667.

Schroder HM, Driver MJ, Streufert S. 1967. *Human Information Processing.* New
York: Holt, Rinehart, and Winston.

Smith J, Plaat F, Fisk NM. 2008. "The Natural Cesarean: A Woman-Centred Technique." *British Journal of Obstetrics and Gynaecology* 115: 1037–1042.

Emotions." *Psychoneuroendocrinology* 23(8): 819–835.

*University of Connecticut Science News.* 2020. "Life-Hack: Rituals Spell Anxiety Relief." *Science Daily*, 30 June. Retrieved 28 October 2022 from https://www.sci
encedaily.com/releases/2020/06/200630111504.html.

# Index

first-time pregnancy considered "high risk," 125
home birth viewed as "extremely risky," 11, 125
involving cesarean section (CB), 173
involving pregnancy. *See under* women
management of, 14, 125, 172, 174, 221, 286, 296–297
*Ritual: What It Is, How It Works* (Davis-Floyd and Laughlin), 23, 42
ritual(s)
  and stages of cognition, 34–35
  as "life-hacks" (Xygalatas), 35, 300–301
  as buffer between cognition and chaos, 35, 280, 294
  as "life hacks" (Xygalatas), 280
  as "mechanisms of resilience" (Xygalatas), 280, 301
  as "mental technology" (Xygalatas), 35
  biomedical ritual and tradition, 32
  defined, 280
  during home birth, 24
  enact a culture's core values, 18
  meditation, 24
  obstetric procedures as, 18, 294
  "rite of passage." *See under* birth
  singing during, 24–25
  summarized, 41–42
Rochat, Line, 138
Rothman, Barbara Katz, 280

Sister Morningstar, 40
"situated knowledges" (Haraway), 150
"situated learning" (Lave and Wenger), 198
Smith, Margaret Charles, 39
social class, 201
social media, 61
Stach, Malgorzata, 60
stages of cognition (Davis-Floyd), 1–3, 23, 186, 279–280
  "4 Stages of Cognition" (Schroder, Driver, and Streufert), 15, 279–280

and birth knowledge systems, 29–34
and home-birth advocates, 29
and intelligence, 28–29
"open" and "closed" thinking, 3, 14, 20, 29, 33, 131, 133, 145–146, 279–280, 283
processing new information and, 15–16, 29, 33
rituals and. *See* rituals
Stage 1, 3, 15–16, 29–32, 5, 186, 280, 283, 296
  fanaticism, 18–19, 29
  fundamentalism, 17, 29, 296
  naïve realism, 16
  only one possible set of interpretations of reality, 16
  "true believer" (Hoffer), 17, 29
  "us" versus "them" mentality, 18
Stage 2 (ethnocentrism), 15, 19, 29–32, 280
  ethnocentric ob/gyns, 30
  "our way is best," 19
Stage 3 (cultural relativism), 20, 32–34, 280
  complex rules for comparing perspectives, 20
  "informed relativism" (Davis-Floyd), 3, 20, 32, 33, 42
Stage 4 (global humanism), 21–22, 32–34, 280
  complex relationships among rules of comparison, 21
  role of social science, 43
  searching for universal standards that work for everyone, 22
Stage 1 versus Stage 4 thinkers, 25
stress and, 34–35
"structural-causal thinking" (McCabe), 216, 218
"substage" (cognitive breakdown, "losing it"), 1, 4, 33–34, 62–63, 280–281, 300
"tunnel vision," 34
summarized, 41
St. John, Gloria, 290
Sung, Lilias, 294
"supervalue" (Davis-Floyd), 272n2

surgery. *See under* medical procedures
Switzerland, 6, 125, 290, 304
  birthing statistics in, 54, 126
  "gentle" cesarean in, 125, 290–292,
    304
  high cesarean rates in, 6, 126
  hospital births in, 126
  Hospital Le Samaritain, 129
  Hospital of Morges, 130
  Hospital Riviera-Chablais (HRC),
    128
  "Parents' Experiences of Surgical
    Birth: A Socio-Anthropological
    Study of Cesarean Culture in
    Switzerland," 140n2
  Swiss Medical Association (FMH),
    130
  Swiss Society of Gynecology and
    Obstetrics (SGGG), 126
  University Hospital of Canton of
    Vaud (CHUV), 130

Taylor, Janelle, 195
technocratic, humanistic, and holistic
    paradigms (Davis-Floyd), 1–3,
    94, 107, 260–261, 286
  as a spectrum of practice, 3
  as belief systems, 15
  challenges of changing the status quo,
    118
  fear of paradigm change. *See* fear
  holistic paradigm, 10, 80. 94
    maxim "change the energy, change
      the outcome," 3
    principles of connection and
      integration, 2–3
    "universalists," 22
  humanistic (bio-psycho-social)
    paradigm, 10, 94, 104–107,
    116, 128, 135–136, 139, 184,
    303
    advantages in the 21st century, 43
    principle of connection, 2
    superficial and deep humanism, 2,
      34, 119
  paradigm (way of knowing), 15
  "paradigm shift," 117–119

redefined as "technocratic-
    superficially humanistic-deeply
    humanistic-holistic," 2, 286
  technocratic paradigm, 52, 75, 88, 117
    "Biomedical Empire" (Rothman),
      280
    birth services in, 52, 117
    "body as a machine," 2
    as "closed" system, 31
    fight to eliminate alternative
      paradigms, 42, 119
    principle of separation, 2
"The Circle Song" (Hudson), 24
*The Global Witch Hunt Plaguing Birth:
  Practitioner Persecution and
  Restorative Resistance* (Davis-
  Floyd, Daviss, Hayes-Klein),
  44n4
*The Power of Ritual* (Davis-Floyd and
  Laughlin), 23
Tully, Kristin, 173

ultrasound. *See under* medical
    procedures
United Kingdom (UK), 31, 261, 265
  Albany Midwifery Practice, 31
  midwifery in, 31, 52
  National Health Service (NHS), 52,
    93, 262
  Royal College of Midwives, 52
  Royal College of Obstetricians and
    Gynecologists, 262, 27
  National Institute for Health and
    Care Excellence (NICE), 259
United Nations, 26
  4th World Congress on Women
    (1995), 27
  Convention on the Elimination of
    Discrimination against Women
    (CEDAW), 71
  Millennium Development Goal, 259
  *Universal Declaration of Human
    Rights*, 27
United States, 7, 98, 215, 239, 262
  Affordable Care Act, 251
  American College of Nurse-
    Midwives, 37

www.ingramcontent.com/pod-product-compliance
Lightning Source LLC
Chambersburg PA
CBHW070907030426
42336CB00014BA/2326